Neoplastic Mimics in Soft Tissue and Bone Pathology

Pathology of Neoplastic Mimics Series
Mark R. Wick and Peter A. Humphrey

Series Editors

Dermatopathology
Mark R. Wick and James W. Patterson

Thoracic and Cardiovascular Pathology
Mark R. Wick and Henry D. Tazelaar

Genitourinary Pathology
Peter A. Humphrey, J. Carlos Manivel, and Robert H. Young

Gastrointestinal and Liver Pathology
Arief A. Suriawinata

Soft Tissue and Bone Pathology
Vickie Y. Jo and Jason L. Hornick

Neoplastic Mimics in Soft Tissue and Bone Pathology

Vickie Y. Jo, MD
Department of Pathology
Brigham and Women's Hospital; and
Assistant Professor of Pathology
Harvard Medical School
Boston, Massachusetts

Jason L. Hornick, MD, PhD
Director of Surgical Pathology
Director, Immunohistochemistry Laboratory
Brigham and Women's Hospital; and
Associate Professor of Pathology
Harvard Medical School
Boston, Massachusetts

demosMEDICAL
New York

Visit our website at www.demosmedical.com

ISBN: 978-1-620700-51-8
e-book ISBN: 978-1-617052-16-3

Acquisitions Editor: Rich Winters
Compositor: diacriTech

Library of Congress Cataloging-in-Publication Data

Jo, Vickie Y., author.
Neoplastic mimics in soft tissue and bone pathology / Vickie Y. Jo, Jason L. Hornick.
p. ; cm.
Includes bibliographical references and index.
ISBN 978-1-62070-051-8—ISBN 978-1-61705-216-3 (e-book)
I. Hornick, Jason L., author. II. Title.
[DNLM: 1. Granuloma, Plasma Cell—pathology. 2. Bone Neoplasms—pathology. 3. Diagnosis, Differential. 4. Soft Tissue Neoplasms—pathology. QZ 140]
QP88.2
612.7'5—dc23

2015026904

Printed in the United States of America by Bradford & Bigelow.
15 16 17 18 / 5 4 3 2 1

Contents

Preface

Central to the practice of surgical pathology is accurate diagnosis of a "tumor." This role is essential for appropriate prognostication and clinical management. Many nonneoplastic and benign lesions can show morphologic features that mimic malignant neoplasms, often requiring clinical correlation and application of ancillary studies to aid the differential diagnosis. Soft tissue and bone pathology is a challenging subspecialty, given the overall rarity of mesenchymal neoplasms, the large number of distinct tumor types, and the increasing use of minimally invasive biopsy techniques. Diagnostic challenges in soft tissue and bone pathology are often encountered by practicing surgical pathologists (with widely varied levels of expertise and experience); misclassification of a tumor with benign behavior as malignant may lead to serious clinical consequences.

Our discussion of "neoplastic mimics" in this book includes reactive and nonneoplastic processes that may simulate defined neoplasms of soft tissue and bone, as well as benign mesenchymal tumors that may mimic tumors with intermediate (locally aggressive or rarely metastasizing) or malignant behavior. For each mimicker, a differential diagnosis is discussed with attention to clinical, morphologic, immunohistochemical, and genetic features, and accompanying photomicrographs highlight characteristic traits of these often rare entities. Key references are also provided. We hope that this monograph will complement existing texts in soft tissue and bone pathology, and will serve the training or practicing pathologist as a useful educational guide to this challenging subspecialty.

Acknowledgments

The authors wish to acknowledge the support of their colleague and mentor, Dr. Christopher D. M. Fletcher at Brigham and Women's Hospital, Harvard Medical School, Boston, Massachusetts.

The authors would also like to recognize the assistance (and patience) provided by David D'Addona (Acquisitions Editor for Demos Medical Publishing), his predecessor Rich Winters, and Norman Graubart (Assistant Editor for Demos Medical Publishing) during all stages of this project.

1

Neoplastic Mimics: General Considerations

INTRODUCTION

"*Pseudotumor*" is an indefinite term that has typically been used to indicate the presence of a mass, which is felt to represent a neoplasm at some level of observation. In most circumstances it is a misnomer, because a mass actually exists; in that situation, the term "neoplastic mimics" or "pseudoneoplasm" would be more appropriate. However, there may still be circumstances in which the term "pseudotumor" is appropriately used; some of those scenarios are presented in the following sections. Nonetheless, this discussion is directed to those lesions that are best designated as "neoplastic mimics." They are typically represented by masses that have been biopsied or resected, but the microscopic slides do not show the presence of a neoplastic process.

From where did the designation of "pseudotumor" arise? Ophthalmology has been cited as the first specialty in which the literature used the descriptor of "pseudotumor" (1); in 1930, Birch-Hirschfeld employed it in discussing orbital lesions that had produced proptosis (2). Thereafter, other authors appended such adjectives as "inflammatory," "lymphoid," "granulomatous," "xanthomatous," and "fibrous" in attempts to subdivide "pseudotumors" into *pathologically* recognizable subgroups (3). The word "pseudotumor" has also been synonymized with such alternatives as "postinflammatory tumor" (4,5), "histiocytoma" (6)," plasma cell granuloma" (7–9), "mast cell granuloma" (10), "xanthoma" (11–14), "xanthogranuloma" (15), "plasma cell/histiocytoma complex" (16), and, in some reports (17), "sclerosing hemangioma" as well.

This brief introductory discussion further considers definitions and presentations of "pseudotumors" or, in a more general term "neoplastic mimics." Because this discussion is especially aimed at pathologists, it will generally be based on the morphologic characteristics of the lesions being considered.

PHILOSOPHICAL AND PRACTICAL ISSUES

The visual images of the same cases that are seen by internists, surgeons, radiologists, and pathologists are potentially quite dissimilar. For example, the surgeon may believe that he or she has identified a palpable mass in the breast, but the radiologist may see little or nothing on mammogram. Similarly, a pathologist examining a fine needle aspiration biopsy of the putative lesion may find nothing that is abnormal. In this scenario, the second and third physicians may question the claims of the surgeon, but unless they physically examine the patient themselves, they can never really determine whether a "tumor" is actually present at a clinical level of assessment. Nonetheless, the palpable lesion is certainly a potential neoplasm in the mind of the surgeon.

Radiologists and pathologists are subject to the same tricks of nature. For example, it is well known that hemorrhages in hemophiliac patients may simulate neoplasms in radiographs, although none is seen through the microscope after excision (18,19). Comparable comments apply to the roentgenographically defined images of "tumefactive biliary sludge" (20), duodenal ampullary "mucosal rosettes" (21), tumor-like musculoskeletal variations (22), and pulmonary "rounded atelectasis" (23–26). From the perspective of the pathologist, adnexal nevi of the skin (27–29), cutaneous reactions to Monsel's reagent (a styptic solution) (30,31), and the presence of the juxtaoral organ of Chievitz (a histologic imitator of squamous carcinoma) in biopsies of the oral mucosa (32–36) are singular neoplastic mimic conditions with no associated clinical or radiographic aberrations. Only by face-to-face collegial interaction can all information on such cases be integrated, to yield a clear delineation of the processes or anatomic variations in question (37). Indeed, practically speaking, interpretative disagreement between specialists—as stressful as that can be—is often the principal clue to the existence of a neoplastic mimic condition.

A considerable number of "pseudotumors" can simulate neoplasms on all levels of analysis— clinical, radiologic, and pathologic— and they consequently represent particular diagnostic pitfalls which can lead to therapeutic misdirection. Those are the entities to which this book is principally directed. In addition, other pathologic conditions are included that histopathologists alone—and not clinicians or radiologists—may uniquely misinterpret as neoplastic in nature.

Certain caveats must be stated in addressing this general topic. First, the lesions known as "inflammatory pseudotumors" (IPs) are generally recognized as representing true neoplasms ("inflammatory myofibroblastic tumors") although sometimes considerable difficulty may still be encountered in separating them from selected inflammatory conditions (38). Similar comments are applicable to angiomyolipomas, certain melanocytic nevi, and proliferative but reactive lymphoid lesions ("pseudolymphomas"). After the application of such techniques as immunohistochemistry, cytogenetics, and gene rearrangement analyses, the majority of true neoplasms in these lesional groups can be defined correctly. Furthermore, as more knowledge continues to accrue from those studies, the classification of "neoplastic mimics" will undoubtedly undergo continuing revision.

TOPOGRAPHIC DISTRIBUTION AND BIOLOGIC NATURE OF NEOPLASTIC MIMICS

Virtually all topographic sites in the human body may play host to lesions that simulate neoplasms. Perhaps because they are especially sensitive to etiologic influences that cause neoplastic mimics, some locations appear to be particularly prone to them. Principal examples are the lungs, urinary tract, and gut. In addition, neoplastic mimic processes are partially overlapping and partly distinctive as seen in various anatomic sites. That observation may again reflect the relative influences of different pathogenetic factors on different tissues, but other variables probably have an effect as well. The following sections consider "neoplastic mimics" as related to their putative causal categories.

IDIOPATHIC NEOPLASTIC MIMICS

True IP has an unknown cause in most cases, and is most commonly seen in the pulmonary parenchyma (38–61). It may conceivably represent a localized remnant of unresolved or organizing pneumonia (62,63).

There are several other IP variants that represent etiologically heterogeneous entities, with at least one variant of each being idiopathic. Examples include nodular lymphoid hyperplasias of the lung, gut, skin, mucosal surfaces, soft tissue, and lymphoreticular system (64–72); and fibro-osseous lesions of craniofacial and small tubular bones (73–76). In these groups of disorders, some potentially identifiable pathogenetic factors may include viral infection or autoimmune diseases (71,72); and fibrous dysplasia or familial "cherubism" (75,77). However, other morphologically-identical IPs are associated with no causal explanations and are therefore classified as idiopathic.

Still other conditions are "quasi-neoplastic," in that they feature etiologically unknown, and, to some extent, autonomous, cellular proliferations in various locations without a definable stimulus. Radial scar of the breast (78–81); urethral (prostatic utricular) polyp (82); fibroepithelial polyp of the urinary bladder (83); some "tumefactive fibroinflammatory lesions" of soft tissue (84,85); metaphyseal fibrous defects ("nonossifying fibromas") of bone (86,87); and aneurysmal bone cysts (88–92) belong to this category. They differ biologically from true neoplasms because they are self-limited or even spontaneously-regressing.

Other neoplastic mimic processes do have a linkage with underlying disease processes, but the ultimate etiology of the latter conditions can be idiopathic. Proliferative Paget's disease of bone (osteitis deformans) (93–96), tumefactive plaques of active multiple sclerosis (97–100), and lymphoma-like Hashimoto's thyroiditis (101,102) are representative examples.

REPARATIVE/POSTTRAUMATIC NEOPLASTIC MIMICS

Exaggerated host responses to tissue insults arguably comprise the most common mechanisms underlying the formation of neoplastic mimics. In many of those instances the injury may have been trivial and subclinical—to wit, unnoticed by the patient—and the resulting reparative process might therefore be regarded initially as idiosyncratic. That situation likely applies to nodular fasciitis (103,104), proliferative fasciitis and myositis (105–108), giant-cell reparative granuloma of bone (109–112), fibrohyaline pleuritis (113,114), and xanthogranulomatous inflammation in several sites (115–120).

Still other pseudoneoplasms are caused by documented episodes of injury, but again with an amplified and idiosyncratically robust reparative response. Pseudocarcinomatous ("pseudoepitheliomatous") hyperplasias of the skin (121,122), acroangiodermatitis (123), myositis ossificans (124,125), "atypical (ischemic) decubital fibroplasia" (126–129), tumefactive synovial chondrometaplasia (130), necrotizing sialometaplasia (131–133), gliosis in the central nervous system (134), nephrogenic urothelial metaplasia (135), inflammatory polyps of the anorectal region (136), colitis cystica profunda (137), florid reactive mesothelial proliferations (138–141), tumor-like chronic pancreatitis (142), therapy-induced tissue reactions (143–146) (which are simultaneously reparative and iatrogenic, causally), and polypoid-papillary cystitis (147) are all examples of lesions in this category. Why some individuals develop exaggerated repair mechanisms and others do not is an open question at present.

DEVELOPMENTAL NEOPLASTIC MIMICS

The most straightforward group of neoplastic mimics relates to individual abnormalities in development or, alternatively, ignorance on the part of pathologists regarding the details of normal organogenesis and embryology. Choristomas (148), hamartomas (149–153), and cutaneous nonmelanocytic nevi are members of the first of those categories, because they are classified as flaws of morphogenesis. Tissue remnants or heterotopias relating to embryologic development constitute another large subgroup in the same cluster, including examples of vaginal adenosis (154–156), cervical mesonephric remnants (157), "adenomyoma" of the duodenum (158), cutaneous "rudimentary meningocele" (159), and glial heterotopias (160,161).

On the other hand, the juxtaoral organ of Chievitz is a normal structure rather than an embryologic vestige or developmental anomaly (32–36). However, it is so uncommonly seen in mucosal biopsies that some observers may fail to recognize it and confuse this inclusion with a malignant neoplasm (squamous carcinoma).

Malformations related to congenital or Mendelian syndromes also may resemble neoplasms. The tumefactive lesions of osseous fibrous dysplasia (94,109,162,163) and the paraventricular glial nodules of tuberous sclerosis (161) are representatives.

"FUNCTIONAL" NEOPLASTIC MIMICS

Some neoplastic mimics are caused by a dysfunctional pathophysiologic state, often relating to endocrine abnormalities. "Dominant" nodules often arise in parenchymal hyperplasias of the thyroid or parathyroid glands (102) and those lesions can simulate adenoma or even carcinoma microscopically. Comparable comments apply to localized unilateral nodular adrenocortical hyperplasia (164). Other neoplastic mimic conditions with endocrine underpinnings include prostatic hyperplasias (165,166), focal nodular hyperplasia of the liver (167–169), ovarian stromal hyperthecosis (170), the Arias-Stella reaction in epithelium of the gynecologic tract (171–173), osteitis fibrosa cystica ("brown tumor" of hyperparathyroidism) (174–178), and uterine cervical microglandular hyperplasia (179).

IATROGENIC NEOPLASTIC MIMICS

Several medical procedures may produce subsequent tissue reactions that imitate the appearance of neoplasms. Most are reparative in nature and could also have been included in section '"Functional" Neoplastic Mimics.' However, because of their clearly iatrogenic nature, they deserve special recognition. Instrumentation or surgery of the genitourinary tract may cause an idiosyncratic tumefaction comprising variably-atypical spindle cells, known simply as "postoperative spindle cell nodules" (180–186). In the same vein, application of the iron salt-based cutaneous styptic, Monsel's solution, has caused idiosyncratic cellular proliferations resembling spindle-cell tumors of the skin and uterine cervix (30,31).

Other neoplastic mimics in this category may be able to imitate an infiltrative or in situ neoplasm. These include urothelial cytotoxicity caused by cyclophosphamide, simulating in situ urothelial carcinoma (187); epithelial atypia in the breast after chemotherapy (188); and florid vaginal adenosis in women whose mothers took diethylstilbestrol during pregnancy (155). Iatrogenic neoplastic mimics are particularly problematic for pathologists (189), because we often are not supplied with pertinent—and sometimes crucial—information concerning prior treatments or interventions.

INFECTIOUS NEOPLASTIC MIMICS

Particularly because of Acquired Immunodeficiency Syndrome (AIDS), tissue reactions to several infectious pathogens have been increasingly recognized that are capable of simulating neoplasms. Conjointly cytopathic and reparative responses to infection with cytomegalovirus, Epstein-Barr virus (EBV), papovavirus, selected species of mycobacteria, and other bacilli can produce proliferations in several organ systems with a histological likeness to sarcomas, gliomas, or lymphomas (71,190–194).

That phenomenon is not restricted to individuals with AIDS. It is also the basis for malakoplakia (195–199), "histoid" cutaneous infections caused by *Mycobacterium leprae* (200,201), and florid lymphoid hyperplasia of the terminal ileum in patients infected with *Yersinia* (202).

As outlined in the foregoing material, neoplastic mimic proliferations are potentially encountered in virtually all the topical areas of anatomic pathology, including cytopathology. Thus, they represent a truly-protean challenge with many possible implications for patient care and case outcome. All pathologists must bear those facts in mind during day-to-day practice in order to guard against misinterpretations.

Table 1.1 presents a synopsis of this discussion in tabular form, separated into organ systems.

This volume, *Neoplastic Mimics in Soft Tissue and Bone Pathology*, provides comprehensive descriptions, discussion, and images of nonneoplastic and reactive processes that mimic neoplastic entities, as well as benign neoplasms that simulate tumors that exhibit either intermediate or malignant behavior. For similar coverage of the other systems and categories of lesions shown in the following table, the reader is referred to the other volumes of the Neoplastic Mimics series of atlases.

TABLE 1.1 Selected Examples of Neoplastic Mimic Lesions and Related Neoplastic Imitators

SKIN
Cutaneous nonmelanocytic nevi and hamartomas (epithelial and mesenchymal neoplasms)
Lymphoid hyperplasias (lymphomas)
Reactions to Monsel's solution (sarcomas; sarcomatoid carcinomas)
Acroangiodermatitis (Kaposi's sarcoma)
Proliferating scars and posttraumatic spindle-cell nodules (mesenchymal tumors; sarcomatoid carcinomas)
Intravascular papillary endothelial hyperplasia (Masson's lesion) (vascular neoplasms)
Pseudocarcinomatous epithelial hyperplasia (squamous cell carcinoma)
"Rudimentary meningocele" (mesenchymal neoplasms)
Ruptured ganglion cyst (acral myxoinflammatory sarcoma)
Mycobacterial pseudotumors (mesenchymal neoplasms)
Bacillary angiomatosis (hemangiomas)
Kimura disease (hypereosinophilic syndrome; eosinophilic leukemia)
SOFT TISSUE
Neuromuscular choristoma (peripheral nerve sheath neoplasms)
Fibrolipomatous hamartoma (lipomas)

(Continued)

TABLE 1.1 Selected Examples of Neoplastic Mimic Lesions and Related Neoplastic Imitators *(Continued)*

Nodular fasciitis (sarcomas)
Proliferative myositis (sarcomas)
Myositis ossificans (osteosarcoma)
"Tumefactive fibroinflammatory lesions" (fibromatoses)
Florid (tumefactive/focal) lymphocytic myositis (lymphoma)
"Atypical decubital" (ischemic) fibroplasia (sarcomas)

BONES AND JOINTS

"Bizarre osteochondromatous proliferations" (Nora's lesion) of digits (cartilaginous neoplasms)
Synovial chondrometaplasia/chondrocalcinosis (cartilaginous neoplasms)
Fibrous dysplasia and "fibro-osseous lesions" (osteosarcoma and fibrosarcoma)
Proliferative-phase Paget's disease of bone (osteosarcoma)
Aneurysmal bone cyst (telangiectatic osteosarcoma)
Giant cell reparative granuloma (giant cell tumor)
Avulsion fractures of ischial tuberosities (osteosarcoma)
"Brown tumor" of hyperparathyroidism (osteitis fibrosa cystica) (giant cell tumor)

BREAST

Radial scar (low-grade ductal adenocarcinoma)
Choristoma (hamartoma) (metaplastic carcinoma)
Proliferative adenosis (low-grade ductal adenocarcinoma)
Extramedullary hematopoiesis (invasive lobular carcinoma)
Collagenous spherulosis (adenoid cystic carcinoma or intraductal carcinoma)
Pseudoangiomatous stromal hyperplasia (angiosarcoma)

NERVOUS SYSTEM

Gliosis (low-grade gliomas)
Active-phase plaques of multiple sclerosis (gliomas)
Progressive multifocal leukoencephalopathy (gliomas)
Paraventricular glial nodules of tuberous sclerosis (gliomas; gangliogliomas)
Viral encephalitides (lymphoma)

ENDOCRINE SYSTEM

Sclerosing and proliferative Hashimoto's thyroiditis (anaplastic carcinomas and lymphomas)
Nodular thyroid hyperplasia (thyroid adenomas and differentiated thyroid carcinomas)
Nodular parathyroid hyperplasia (parathyroid adenoma)
Nodular adrenal hyperplasia (adrenocortical adenoma)
Adrenal myelolipoma (liposarcoma)

LYMPHORETICULAR SYSTEM

Selected lymphoid hyperplasias (lymphomas)
Florid oligoclonal hyperplasia in bone marrow recovery (myelodysplasia; leukemia)

(Continued)

TABLE 1.1 Selected Examples of Neoplastic Mimic Lesions and Related Neoplastic Imitators *(Continued)*

Infection-related hemophagocytic syndrome (T-cell lymphoma)
EBV-related atypical lymphoid hyperplasias (large-cell lymphoma)
Mycobacterial pseudotumors (dendritic-cell tumors)

UPPER AIRWAY

Pseudocarcinomatous epithelial hyperplasia (squamous cell carcinoma)
Juxtaoral organ of Chievitz (low-grade squamous or mucoepidermoid carcinoma)
Necrotizing sialometaplasia (squamous or mucoepidermoid carcinoma)
Radiation effects on mucosal epithelia (squamous carcinoma)
Benign lymphoepithelial lesion of salivary gland (lymphomas)
Traumatized antral/choanal polyps (polypoid sarcomatoid carcinomas)
Glial heterotopias (peripheral nerve sheath tumors)
Benign fibro-osseous lesions (low-grade fibrosarcoma or osteosarcoma)

LOWER AIRWAY

Pseudocarcinomatous epithelial hyperplasia (squamous cell carcinoma and adenocarcinoma)
Atypical bronchiolar and alveolar epithelial hyperplasia (carcinomas)
Fibrohyaline plaques of pleura and fibrohyaline pleuritis (desmoplastic mesothelioma)
Florid mesothelial hyperplasia (epithelial mesothelioma)
Localized tumefactive organizing pneumonia (inflammatory sarcomatoid carcinoma)
Selected examples of lymphocytic interstitial pneumonia (lymphoma)
Pulmonary chondroid/lipomatous/muscular hamartomas (metaplastic carcinomas)

MEDIASTINUM

Sclerosing mediastinitis (sclerosing carcinomas, lymphomas, or germ-cell tumors)
Thymic dysplasia (thymoma)
Proliferating thymic cyst (thymic squamous carcinoma)
Benign mesothelial inclusions in mediastinal lymph nodes (metastatic carcinoma)

GASTROINTESTINAL TRACT

Pseudocarcinomatous epithelial hyperplasia (adenocarcinoma)
Enteritis/colitis cystica profunda (adenocarcinoma)
"Adenomyoma" of duodenum (well-differentiated adenocarcinoma)
Tumefactive chronic pancreatitis (well-differentiated ductal adenocarcinoma or lymphoma)
Florid lymphoid hyperplasia (lymphomas)
Hepatic bile duct hamartoma (metastatic adenocarcinoma)
Hepatic focal nodular hyperplasia (fibrolamellar hepatocellular carcinoma)
Inflammatory "cloacogenic" polyp (tubulovillous adenoma)
Chronic tumefactive pancreatitis (low-grade pancreatic ductal adenocarcinoma)
Xanthogranulomatous cholecystitis (sarcomatoid carcinoma)

(Continued)

TABLE 1.1 Selected Examples of Neoplastic Mimic Lesions and Related Neoplastic Imitators *(Continued)*

GENITOURINARY TRACT (MALE AND FEMALE)

Pseudocarcinomatous epithelial hyperplasia (carcinomas)
Postoperative spindle cell nodules (sarcomas; sarcomatoid carcinoma)
Drug effects (eg, Cytoxan cystitis mimicking carcinoma in situ) (urothelial carcinoma)
Proliferative prostatic urethral (utricular) polyp (adenocarcinoma)
Paratesticular mycobacterial pseudotumor (sarcomas)
Lymphoplasmacytic orchitis (lymphoma)
Xanthogranulomatous nephritis/cystitis/orchitis/endometritis/oophoritis (carcinomas)
Adenomatous and basal-cell prostatic hyperplasia (adenocarcinoma)
Cribriform intraductal prostatic hyperplasia (adenocarcinoma)
Nodular stromal prostatic hyperplasia (low-grade sarcoma)
Prostatic sclerosing adenosis (adenocarcinoma)
Radiation effect on prostatic epithelium (residual adenocarcinoma)
Granulomatous prostatitis/orchitis (sclerosing carcinoma and sclerosing seminoma)
Vaginal adenosis (adenocarcinoma)
Uterine cervical mesonephric remnants (adenocarcinoma)
Uterine cervical microglandular adenosis (adenocarcinoma)
Ovarian stromal hyperplasia/hyperthecosis (ovarian stromal neoplasms)
Nephrogenic metaplasia of bladder and urethra (adenocarcinoma)
Endometriosis (adenocarcinoma)

CARDIOVASCULAR SYSTEM

Rhabdomyomatous hamartomas of myocardium (true "adult" rhabdomyoma)
Endodermal choristoma of interatrial cardiac septum (metastatic adenocarcinoma)
Lipomatous hypertrophy of the heart (lipoma)
Mesothelial-monocytic intracardiac excrescences (metastatic adenocarcinoma or mesothelioma)
Endocardial and myocardial lymphocytic infiltrates after transplantation (lymphomas)
Florid pericardial mesothelial hyperplasia (epithelial mesothelioma and metastatic adenocarcinoma)

2

General Considerations in Soft Tissue and Bone Pathology

Neoplasms of soft tissue and bone comprise numerous and diverse tumor types. Owing to their rarity and significant morphologic overlap, mesenchymal neoplasms often present diagnostic challenges in surgical pathology practice. The classification of soft tissue and bone tumors has evolved considerably over the past two decades with rapid advances in molecular genetics; for many tumor types, this has led to the development of useful diagnostic tools (including novel immunohistochemical markers). Accurate classification is critical for proper prognostication and patient management. The approach to any soft tissue and bone tumor requires correlation with clinical and radiologic data (the latter especially for bone tumors); clinical features help inform differential diagnosis.

The biologic behavior of soft tissue and bone tumors is stratified into four managerial categories: (a) benign; (b) intermediate, locally aggressive; (c) intermediate, rarely metastasizing; and (d) malignant (ie, sarcoma). "Locally aggressive" tumors may show infiltrative and destructive growth patterns, often with high local recurrence rates, but do not metastasize. Relatively common examples of locally aggressive mesenchymal neoplasms include desmoid fibromatosis and atypical lipomatous tumor (well-differentiated liposarcoma). In contrast, "rarely metastasizing" tumors may also be locally aggressive (though not necessarily), and harbor low metastatic potential (<2%), which for most such tumor types is not predictable on histologic grounds. Examples of rarely metastasizing tumors include solitary fibrous tumor and plexiform fibrohistiocytic tumor. While marginal excision is sufficient for benign tumors, complete surgical resection with negative margins is attempted for many neoplasms of intermediate biologic potential, similar to sarcomas.

The major categories of soft tissue and bone tumors according to the World Health Organization Classification are listed in **Table 2.1**. Most of these categories

TABLE 2.1 WHO Classification of Tumor Types in Soft Tissue and Bone

SOFT TISSUE
Adipocytic Tumors
Fibroblastic/myofibroblastic Tumors
So-called Fibrohistiocytic Tumors
Smooth Muscle Tumors
Pericytic Tumors
Skeletal Muscle Tumors
Vascular Tumors
Chondro-osseous Tumors
Gastrointestinal Stromal Tumors
Nerve Sheath Tumors
Tumors of Uncertain Differentiation
Undifferentiated/unclassified Sarcomas
BONE
Chondrogenic Tumors
Osteogenic Tumors
Fibrogenic Tumors
Fibrohistiocytic Tumors
Ewing Sarcoma
Osteoclastic Giant-cell Rich Tumors
Notochordal Tumors
Vascular Tumors
Myogenic, Lipogenic, and Epithelial Tumors
Tumors of Undefined Neoplastic Potential
Undifferentiated High-grade Pleomorphic Sarcoma

are based on shared lines of differentiation, determined largely by morphologic and immunohistochemical features, though groups of undifferentiated tumors and those of "uncertain differentiation" exist (and will likely persist). While some tumor categories include tumors that largely share morphologic features (such as smooth muscle tumors), other categories, such as fibroblastic/myofibroblastic and vascular neoplasms, are comprised of tumors showing a wide range of morphologic appearances. Immunohistochemical stains are often useful in determining line of differentiation; examples are included in **Table 2.2**. Additionally, many clinically useful relatively tumor-specific diagnostic markers are increasingly available, which have been developed from gene expression profiling studies or following the identification of specific

TABLE 2.2 Select Immunohistochemical Markers for Determining Line of Differentiation or Tumor Type

LINE OF DIFFERENTIATION	IMMUNOHISTOCHEMICAL MARKERS
Smooth Muscle	Smooth muscle actin (SMA), desmin, caldesmon
Skeletal Muscle	Desmin, muscle-specific actin, myogenin
Endothelial	CD34, CD31, ERG
Fibroblastic/Myofibroblastic	CD34, SMA, desmin
Myoepithelial	Cytokeratin, EMA, S-100, GFAP
Neural crest	S-100, GFAP, SOX10
Perineurial	EMA, CD34, claudin-1
Gastrointestinal stromal	KIT, DOG1
Osteoblastic	SATB2
Melanocytic	S-100, Mart-1/Melan-A, HMB-45
Histiocytic	CD68, CD163

gene fusions or other genetic alterations. For instance, MDM2 and CDK4 are useful immunohistochemical markers for well-differentiated liposarcoma and dedifferentiated liposarcoma, which are characterized by amplification of the chromosome 12q13-15 region (containing these genes) in the form of ring or giant marker chromosomes.

Molecular genetic advances over the past two decades have led to the development of new diagnostic tests in soft tissue and bone pathology. Many sarcomas harbor recurrent chromosomal rearrangements, and cytogenetic and molecular assays allow for confirmation of challenging diagnoses. An increasing number of tumors of benign or intermediate biologic potential have also been characterized by genetic means, including nodular fasciitis (now considered a "self-limiting" neoplasm having *MYH9-USP6* gene fusion) and myxoma (which harbors *GNAS* gene mutations). While fresh tissue in many large tumors can be allocated for conventional cytogenetic studies in large practice settings, molecular diagnostic assays may be applied routinely to formalin-fixed, paraffin-embedded tissue, including more limited samples (such as fine-needle aspiration and core biopsies).

Despite the many immunohistochemical and molecular genetic advances, numerous diagnostic pitfalls remain in soft tissue and bone pathology. There is frequent overlap in clinicopathologic and morphologic features between benign, intermediate, and malignant tumors, and reactive processes can also mimic neoplasms of any biologic potential. Many soft tissue and bone tumors have heterogeneous morphologic appearances, and may therefore be particularly difficult to recognize in small biopsy samples or if a large tumor is inadequately sampled. Increasing numbers of relatively specific immunohistochemical markers are being developed; immunohistochemistry is more widely available than more costly molecular diagnostic assays (which require specialized molecular laboratories). However, no single marker is perfectly sensitive or specific. For example, MDM2 is positive in nearly all well-differentiated liposarcomas and dedifferentiated liposarcomas; however, MDM2 is also expressed in many cases of malignant peripheral nerve sheath tumor and is often positive in histiocytes, which may be a pitfall when evaluating adipocytic lesions with fat necrosis. Genetic studies should also be used with caution: fluorescence in situ hybridization (FISH) for *EWSR1* can confirm the presence of *EWSR1* gene rearrangement, but many tumor types of varying biologic potential harbor *EWSR1* translocations, including the benign tumor myoepithelioma, angiomatoid fibrous histiocytoma (a rarely metastasizing tumor), and Ewing sarcoma, to name a few.

Our discussion of "neoplastic mimics" in soft tissue and bone pathology addresses nonneoplastic and reactive processes that morphologically mimic defined neoplastic entities, including lesions that pursue a benign clinical course but have defining cytogenetic alterations. Benign neoplasms with morphologic features simulating tumors that exhibit either intermediate or malignant behavior are also addressed, given the major differences in treatment and prognosis. The overlapping and discriminatory clinicopathologic, morphologic, immunohistochemical, and genetic features will be discussed for each differential diagnosis, organized by the major categories of soft tissue tumor types and as cartilaginous and osseous bone tumors.

3 Mimics of Adipocytic Neoplasms

- FAT NECROSIS
- INTRAMUSCULAR ANGIOMA
- SCLEROSING MESENTERITIS
- SILICONE REACTION
- MASSIVE LOCALIZED LYMPHEDEMA
- PROLAPSED ORBITAL FAT
- MYELOLIPOMA
- LIPOMA (INCLUDING INTRAMUSCULAR LIPOMA AND LIPOMATOSIS)
- SPINDLE CELL LIPOMA/PLEOMORPHIC LIPOMA
- HIBERNOMA
- LIPOBLASTOMA

Adipocytic neoplasms are often considered in the differential diagnosis for lesions showing variation in adipocyte size or containing cells resembling lipoblasts. Mature fat (that has not been subjected to trauma) is characterized by an adipocyte population that is uniform in size with widely spaced, thin indistinct nuclei typically compressed at the edges of the cells (**Figure 3.1**). The nucleus of a fat cell has a central vacuole (*lochkern*) that may be seen on histologic cross section, but is not hyperchromatic and lacks distinct nucleoli (**Figure 3.2**). In subcutaneous tissue, normal fat is arranged in a lobular architecture with individual lobules demarcated by thin bands of collagen. True lipoblasts typically show variation in size, and have single or multiple optically clear cytoplasmic vacuoles that indent an enlarged hyperchromatic nucleus, creating a scalloped appearance (**Figure 3.3**). Additionally, several adipocytic tumors characterized by benign biologic behavior (lipoma, spindle cell lipoma/pleomorphic lipoma, and lipoblastoma) may show considerable morphologic overlap with liposarcoma subtypes, and are thus also discussed in this section.

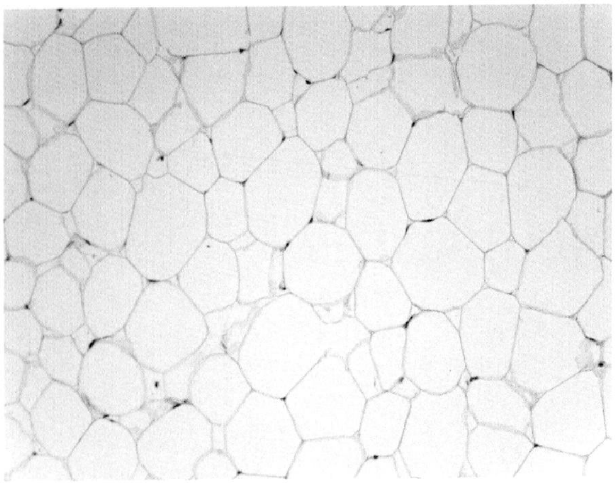

FIGURE 3.1 Mature fat comprised of uniformly sized adipocytes with thin compressed nuclei.

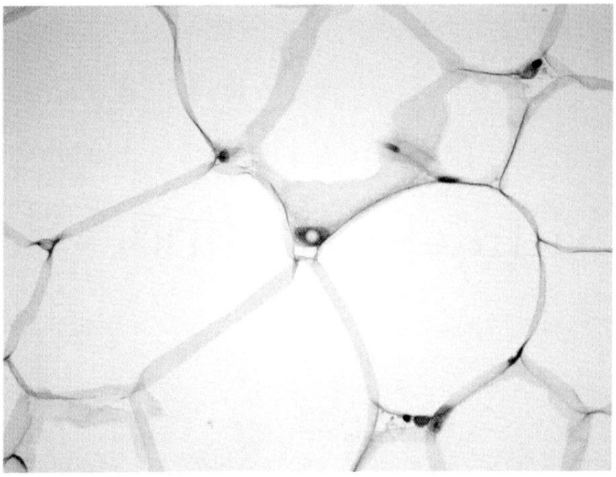

FIGURE 3.2 The central vacuole (*lochkern*) of the adipocyte nucleus can be seen on cross-section.

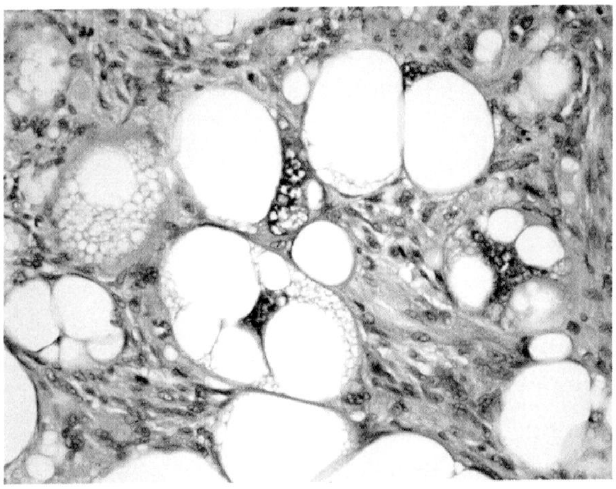

FIGURE 3.3 True lipoblasts vary in size, and have enlarged hyperchromatic nuclei that appear "scalloped" from indentation by single or multiple cytoplasmic vacuoles.

FAT NECROSIS

Fat necrosis involving either normal adipose tissue or a benign adipocytic neoplasm (such as a lipoma; see section "*Lipoma*") may impart worrisome features of malignancy, both to the clinician and pathologist. Superficial lesions may be palpable, and a history of trauma may not be documented or known. Adipocytic tissue affected by fat necrosis appears more cellular, with infiltration by histiocytes, occasional multinucleated giant cells, and variation in adipocyte size (**Figure 3.4A**). The histiocytes often have cytoplasmic vacuolization and may therefore resemble lipoblasts, but lack the characteristic scalloped, hyperchromatic nuclei (**Figure 3.4B**). The multinucleated giant cells likewise lack worrisome features of malignancy upon closer histologic examination. However, the constellation of findings in fat necrosis may be misinterpreted as atypical lipomatous tumor (ALT)/well-differentiated liposarcoma (WDLPS) (**Figure 3.5**). This distinction is important, as ALT/WDLPS requires complete surgical resection given its risk of recurrence and potential to progress to dedifferentiated liposarcoma (DDLPS), which is associated with an acquisition of metastatic potential. ALT/WDLPS/DDLPS are characterized by amplification of 12q13-15 in the form of supernumerary ring and giant marker chromosomes, which contain the cell cycle regulatory genes *MDM2* and *CDK4*, among others (203,204). This results in high-level expression of the MDM2 and CDK4 proteins. Immunohistochemistry for MDM2 and CDK4 is a useful marker for ALT/WDLPS/DDLPS, which shows a nuclear staining pattern (**Figure 3.5C**). However, an important pitfall is that histiocytes can also show nuclear staining for MDM2 (**Figure 3.4C**) (205). Careful histologic examination for the

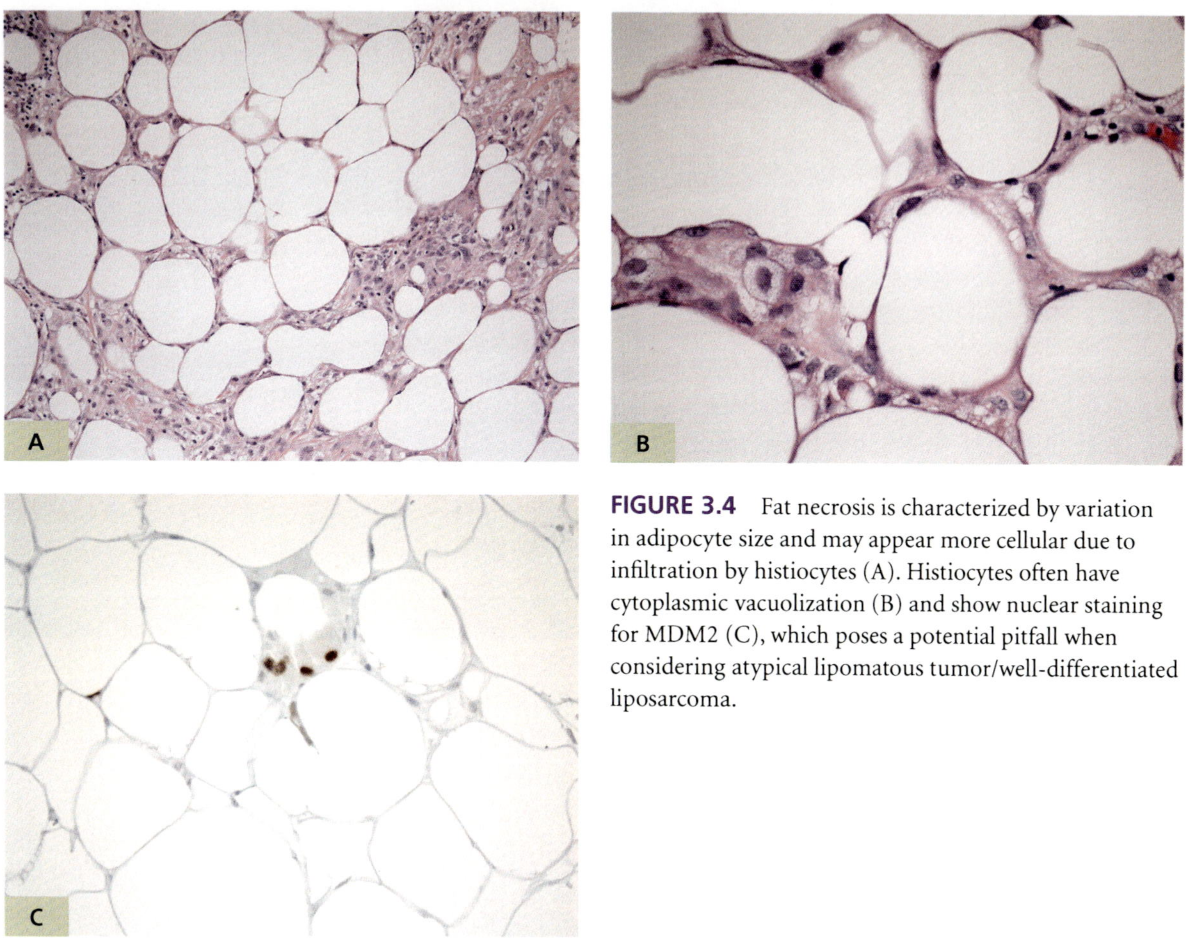

FIGURE 3.4 Fat necrosis is characterized by variation in adipocyte size and may appear more cellular due to infiltration by histiocytes (A). Histiocytes often have cytoplasmic vacuolization (B) and show nuclear staining for MDM2 (C), which poses a potential pitfall when considering atypical lipomatous tumor/well-differentiated liposarcoma.

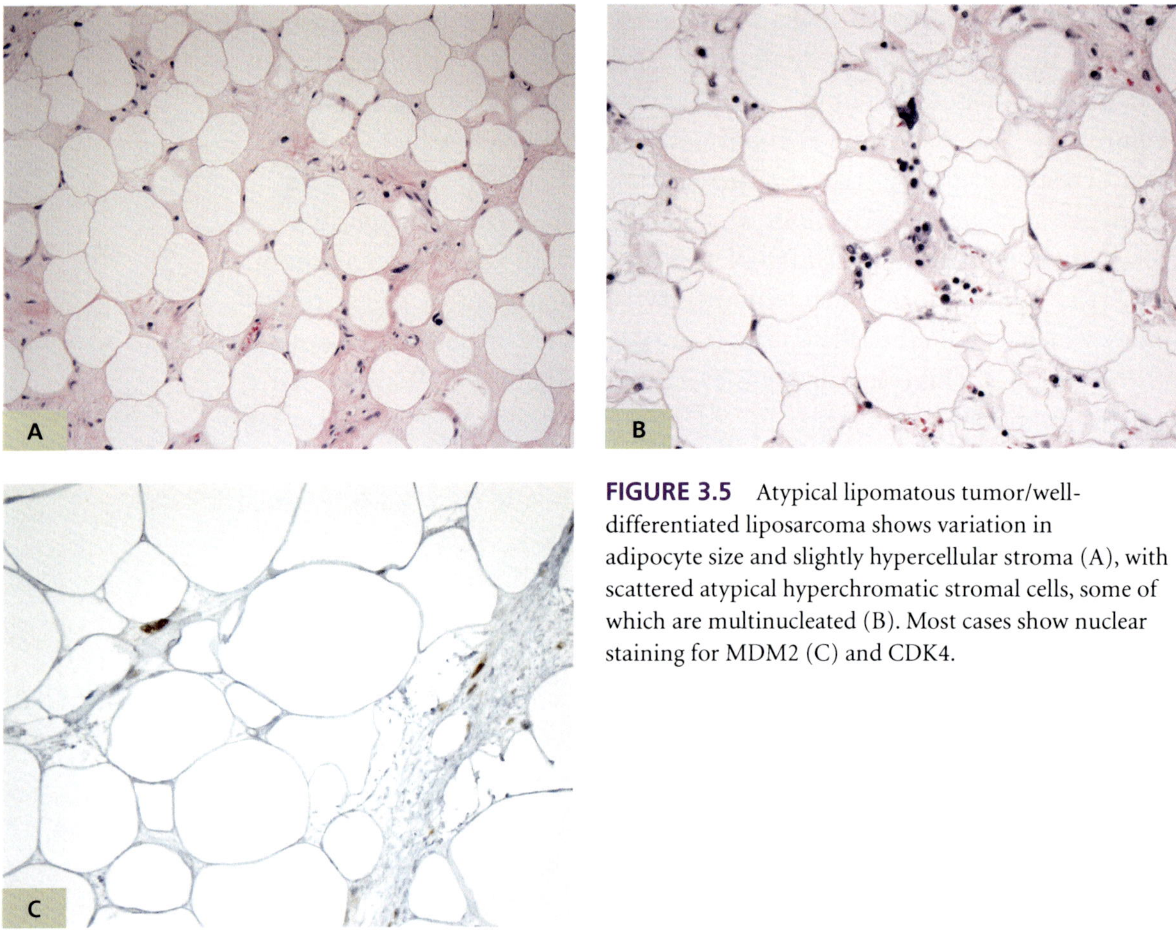

FIGURE 3.5 Atypical lipomatous tumor/well-differentiated liposarcoma shows variation in adipocyte size and slightly hypercellular stroma (A), with scattered atypical hyperchromatic stromal cells, some of which are multinucleated (B). Most cases show nuclear staining for MDM2 (C) and CDK4.

hyperchromatic atypical stromal cells of ALT/WDLPS is necessary, especially for large lipomas that have been traumatized with resultant fat necrosis. Immunohistochemistry for histiocytic markers such as CD68 or CD163 may be useful to confirm the identity of the MDM2-positive cells in such cases.

INTRAMUSCULAR ANGIOMA

Intramuscular angioma occurs over a wide age range and arises in the lower limbs, head and neck, and trunk (206). This tumor type arises within skeletal muscle and consists of a vascular proliferation, comprised of a combination of large thick-walled vessels, cavernous vascular spaces, and small capillaries in varying proportions, associated with variable amounts of fat (which can predominate in some cases) (**Figure 3.6A**). These lesions are poorly circumscribed with infiltration into adjacent skeletal muscle, often leading to myocyte atrophy

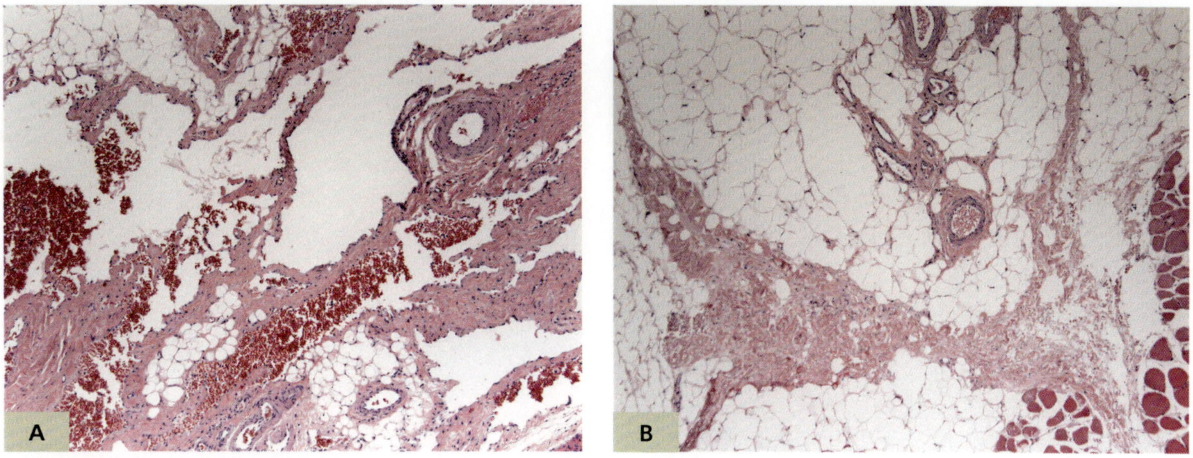

FIGURE 3.6 Intramuscular angioma. Lesions are comprised of varying proportions of fat and a vascular component characterized by thick-walled vessels, cavernous vascular spaces, or small capillaries (A), with frequent infiltration into adjacent skeletal muscle (B).

(**Figure 3.6B**). Complete resection may be challenging due to this infiltrative growth pattern; at least half of intramuscular angiomas recur secondary to incomplete resection (206). The chief alternative diagnostic consideration is an intramuscular lipoma. However, in some cases the atrophic skeletal muscle cells may be confused with the atypical multinucleated cells of ALT/WDLPS. Recognition of the prominent vascular component and infiltrative growth into skeletal muscle will assist in proper recognition of intramuscular angioma, and immunohistochemistry for MDM2 and CDK4 is negative. A desmin stain will be positive in the atrophic myocytes.

SCLEROSING MESENTERITIS

Idiopathic fibroinflammatory lesions characterized by varying combinations of fibrosis, chronic inflammation, and fat necrosis can present as abdominal masses (sclerosing mesenteritis) (**Figure 3.7**) or in the retroperitoneum (retroperitoneal fibrosis). Given the anatomic locations, inflammatory or sclerosing types of WDLPS may be considered, particularly because in these subtypes the atypical stromal cells characteristic of WDLPS are often obscured by chronic inflammation (in the case of the inflammatory type) and may be few in number (**Figure 3.8**). Sclerosing mesenteritis, which encompasses the entities previously known as sclerosing lipogranuloma, mesenteric panniculitis, and mesenteric lipodystrophy, presents in older adults usually as a single mass (more rarely as multiple masses or a more diffuse process) measuring up to 40 cm in greatest

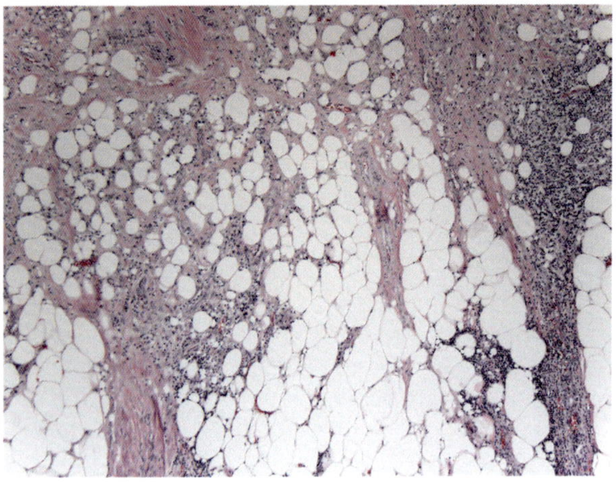

FIGURE 3.7 Sclerosing mesenteritis is characterized by fibrosis, chronic inflammation, and fat necrosis.

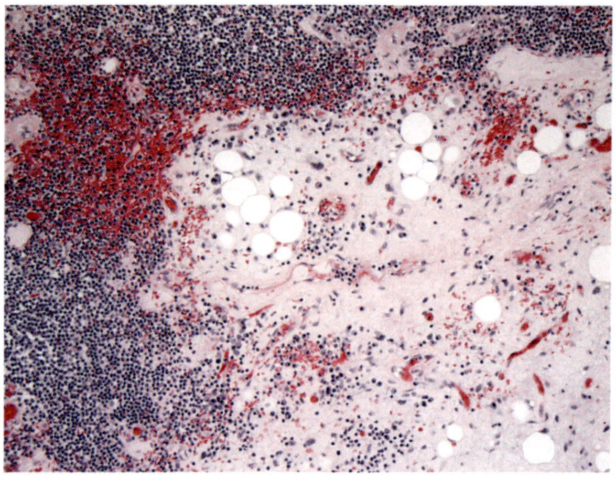

FIGURE 3.8 In the inflammatory subtype of well-differentiated liposarcoma, the atypical stromal cells may be obscured and few in number.

dimension (207). The fibrosis, chronic inflammation, and fat necrosis may be variable in proportion within a given lesion, and while reactive in nature, can lead to significant morbidity secondary to mass-related symptoms and complications such as bowel obstruction. The inflammatory infiltrate is typically a mixture of B and T lymphocytes. Proper diagnosis of either sclerosing mesenteritis or retroperitoneal fibrosis is particularly challenging in small core biopsy samples, given the clinical concern for liposarcoma. Immunohistochemistry for MDM2 or fluorescence in situ hybridization (FISH) to confirm the presence of *MDM2* amplification can be helpful to identify challenging cases of WDLPS (205).

SILICONE REACTION

Lipogranulomatous inflammation may manifest as "masses" in more superficial somatic soft tissue sites following liquid or gel silicone injection for cosmetic or reconstruction purposes. Most common sites include breast, lip, chin, and buttock. Silicone reactions result in sheets of histiocytes containing multivacuolated cytoplasm, with giant cells and chronic inflammation (**Figure 3.9**). The multivacuolated histiocytes are a caricature of lipoblasts, and their presence may raise suspicion for a liposarcoma in the absence of clinical history. However, in silicone reactions, the histiocytes are typically uniformly small in size, the nuclei contain fine chromatin (as opposed to the hyperchromatic nuclei of lipoblasts), and

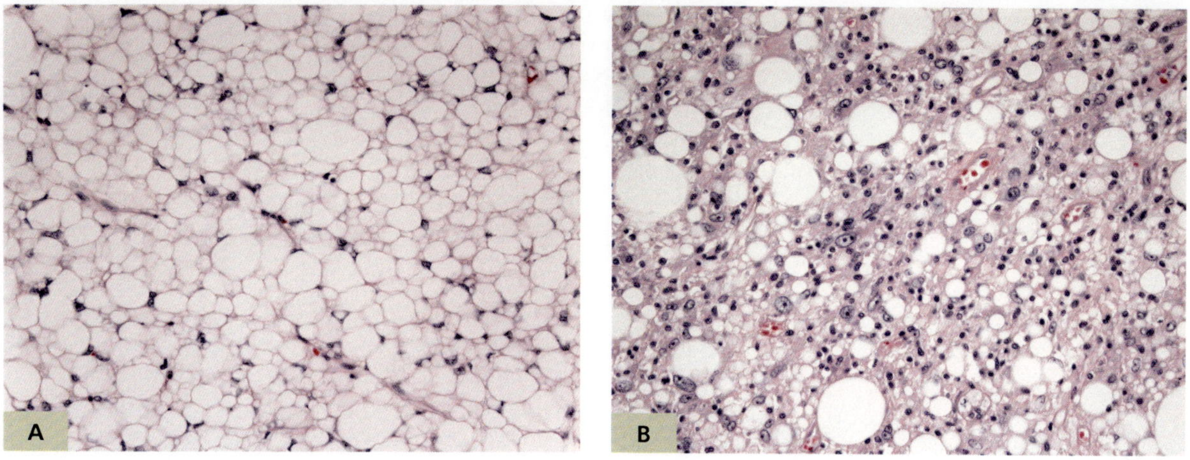

FIGURE 3.9 Silicone reaction. Sheets of histiocytes with vacuolated cytoplasm may mimic lipoblasts (A), but the histiocytes lack atypical nuclei and are often accompanied by chronic inflammation (B).

atypical stromal cells are absent. Lipoblasts are rarely present in such abundance in true liposarcomas. As discussed previously, histiocytes can show nuclear reactivity for MDM2 (a potential diagnostic pitfall), but CD163 and CD68 will be consistently positive, confirming the identity of histiocytes.

MASSIVE LOCALIZED LYMPHEDEMA

Massive localized lymphedema typically occurs in the proximal extremities of morbidly obese patients, presenting as huge masses measuring 20 to 30 cm or greater (208). These lesions are considered to be reactive in nature (likely developing secondary to lymphedema). Diagnosis on small biopsy specimens may be challenging, as many histologic changes are observed in massive localized lymphedema: there is dermal fibrosis overlying subcutaneous lobules of mature adipose tissue separated by expanded edematous fibrous septa (**Figure 3.10A,B**). Fibroblasts, including reactive enlarged forms, are present in the septa and may resemble the atypical stromal cells of ALT/WDLPS; however, the fibroblasts lack atypia and hyperchromatic nuclei (**Figure 3.10C**). Careful attention to the zonal appearance of the lobules will help distinguish massive localized lymphedema, in which capillary proliferation is often found at the interface between the septa and adipose tissue, from ALT/WDLPS. Despite being a benign and reactive lesion, massive localized lymphedema may recur, presumably due to the continued accumulation of lymph.

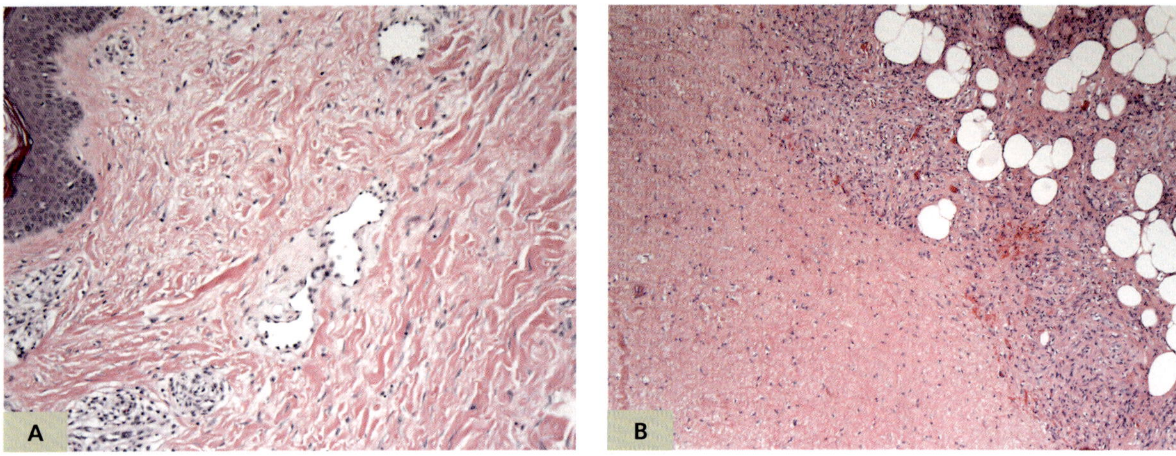

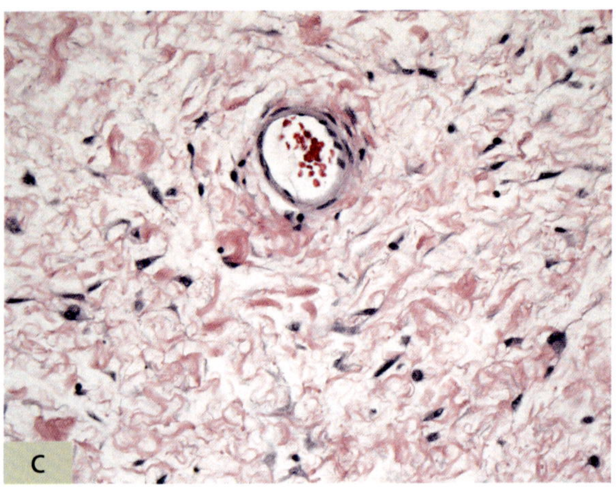

FIGURE 3.10 Massive localized lymphedema is characterized by dermal fibrosis with dilated lymphovascular spaces (A) overlying expanded edematous fibrous septa separating mature adipose tissue; a capillary proliferation is common at the interface with the fat (B). Benign-appearing fibroblasts are present in the septa (C).

PROLAPSED ORBITAL FAT

Rarely, intraconal orbital fat may herniate (secondary to aging or trauma) into the subconjunctival space, typically in the superotemporal region. Such lesions may be unilateral or bilateral and range in size from 0.6 to 2.3 cm (209). Histologically, prolapsed orbital fat contains thin fibrovascular septa separating lobules of mature fat, in which multinucleated floret-like cells are dispersed (**Figure 3.11**). A variable inflammatory infiltrate of lymphocytes, plasma cells, and histiocytes is a common feature. While WDLPS may be considered, prolapsed orbital fat lacks atypical hyperchromatic stromal cells, and immunohistochemistry for MDM2 and CDK4 is negative. The floret-like stromal cells are morphologically similar to those seen in spindle cell lipoma/pleomorphic

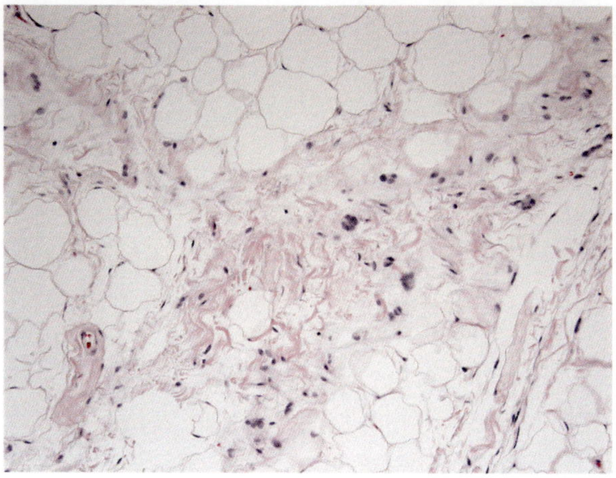

FIGURE 3.11 Prolapsed orbital fat. Multinucleated floret-like cells are dispersed within lobules of mature fat.

lipoma. However, prolapsed orbital fat also lacks the prominent spindle cell component and wiry stromal collagen characteristic of spindle cell lipoma/pleomorphic lipoma (see section "*Spindle Cell Lipoma/Pleomorphic Lipoma*"). Recurrence of prolapsed orbital fat is rare after complete excision.

MYELOLIPOMA

Myelolipoma is a benign lesion that most frequently arises in the adrenal gland in adult patients, but may also present as an extra-adrenal retroperitoneal mass. Tumors are frequently asymptomatic and are detected incidentally on imaging studies. The radiographic features of myelolipoma are usually sufficiently distinctive that the diagnosis can be rendered radiologically in the majority of cases; lesions are not resected unless there are equivocal radiologic features and a concern for malignancy. Lesions that are large retroperitoneal masses are frequently biopsied or resected out of concern for WDLPS. Myelolipomas can be extremely large, and may contain necrosis, hemorrhage, calcification, or osseous metaplasia, which may be concerning on radiology or gross examination. Myelolipoma is comprised of mature fat in which islands of hematopoietic marrow elements are scattered (**Figure 3.12**). Myeloid and erythroid precursor elements may be overlooked as mixed inflammation, and megakaryocytes may be mistaken for multinucleated atypical stromal cells and thus raise concern for WDLPS. Immunohistochemistry for MDM2 and CDK4 is negative, and markers are available to identify the different hematopoietic elements; CD61 in particular is helpful to identify megakaryocytes. While long considered to be

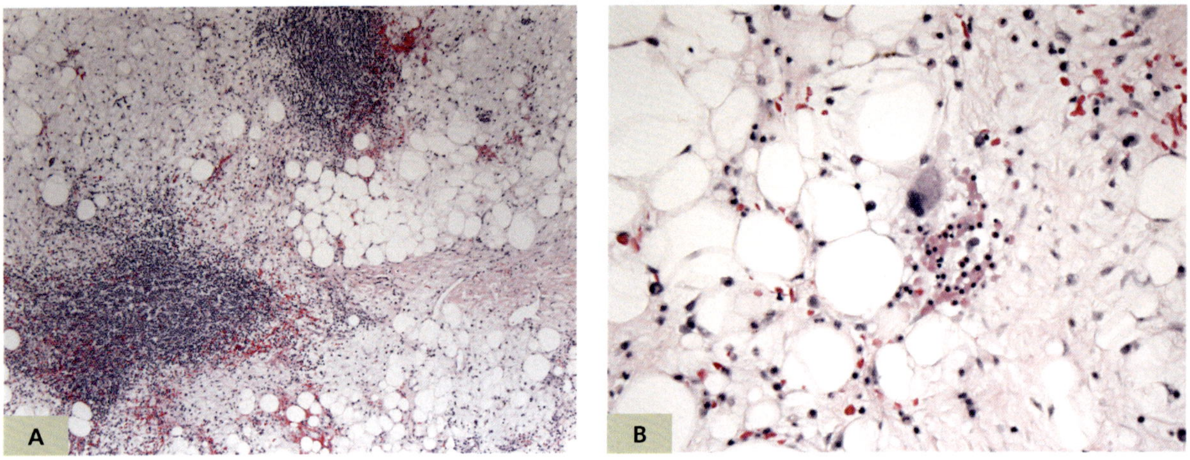

FIGURE 3.12 Myelolipoma. Islands of hematopoietic marrow elements are scattered in mature fat (A); megakaryocytes are commonly found (B).

a reactive process, nonrandom X-chromosome inactivation in myelolipomas of female patients has been demonstrated, suggesting that these lesions may be monoclonal (210).

LIPOMA (INCLUDING INTRAMUSCULAR LIPOMA AND LIPOMATOSIS)

Lipoma, the most common adipocytic tumor, most frequently presents as a subcutaneous mass in somatic soft tissue sites. Tumors may also occur in intramuscular sites, such as in the limbs and in the head and neck (*intramuscular lipoma*); such lesions typically have a more infiltrative growth pattern. Rarely lipomas may even occur in the retroperitoneum (211,212). Conventional lipomas follow a benign clinical course and very rarely recur, although intramuscular lipomas have higher recurrent potential. Several recurrent chromosomal alterations are known in lipoma, most frequently rearrangements involving 12q13-15, 13q, or 6p21-23. The diagnosis of benign lipoma is typically straightforward, but adipocytic (lipoma-like) ALT/WDLPS may be considered when lipomas are large (in excess of 10 cm) or located in subfascial soft tissue or the retroperitoneum. Confirmation of the absence of 12q13-15 (*MDM2* and *CDK4*) amplification by immunohistochemistry or FISH is advisable in these instances, especially for retroperitoneal sites where WDLPS is statistically much more likely. Lipomas containing extensive microscopic fat necrosis can mimic WDLPS, as described previously.

Intramuscular lipoma may show such prominent skeletal muscle infiltration (**Figure 3.13**) that the entrapped and atrophic myocytes may resemble the atypical stromal cells of WDLPS. Its propensity for recurrence may also be clinically worrisome. Lipomatosis is more concerning for a malignant neoplasm from a clinical standpoint, given that the massive accumulation of fat can present as a symptomatic and obvious mass, often resulting in compressive symptoms of adjacent structures. Despite having the histologic appearance of lobulated benign fat, recurrence is frequent after surgical resection and lesions are therefore often associated with high morbidity.

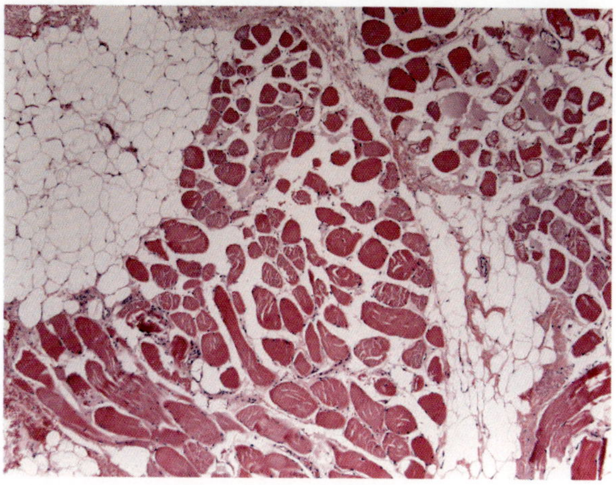

FIGURE 3.13 Intramuscular lipoma typically has a more infiltrative growth pattern with mature adipocytes admixed with skeletal muscle fibers.

SPINDLE CELL LIPOMA/PLEOMORPHIC LIPOMA

Spindle cell lipoma/pleomorphic lipoma frequently harbors rearrangements or deletion of 13q14, similar to mammary-type myofibroblastoma and cellular angiofibroma (213,214). Spindle cell lipoma/pleomorphic lipoma typically presents as subcutaneous masses in the posterior neck, back, or shoulder; such tumors arising in the skin show a broader anatomic distribution. Tumors are comprised of mature fat admixed with a benign-appearing spindled and ovoid cell population embedded in a variably collagenous or myxoid matrix with prominent thick collagen fibers (**Figure 3.14**). Multinucleated stromal cells are common (in pleomorphic lipoma), with nuclei arranged in a floret-like pattern (**Figure 3.15**). Nuclei are bland and lack atypia, and mitoses are rare. Lipoblasts may be present in spindle cell lipoma/pleomorphic lipoma, and, when identified in conjunction with multinucleated floret-like cells, a diagnosis of WDLPS may be considered. The presence of ropy collagen bundles, sharp circumscription, and the absence of nuclear atypia are features that favor spindle cell lipoma. Immunohistochemistry or cytogenetic studies can be used to identify *MDM2* amplification (or overexpression) in WDLPS. The 13q14 locus that is frequently rearranged in spindle cell lipoma/pleomorphic lipoma (as well as mammary-type myofibroblastoma and cellular angiofibroma) includes the tumor suppressor gene *retinoblastoma* (Rb).

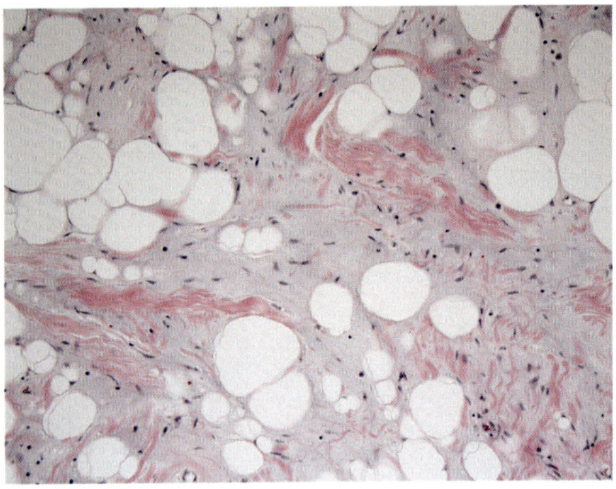

FIGURE 3.14 Spindle cell lipoma/pleomorphic lipoma is characterized by ovoid and spindled cells embedded in a variably collagenous or myxoid matrix, with prominent thick ropy collagen fibers and admixed adipocytes.

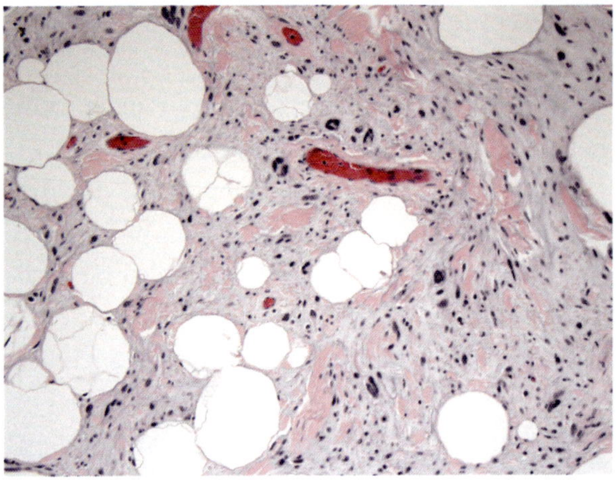

FIGURE 3.15 Multinucleated floret-like stromal cells are characteristic of pleomorphic lipoma.

Immunohistochemistry for Rb may be a helpful diagnostic adjunct in spindle cell lipoma/pleomorphic lipoma, as nuclear expression is absent (ie, lost) in tumor cells (215) (**Figure 3.16**).

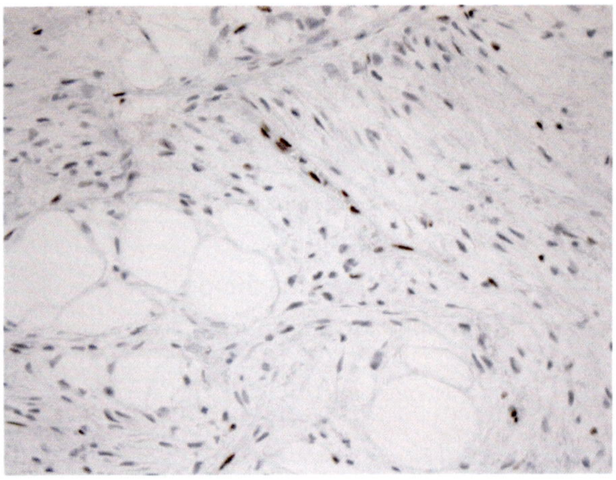

FIGURE 3.16 Loss of nuclear expression of the retinoblastoma protein is characteristic of spindle cell lipoma/pleomorphic lipoma.

HIBERNOMA

Hibernoma is an adipocytic tumor characterized by 11q13 rearrangement (216) that may occasionally be mistaken for a lipoblast-forming malignant neoplasm. Tumors most frequently occur on the thigh, trunk, and head and neck, and may present as masses as large as 24 cm (average 9.3 cm)(217). Hibernomas are comprised of an admixture of white fat and "brown fat" cells: polygonal adipocytes with multivacuolated cytoplasm ranging from eosinophilic-to-clear in appearance (**Figure 3.17**). While the brown fat cells may mimic lipoblasts, they lack the characteristic hyperchromatic scalloped nuclei. Careful histologic examination and adequate sampling is mandatory, as occasional brown fat cells may be present in liposarcoma, including both myxoid liposarcoma and WDLPS. Tumors with predominantly eosinophilic morphology may also mimic skeletal muscle tumors (see Chapter 5).

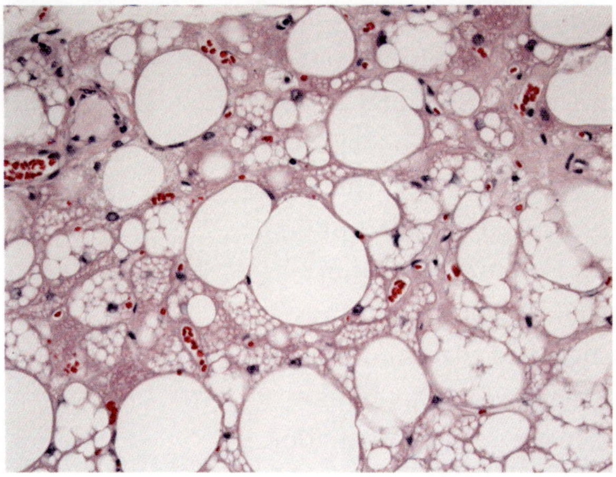

FIGURE 3.17 Hibernomas show an admixture of white fat and brown fat. The brown fat cells have abundant multivacuolated eosinophilic-to-clear cytoplasm.

LIPOBLASTOMA

Lipoblastoma, a tumor of infancy, is a multilobulated tumor comprised of lipoblasts in varying maturation stages embedded in a prominent myxoid stroma. Tumors typically occur on the limbs in patients 3 years of age or younger, although a wide anatomic distribution may be seen, and occasional tumors are detected in older children and adolescents. Lipoblastoma frequently harbors 8q11-13 rearrangements (218,219). These tumors are benign with no risk of metastasis; surgical resection is usually curative, with recurrence observed in up to 46% of cases typically after incomplete resection (220). Tumors can either be well-circumscribed or infiltrative (though recurrence is seen for tumors showing either growth pattern), and usually present as slow-growing masses 2 to 5 cm in greatest dimension. A wide histologic spectrum of adipocytic maturation is seen, both within a given lesion and between tumors. The tumor cell population includes a primitive spindled-to-stellate mesenchymal cell component, lipoblasts varying from signet-ring-cell type to multivacuolated, and mature adipocytes (**Figure 3.18**). Cytologic atypia and mitotic activity are absent. Lipoblastoma may contain a proliferation of thin-walled branching capillaries. Owing to the abundant myxoid

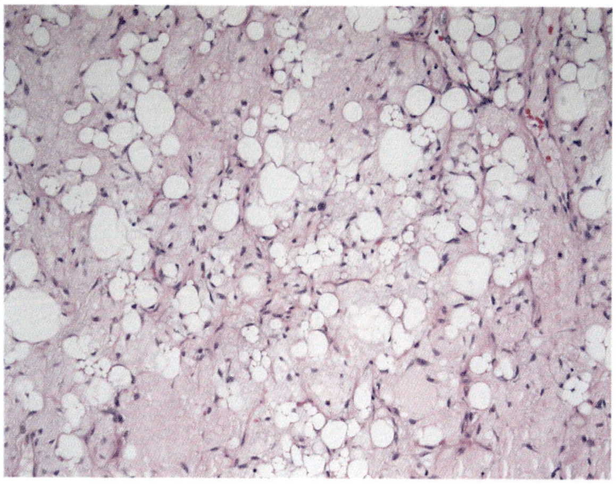

FIGURE 3.18 Lipoblastoma is comprised of a spindled-to-stellate mesenchymal cell population admixed with lipoblasts and mature adipocytes; cytologic atypia and mitotic activity are absent.

stroma, vascular pattern, and lipoblast population, distinction between lipoblastoma and myxoid liposarcoma may be challenging. The clinical context is usually discriminatory: lipoblastoma rarely occurs outside of infancy and early childhood, whereas myxoid liposarcoma is rare in children. Lipoblastoma lacks cytologic atypia, hyperchromatic nuclei, and hypercellular foci, which are features observed in most myxoid liposarcomas (even in low-grade tumors) (**Figure 3.19**). In challenging cases, cytogenetic or FISH studies for confirmation of the t(12;16) translocation (resulting in *FUS-DDIT3* fusion) is diagnostic of myxoid liposarcoma (221). Recent studies have suggested that immunohistochemistry for PLAG1 may be helpful to support a diagnosis of lipoblastoma (222). Of note, myxoid liposarcoma may show extensive cytodifferentiation in response to chemotherapy (**Figure 3.20**); thus, careful clinical correlation is required.

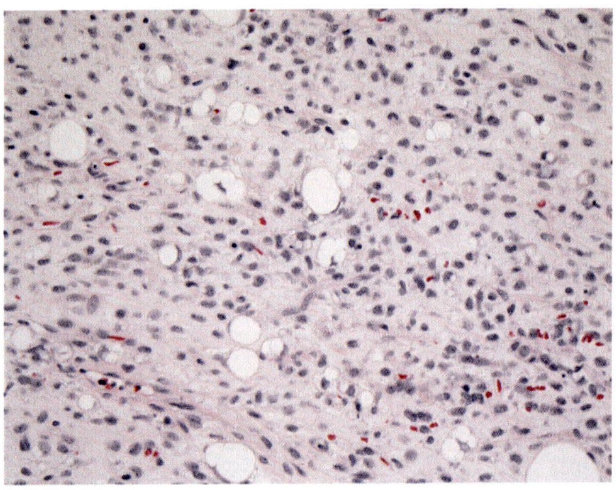

FIGURE 3.19 Myxoid liposarcoma shows hypercellularity, characteristic lipoblasts, and thin-walled branching capillaries.

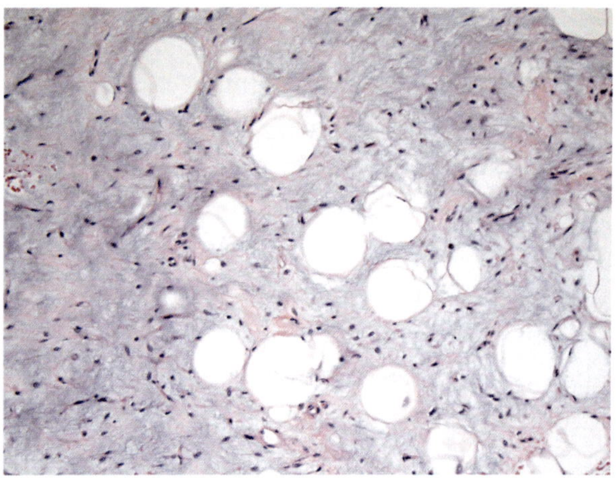

FIGURE 3.20 Postchemotherapy, myxoid liposarcoma may show extensive cytodifferentiation, with abundant mature fat and an absence of lipoblasts.

4

Mimics of Fibroblastic/ Myofibroblastic and Fibrohistiocytic Neoplasms

- MIMICS OF FIBROBLASTIC/ MYOFIBROBLASTIC NEOPLASMS
  - *Nodular Fasciitis*
  - *Proliferative Fasciitis/Proliferative Myositis*
  - *Ischemic Fasciitis*
  - *Fibroma of Tendon Sheath*
  - *Desmoid Fibromatosis*
  - *Pseudosarcomatous Myofibroblastic Proliferation*
  - *Dermatomyofibroma*
  - *Cellular Benign Fibrous Histiocytoma*
  - *Mammary-Type Myofibroblastoma*
  - *Cellular Angiofibroma*
  - *Soft Tissue Perineurioma*
  - *Superficial Angiomyxoma*
  - *Intramuscular Myxoma (Including Cellular Myxoma)*
- SELECTED MIMICS OF PEDIATRIC FIBROBLASTIC/MYOFIBROBLASTIC NEOPLASMS
  - *Fibrous Hamartoma of Infancy*
  - *Infantile Myofibromatosis*
- MIMICS OF FIBROHISTIOCYTIC NEOPLASMS
  - *Reactive and Inflammatory Processes*
  - *Cellular Neurothekeoma*
  - *Cellular Benign Fibrous Histiocytoma*

Fibroblasts are constituents of normal stroma and can proliferate in many reactive settings (myofibroblasts). Fibroblasts and myofibroblasts likely represent a biologic and functional spectrum of a single cell type, thus tumors classified as "fibroblastic/myofibroblastic" represent an extremely diverse group of neoplasms. By immunohistochemistry, fibroblasts are generally positive for CD34; myofibroblasts demonstrate variable expression of smooth muscle actin (SMA), desmin, and cytokeratin.

The classification of tumors as "fibrohistiocytic" in type is based on histologic grounds rather than line of differentiation, referring to the presence of cells that resemble fibroblasts and cells appearing histiocytoid. The category of so-called "fibrohistiocytic tumors" as designated by the World Health Organization (WHO) includes tenosynovial giant cell tumor (localized and diffuse types), deep benign fibrous histiocytoma, plexiform fibrohistiocytic tumor, and giant cell tumor of soft tissue. Plexiform fibrohistiocytic tumor and giant cell tumor of soft tissue have risk for metastasis (which cannot be predicted by histopathologic features), although all tumor types in this group are associated with some rate of recurrence.

MIMICS OF FIBROBLASTIC/MYOFIBROBLASTIC NEOPLASMS

NODULAR FASCIITIS

Nodular fasciitis, historically considered to be a myofibroblastic pseudotumor, follows a distinctive clinical course of rapid growth of a solitary, tender, usually subcutaneous mass and subsequent spontaneous regression. It is now known that nodular fasciitis is a "transient" neoplasm characterized by a recurrent translocation involving the *USP6* gene on chromosome 17p13 and *MYH9* on chromosome 22q.3-q13 (223). Most affected patients are adults, with no gender predilection. Lesions are most common on the upper limb and chest/trunk; in children, head and neck sites (including cranial-based) are more common. Rarely, intravascular, intradermal, fascial, and cranial lesions occur. Patients typically report between 1 and 3 months of rapid growth, and lesions rarely exceed 5 cm in greatest dimension. Recurrence apart from incomplete resection during the active growth phase is exceedingly rare.

Nodular fasciitis is a well-circumscribed lesion comprised of plump, predominantly spindled, myofibroblasts arranged in loose fascicular and storiform patterns (**Figure 4.1A**). In the early "active" phase, lesions tend to be more cellular and can show mitotic activity (**Figure 4.1B**), which may be concerning for a malignant neoplasm. The background stroma may be variably loosely collagenous, myxoid and microcystic, with frequent lymphocytes and extravasated red blood cells. Intravascular and cranial variants tend to show a greater number of osteoclast-like giant cells and occasionally osseous metaplasia (**Figure 4.1C**). As nodular fasciitis progresses, "maturing" lesions show increased stromal collagen, sometimes including keloidal collagen fibers (**Figure 4.1D**). On close histologic examination, the myofibroblasts show bland nuclei with delicate nucleoli and stellate-to-elongated cell processes (these cells are often described as "tissue culture-like"). Significant pleomorphism and nuclear atypia are absent. While mitoses may be readily found, atypical mitotic forms are exceptional. Alternative diagnosis should also be considered if there is tumor necrosis or if the lesion exceeds 5 cm in size.

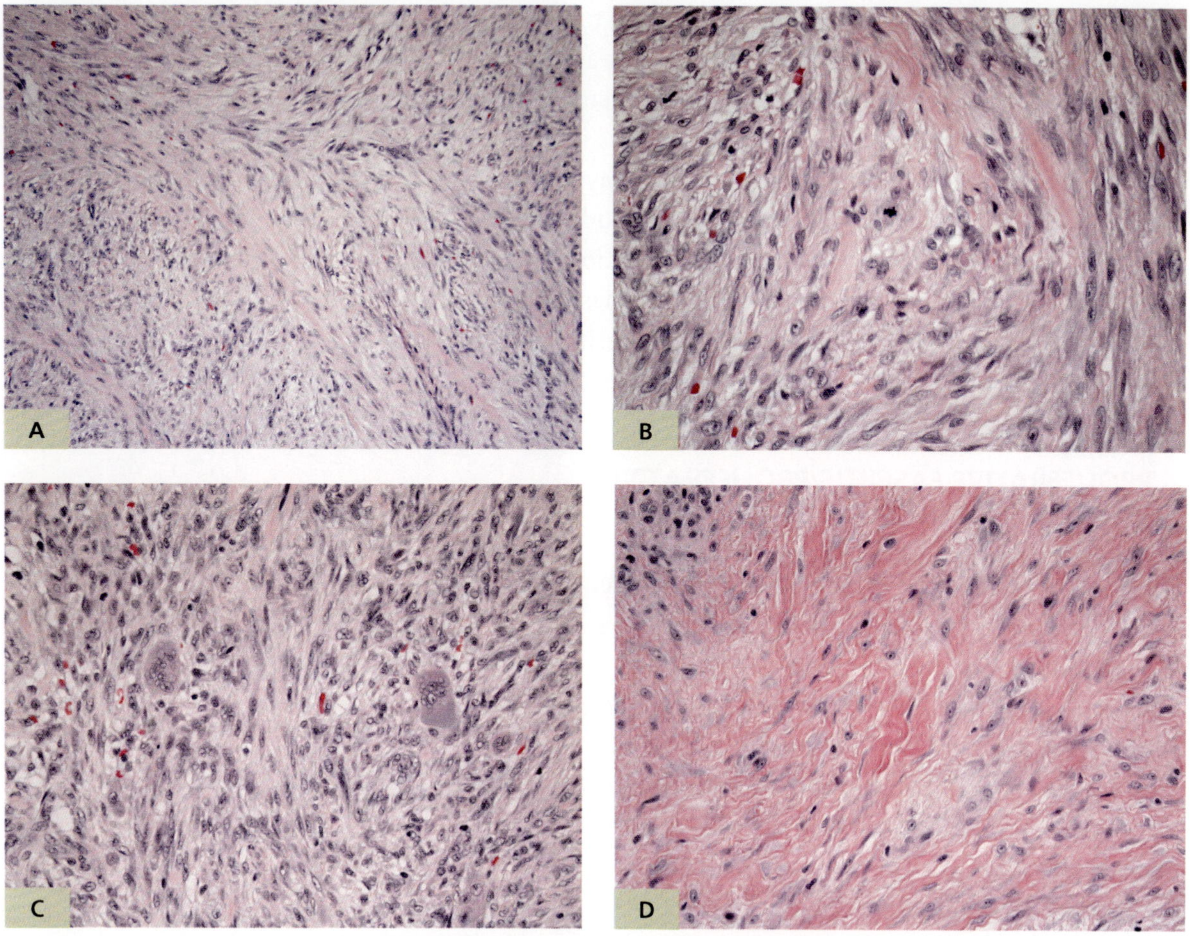

FIGURE 4.1 Nodular fasciitis. Plump spindled myofibroblasts arranged in a loose fascicular and storiform growth pattern with varying collagenous and myxoid stroma (A). Lesions often appear cellular and mitotic figures may be seen (B); however, cytologic atypia and atypical mitotic forms are not observed. Osteoclast-like giant cells are a common finding (C). As nodular fasciitis progresses and matures, the stroma shows increased collagen and frequent keloid-type fibers (D).

Given its pathognomonic clinical course, appropriate diagnosis is helpful in avoiding unnecessary surgical intervention or more aggressive postsurgical management, such as radiation therapy. Variable SMA and rare desmin immunoreactivity is seen in nodular fasciitis; however, these findings are nonspecific when considering most low-grade fibroblastic/myofibroblastic sarcomas in the differential diagnosis. Most commonly, lesions may show overlapping histologic features with desmoid fibromatosis (see section "*Desmoid Fibromatosis*"), which has a potential for recurrence and is often treated with surgical resection. Desmoid fibromatosis is typically composed of longer fascicles of myofibroblasts embedded in a more uniformly collagenous stroma, and lesions tend to be more infiltrative. Approximately 80% of tumors show nuclear positivity for β-catenin, reflecting underlying mutation in

CTNNB1 or *APC*. Clinical history for the subset of tumors arising in the setting of familial adenomatous polyposis (FAP) syndrome is also helpful.

Late-stage cases of nodular fasciitis may resemble desmoplastic fibroblastoma, a benign lesion that typically affects adults in a wide range of anatomic sites, often centered on fascial planes. Lesions are hypocellular, with cytologically benign-appearing spindle and stellate cells embedded in a variably myxoid and collagenous stroma (**Figure 4.2**). Clinical correlation is helpful, as desmoplastic fibroblastoma often presents as a slow-growing mass and does not regress spontaneously. Desmoplastic fibroblastoma is characterized by 11q12 rearrangement, which correlates with *FOSL1* upregulation (224).

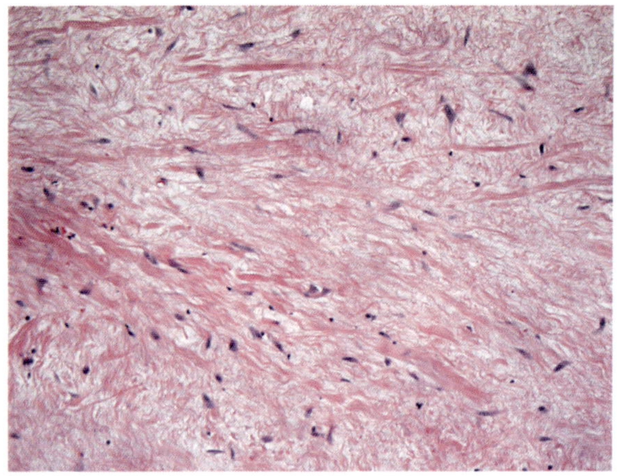

FIGURE 4.2 Desmoplastic fibroblastoma is typically hypocellular with benign-appearing spindled and stellate myofibroblasts embedded in a hyalinized collagenous stroma.

PROLIFERATIVE FASCIITIS/PROLIFERATIVE MYOSITIS

Proliferative fasciitis and proliferative myositis are benign lesions that are similar in clinical presentation as nodular fasciitis, with rapid emergence of a lesion; however, both entities lack recurrent *USP6* gene rearrangements (223). Adults are most commonly affected, and lesions are most common in the proximal extremities, limb girdle, and truncal regions; proliferative myositis refers to lesions in intramuscular sites. Recurrence is rare after complete excision. Both proliferative fasciitis and proliferative myositis are comprised of an admixture of a bland spindle cell component that is morphologically similar to nodular fasciitis, and a population of cells resembling ganglion cells, which are sometimes bi- and trinucleated, with prominent eosinophilic nucleoli (**Figure 4.3**). The ganglion-like cells have a low nuclear-to-cytoplasmic ratio, and the nuclei are not hyperchromatic and have smooth nuclear contours. In proliferative myositis, the entrapped skeletal muscle fibers remain intact and osseous metaplasia may be present (**Figure 4.4**). Mitoses are often present, and the impression of skeletal muscle infiltration of proliferative myositis may appear worrisome for malignancy. However, the absence of atypical mitotic figures and significant cytologic

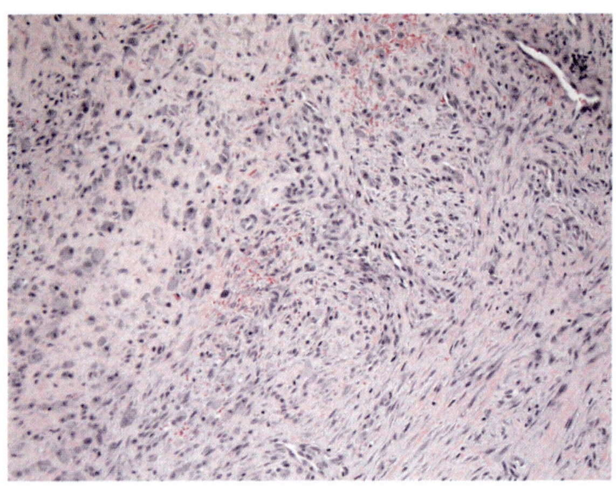

FIGURE 4.3 Proliferative fasciitis is comprised of a myofibroblastic spindle cell population (that resembles nodular fasciitis) admixed with a population of ganglion-like cells that may be bi- and trinucleated.

atypia should be reassuring. While SMA and desmin may be positive in the spindle cell component, the ganglion-like cells are negative.

The enlarged ganglion-like cells, spindle cell component, mitotic activity, and infiltrative growth may raise general concern for a malignant neoplasm. Specifically, proliferative myositis may mimic low-grade myofibroblastic sarcoma. Low-grade myofibroblastic sarcoma is comprised of fascicular growth of mildly atypical myofibroblasts infiltrating between skeletal muscle fibers (**Figure 4.5A**). In contrast to the fasciitis-like component of proliferative myositis, the fascicles of low-grade myofibroblastic sarcoma are more densely cellular and frequently overlap and intersect, and the ganglion cell-like component is absent (**Figure 4.5B**). The neoplastic myofibroblastic cells demonstrate nuclear hyperchromasia and recognizable cytologic atypia. β-catenin immunoreactivity has been reported in up to a third of low-grade myofibroblastic sarcomas (225), which may be helpful given its variable expression of SMA and desmin.

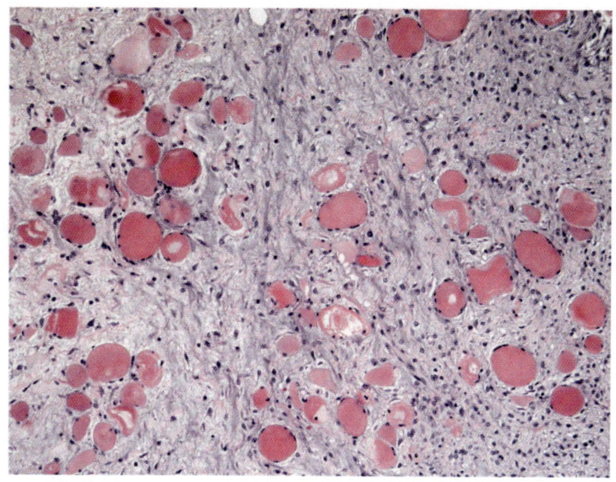

FIGURE 4.4 Proliferative myositis is similar to proliferative fasciitis, with admixed populations of spindled myofibroblastic cells and ganglion-like cells, but shows skeletal muscle infiltration imparting a "checkerboard" appearance.

ISCHEMIC FASCIITIS

Ischemic fasciitis is a reactive process that often occurs in older adults. Lesions are centered in deep subcutis over bony prominences in the hip and sacral regions. Tumor size is on average 4 to 5 cm.

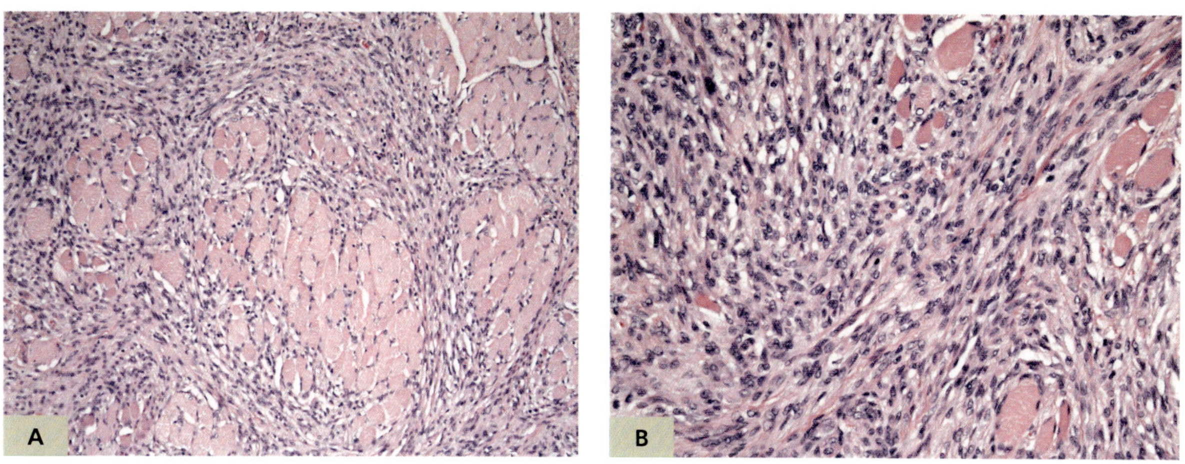

FIGURE 4.5 Low-grade myofibroblastic sarcoma is characterized by fascicular growth of atypical spindle cells with infiltration between skeletal muscle fibers (A). The fascicles are densely cellular and tumor cells show mild but appreciable cytologic atypia (B).

While most early descriptions of ischemic fasciitis reported a strong association with decubitus ulcers in immobile patients (226), not all lesions are associated with debilitation (227). Ischemic fasciitis is a benign lesion; tumors that persist or recur after resection are likely secondary to continued immobility. Ischemic fasciitis shows zonation of large areas of fibrinoid necrosis, granulation tissue, chronic inflammation, fat necrosis, and plump and rounded fibroblasts and myofibroblasts (**Figure 4.6**). Particularly in biopsy specimens or variably present components in tissue sections, the population of enlarged fibroblasts and myofibroblasts may be worrisome for a malignant neoplasm. While mitoses are frequent, atypical mitotic forms and cytologic atypia are absent. A broad range of sarcomas may enter the differential diagnoses, including rhabdomyosarcoma and pseudomyogenic hemangioendothelioma. The myofibroblasts are negative for myogenin (excluding rhabdomyosarcoma); despite possibly showing keratin expression, the lesional cells will be negative for the endothelial markers ERG and CD31 (excluding pseudomyogenic hemangioendothelioma). Thorough sampling and clinical correlation will assist in recognition of ischemic fasciitis.

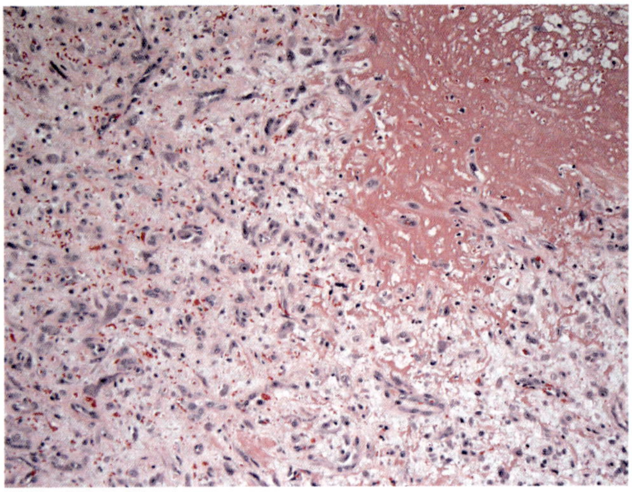

FIGURE 4.6 Ischemic fasciitis shows zonation of large areas of fibrinoid necrosis and granulation tissue with chronic inflammation and plump and rounded fibroblasts/myofibroblasts.

FIBROMA OF TENDON SHEATH

Fibroma of tendon sheath occurs most commonly in adults with a male predominance, and presents as a single firm nodule most frequently on the fingers (often associated with a tendon). 11q12 rearrangement has been identified in fibroma of tendon sheath, which correlates with *FOSL1* upregulation (228). Lesions are well-circumscribed lobular proliferations of bland-appearing fibroblasts and myofibroblasts showing a variably fascicular growth pattern (**Figure 4.7A**). The stroma is collagenous with frequent slit-like vessels (**Figure 4.7B**). While often resembling nodular fasciitis or myofibroma, some cases of fibroma of tendon sheath may resemble desmoid fibromatosis. Complete resection of fibroma of tendon sheath is curative, in contrast to the high recurrence propensity of desmoid fibromatosis. Sharp circumscription and the distinct slit-like vascular pattern of fibroma of tendon sheath

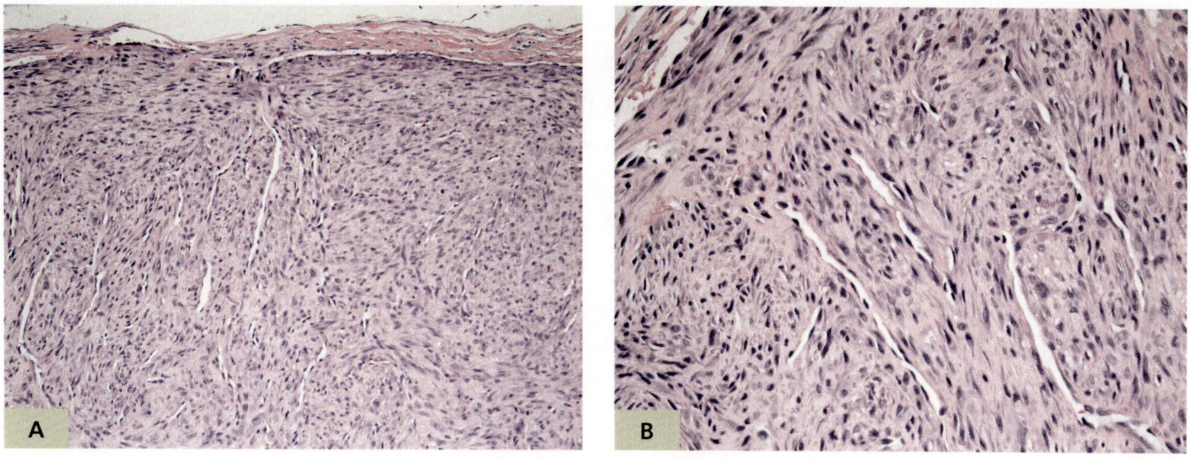

FIGURE 4.7 Fibroma of tendon sheath is a well-circumscribed nodule comprised of fascicles of nondescript spindle cells (A) and frequent slit-like vessels (B).

aid in recognition, and β-catenin will be positive in the majority of desmoid fibromatosis.

DESMOID FIBROMATOSIS

Desmoid fibromatosis, referring to fibromatosis in deep-seated locations, occurs most commonly in young adults and affects women twice as often as men. Desmoid fibromatosis is considered to be a fibroblastic/myofibroblastic neoplasm that can be locally aggressive, with frequent recurrences, but lacks metastatic potential. Tumors arise in extra-abdominal, anterior abdominal wall, and intra-abdominal sites, and are often large (greater than 5 cm). Most tumors show infiltrative growth into adjacent structures, which can lead to significant morbidity especially when surgical resection with adequate margins is sought. However, it has been demonstrated that margin status does not predict recurrence (229,230). Sporadic desmoid tumors are mostly extra-abdominal and associated with *CTNNB1* mutation (231,232), while tumors associated with FAP (which are often intra-abdominal and multicentric, occasionally arising after prophylactic colectomy) are characterized by *APC* gene mutations (233). Both *CTNNB1* and *APC* gene mutations lead to upregulation of β-catenin protein. Desmoid tumors also may arise in the anterior abdominal wall in pregnancy or post-Cesarean section settings, or in association with scar or in a radiation field.

On histologic examination, desmoid tumors are comprised of palely eosinophilic myofibroblasts with tapering vesicular nuclei arranged in long, usually hypocellular fascicles (**Figure 4.8A, B**). Tumor cells are embedded in a collagenous or myxoid stroma, with thicker-walled vessels often associated with edematous changes. Significant cytologic atypia is absent, and while mitotic activity is common in desmoid tumors, atypical mitotic figures are absent. SMA is positive, and nuclear β-catenin reactivity is observed in 80% of cases (**Figure 4.8C**).

One significant diagnostic challenge arises in patients who have undergone multiple prior resections, in which scar tissue is difficult to distinguish from desmoid fibromatosis. Scar tissue is also comprised of myofibroblasts, and sometimes distinction relies on β-catenin immunohistochemistry.

Desmoid fibromatosis may mimic low-grade myofibroblastic sarcoma, which is β-catenin positive in up to a third of cases (225). Low-grade myofibroblastic sarcoma is most common in somatic soft tissue sites, especially in the limbs and head and neck. Tumors are comprised of more cellular fascicles of myofibroblasts, which exhibit appreciable cytologic atypia. In contrast to desmoid fibromatosis, tumor cells of low-grade myofibroblastic sarcoma have hyperchromatic nuclei with irregular and angulated nuclear contours.

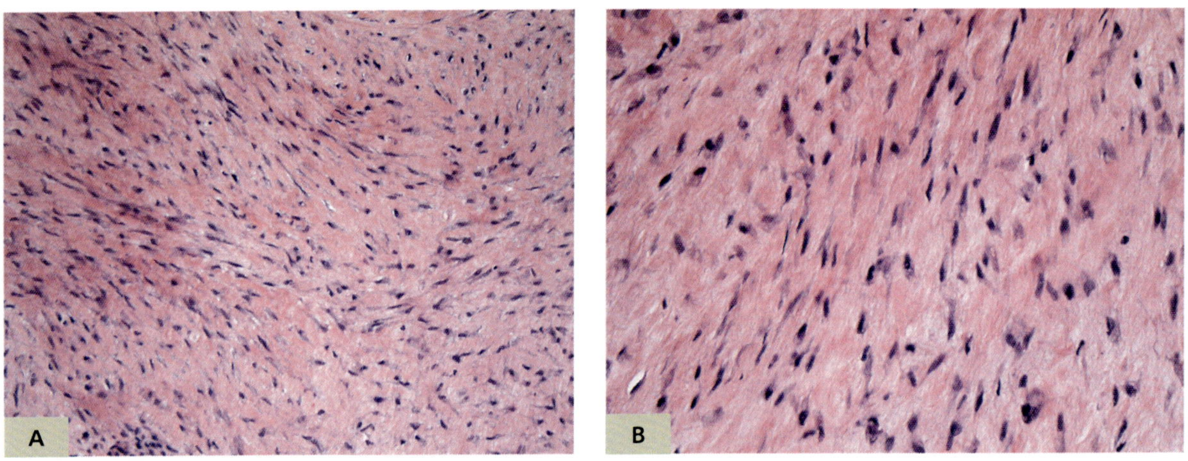

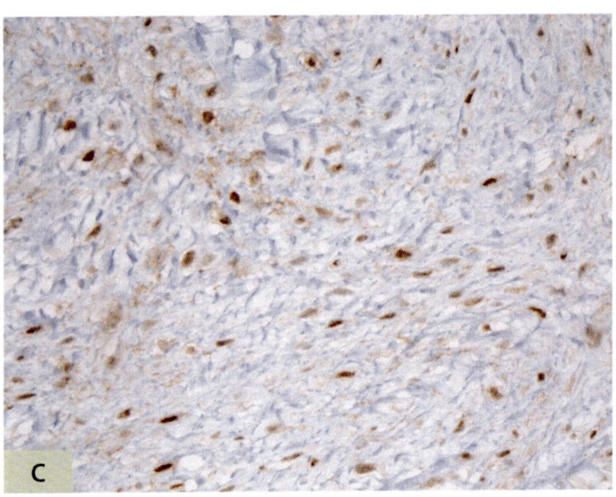

FIGURE 4.8 Desmoid fibromatosis. Tumors are hypocellular with fascicular growth of palely eosinophilic myofibroblasts embedded in a collagenous or myxoid stroma (A). The spindled tumor cells have tapering vesicular nuclei and palely eosinophilic cytoplasm and lack cytologic atypia (B). Nuclear β-catenin is present in up to 80% of cases (C).

In combination with correlation with clinical data, recognition of malignant cytologic features will assist in distinction.

Some cases of intra-abdominal desmoid fibromatosis may mimic inflammatory myofibroblastic tumor (IMT), which presents most commonly in young patients in the abdominal cavity (but can arise at any site). Tumors are often large (up to 10 cm), and repeated recurrences often follow initial resection; a very small risk of metastasis exists. IMT is comprised of cellular fascicles of myofibroblasts accompanied by an inflammatory infiltrate, chiefly of plasma cells and lymphocytes (**Figure 4.9A**). The myofibroblasts are spindled with plump mildly atypical nuclei, and the cytologic atypia would not be expected in desmoid tumor (**Figure 4.9B**). Mitotic activity is common. Immunohistochemistry is positive for SMA and variably positive for desmin and cytokeratin; anaplastic lymphoma kinase (ALK) is positive in approximately half of cases (**Figure 4.9C**). ALK overexpression is secondary to *ALK* gene rearrangement (most frequently in pediatric cases), and the heterogeneous

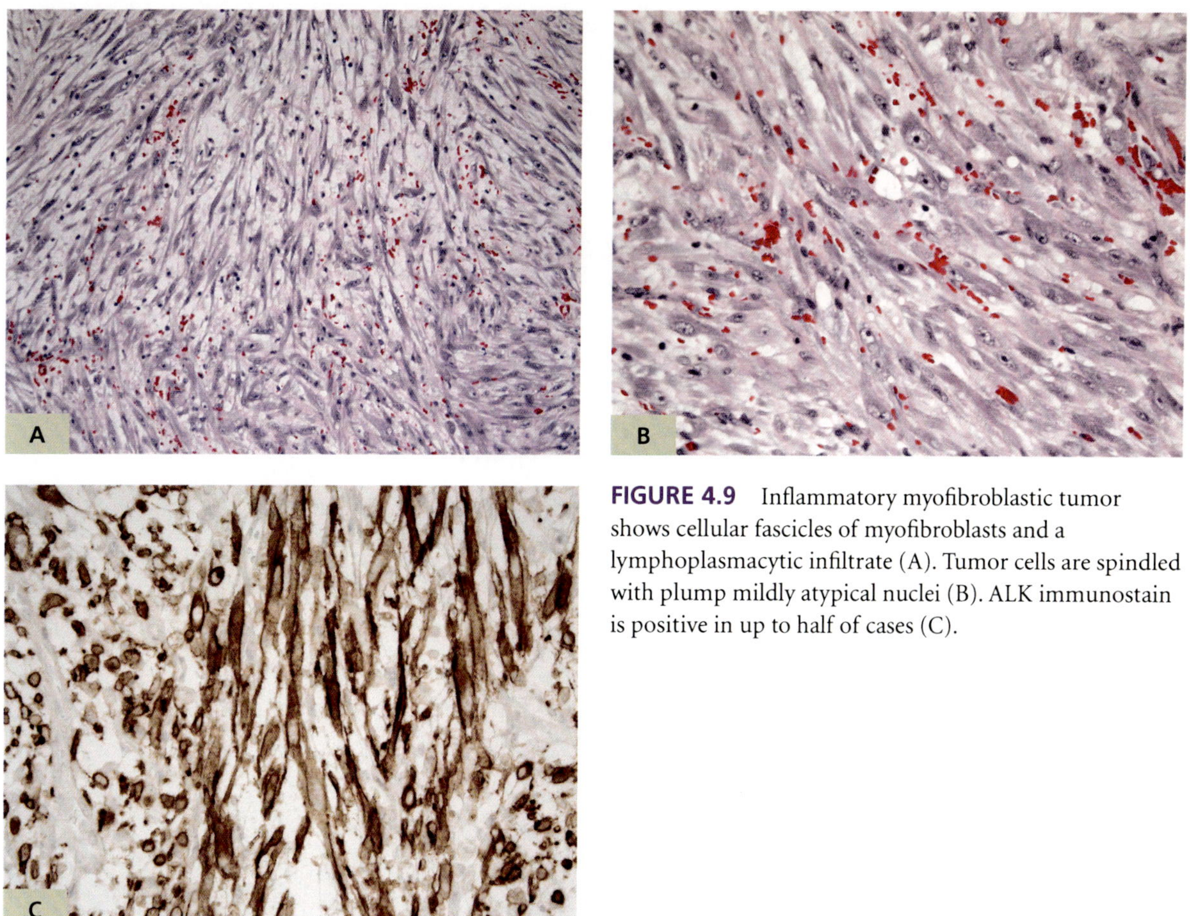

FIGURE 4.9 Inflammatory myofibroblastic tumor shows cellular fascicles of myofibroblasts and a lymphoplasmacytic infiltrate (A). Tumor cells are spindled with plump mildly atypical nuclei (B). ALK immunostain is positive in up to half of cases (C).

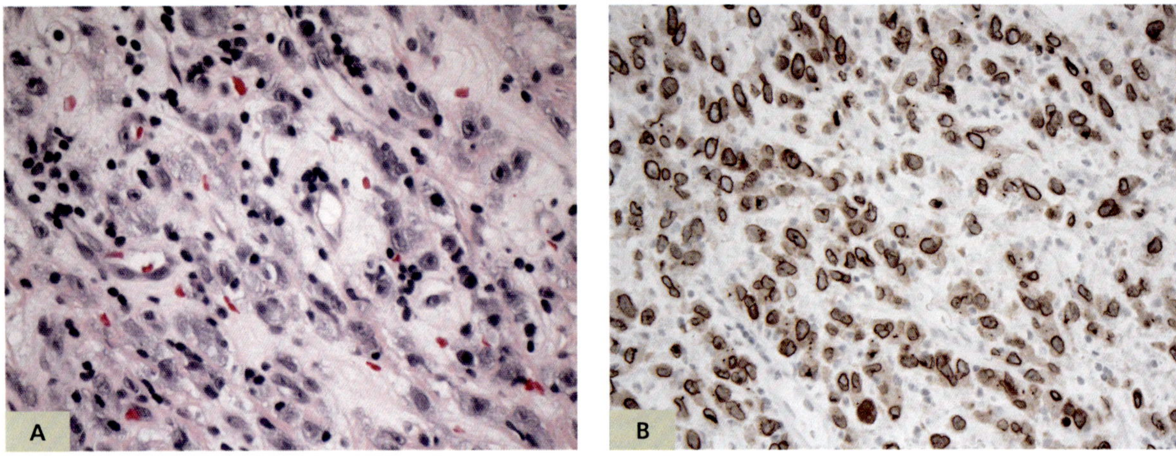

FIGURE 4.10 The epithelioid variant of inflammatory myofibroblastic tumor is associated with more aggressive behavior, and is characterized by plump epithelioid and histiocytoid tumor cells embedded in a myxoid stroma (A). Note the nuclear membrane pattern of ALK staining (as the fusion partner *RANBP2* encodes a nuclear pore protein) (B).

group of fusion partners include *TPM3*, *TPM4*, *CLTC*, and *RANBP2* (234–236). Notably, *ALK-RANBP2* fusion characterizes an "epithelioid" variant which is comprised of plump epithelioid and histiocytoid cells, often contains myxoid stroma, and shows nuclear membrane pattern of ALK staining (as *RANBP2* is a nuclear pore protein)(**Figure 4.10**). The epithelioid variant of IMT is associated with a more aggressive clinical behavior (236).

PSEUDOSARCOMATOUS MYOFIBROBLASTIC PROLIFERATION

Pseudosarcomatous myofibroblastic proliferation (PMP) and postoperative spindle cell nodule (the latter arising after surgery or instrumentation, most frequently in the bladder) are benign tumors that affect adults and arise most commonly in genitourinary sites. Most authors consider PMP to be a clinicopathologically distinct entity from IMT (237). PMP often arises spontaneously without a history of trauma and may present as a large mass (up to 10 cm). PMP is a benign tumor with minimal risk of recurrence and no metastatic risk. Microscopically, PMP is characterized by infiltrative fascicular growth of spindled-to-stellate myofibroblastic cells arranged loosely in a myxoid stroma (**Figure 4.11A**); postoperative spindle cell nodules are small well-circumscribed lesions with identical cytomorphologic features. A sparse lymphocytic infiltrate is common, but plasma cells are generally absent. Slit-like vessels and large epithelioid cells resembling rhabdomyoblasts are frequent (237) (**Figure 4.11B**). The presence of myxoid stroma, absence of plasma cells, and present of pseudorhabdomyoblasts are morphologic features that distinguish PMP from IMT.

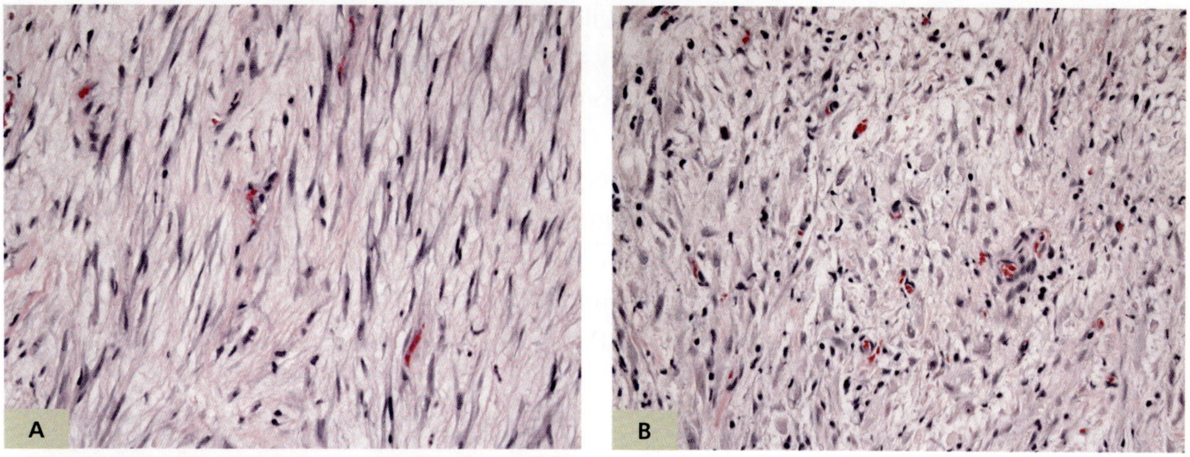

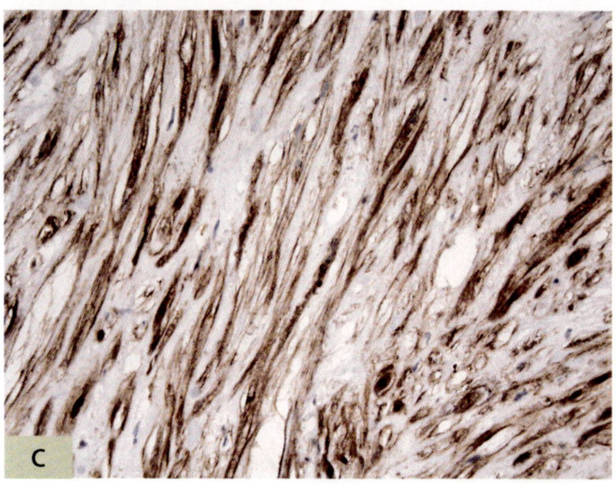

FIGURE 4.11 Pseudosarcomatous myofibroblastic proliferation shows infiltrative fascicular growth of spindled-to-stellate myofibroblasts arranged loosely in a myxoid stroma (A). Tumors may have large cells with brightly eosinophilic cytoplasm resembling rhabdomyoblasts (B). ALK is often positive (C), but *ALK* gene rearrangements are not typically identified.

Immunohistochemistry is less useful for the distinction between PMP and IMT: both show positivity for SMA, desmin, and ALK (**Figure 4.11C**). Focal cytokeratin positivity is also a feature of both tumors (but is more frequent in PMP). However, IMT demonstrating ALK overexpression is associated with *ALK* gene rearrangements, while *ALK* gene rearrangements are typically absent in PMP despite ALK positivity (238). Clinical correlation (as PMP occurs in older patients) and genetic studies are helpful in most contexts.

DERMATOMYOFIBROMA

Dermatomyofibroma occurs most commonly in patients during adolescence and young adulthood. Females are more frequently affected. Lesions may grow slowly over years, and appear as flesh-colored plaque-like growths on the trunk up to 5 cm in greatest dimension. Histologically, dermatomyofibroma appears as a band-like fascicular growth of bland-appearing myofibroblasts centered in the reticular dermis; notably the fascicles run parallel to the overlying epidermis (**Figure 4.12**). Tumors do not show a propensity for recurrence once excised. SMA and desmin are variably positive. Some lesions may mimic dermatofibrosarcoma protuberans (DFSP) in the plaque stage (**Figure 4.13A**). Distinction is added by careful examination for the foci showing the characteristic storiform growth of DFSP (**Figure 4.13B**), and CD34 immunostain will be negative in dermatomyofibroma but positive in DFSP. Most challenging cases of DFSP can be confirmed by molecular testing for the fusion product *COL1A1-PDGFB* secondary to translocation t(17;22)(q21.3;q13.1) (239,240).

CELLULAR BENIGN FIBROUS HISTIOCYTOMA

The cellular variant of benign fibrous histiocytoma (CBFH), also known as dermatofibroma, may mimic several neoplasms secondary to its hypercellularity and fascicular growth. CBFH affects adults most commonly as a lesion on the extremity or trunk, and appears as a dermal-based proliferation of spindle cells arranged in a fascicular architecture with entrapped peripheral dermal collagen (**Figure 4.14A, B**). Foamy macrophages and osteoclast-like giant cells may be present (which may be reminiscent of giant cell tumor of soft tissue; see the section *"Cellular Benign Fibrous Histiocytoma"*

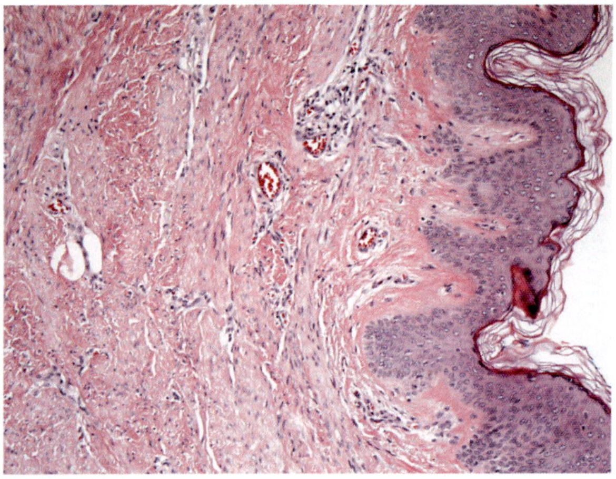

FIGURE 4.12 Dermatomyofibroma is comprised of a band-like fascicular growth of benign myofibroblasts centered in the reticular dermis; the bands appear to run parallel to the overlying epidermis.

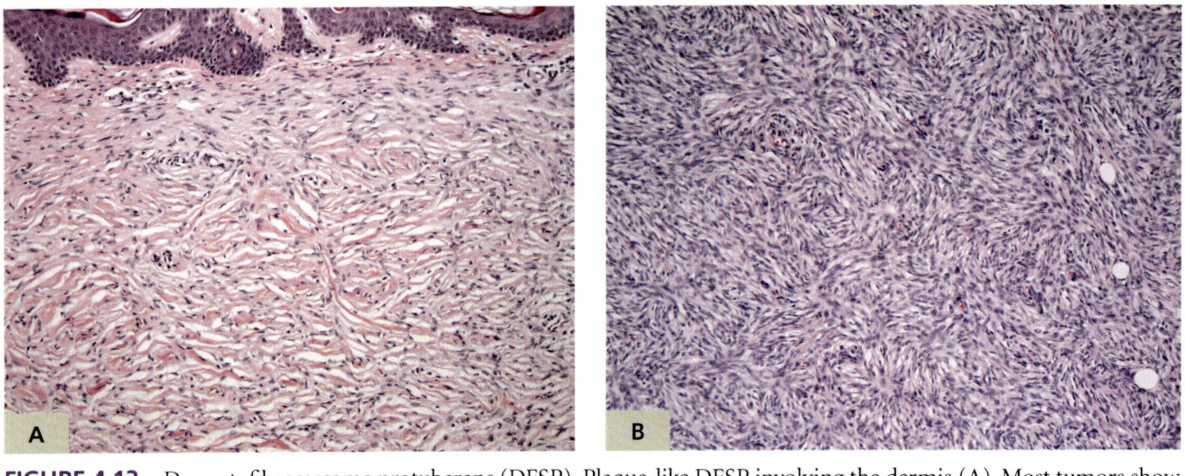

FIGURE 4.13 Dermatofibrosarcoma protuberans (DFSP). Plaque-like DFSP involving the dermis (A). Most tumors show the characteristic features of storiform arrangement of uniform spindled cells and infiltration into subcutaneous fat (B).

in "*Mimics of Fibrohistiocytic Neoplasms*"). The entrapped collagen may occasionally appear keloidal. The presence of necrosis in up to one-fifth of cases may also seem worrisome as a sign of malignancy.

CBFH may be difficult to distinguish from DFSP, which is more common on truncal sites. DFSP shows more storiform architecture and infiltrative growth, with frequent entrapment of adnexal structures and diffuse infiltration of subcutaneous adipose tissue (**Figure 4.15**). Stromal collagen in DFSP is uncommon. In contrast, CBFH rarely entraps adnexal structures and extension into subcutaneous fat is focal at most. Immunohistochemistry may be helpful, as CBFH shows frequent multifocal positivity for SMA (**Figure 4.14C**) and variable staining for CD34. DFSP is typically positive for CD34 and negative for SMA, and FISH studies can be conducted to identify *COL1A1-PDGFB*. Distinction between CBFH and DFSP has important clinical implications: while a subset (20%) of CBFH may recur, DFSP often recurs following incomplete excision and may undergo fibrosarcomatous transformation (**Figure 4.16**).

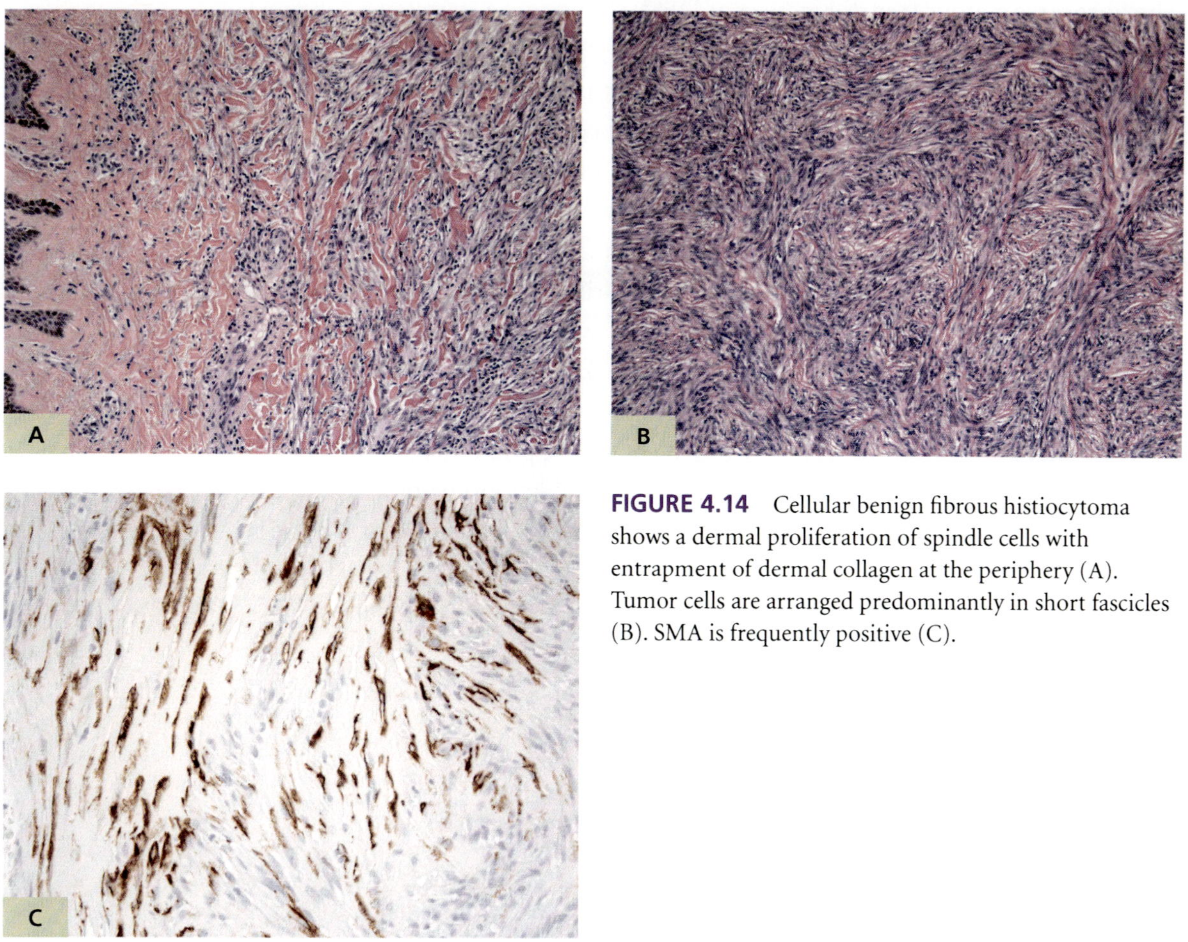

FIGURE 4.14 Cellular benign fibrous histiocytoma shows a dermal proliferation of spindle cells with entrapment of dermal collagen at the periphery (A). Tumor cells are arranged predominantly in short fascicles (B). SMA is frequently positive (C).

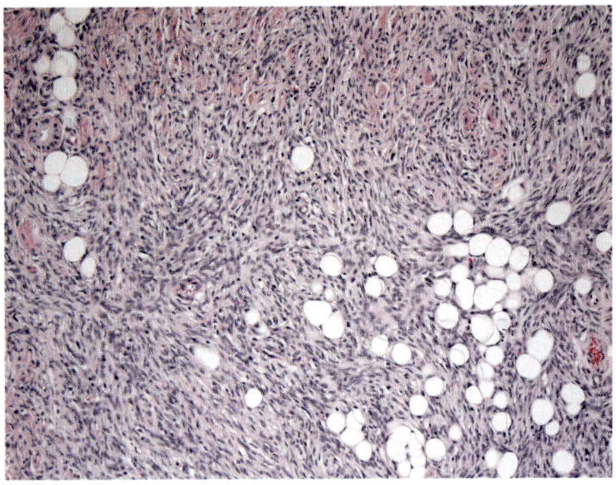

FIGURE 4.15 Dermatofibrosarcoma protuberans shows storiform ("cartwheel"-like) architecture and infiltrative growth, with frequent entrapment of adnexal structures and infiltration of subcutaneous adipose tissue.

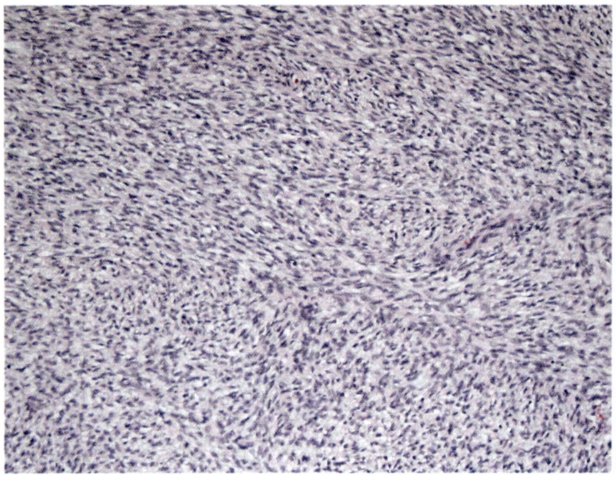

FIGURE 4.16 Fibrosarcomatous transformation of dermatofibrosarcoma protuberans resembles a spindle cell sarcoma, with atypical tumor cells arranged in fascicles.

The fibrosarcomatous transformation of DFSP shows more aggressive behavior with a 15% risk of metastasis.

Rarely, benign fibrous histiocytoma may occur as a subcutaneous or deep soft tissue lesion; these deep-seated lesions arise most commonly on the extremities and are typically well-circumscribed lesions with a fibrous pseudocapsule. Deep CBFH often has collagenous stroma, and may show hemangiopericytoma-like vessels and occasional CD34 positivity, thus mimicking solitary fibrous tumor (SFT). CBFH typically shows more uniformly storiform growth and more even cellularity throughout the lesion than seen in SFT, which characteristically shows varying hypercellular and hypocellular foci (**Figure 4.17A**). SFT is characterized by *NAB2-STAT6* fusion secondary to an intrachromosomal rearrangement on 12q13 (241,242); notably the involved genes are located in close proximity and the resulting rearrangement cannot be detected by conventional karyotype or FISH methods. Immunohistochemistry to identify resultant nuclear expression of STAT6 is diagnostic for SFT (243,244) (**Figure 4.17B**). The biologic behavior of SFT is difficult to predict, as benign-appearing tumors may recur and occasionally metastasize while malignant-appearing tumors can show an indolent course. The best identified histologic predictors of malignancy are hypercellularity, pleomorphism, necrosis, and mitotic counts of 4 or greater per 10 high-power fields (245,246).

MAMMARY-TYPE MYOFIBROBLASTOMA

Mammary-type myofibroblastoma, first described as a tumor of the breast but now known to occur across a wide anatomic range, is related to spindle cell lipoma and

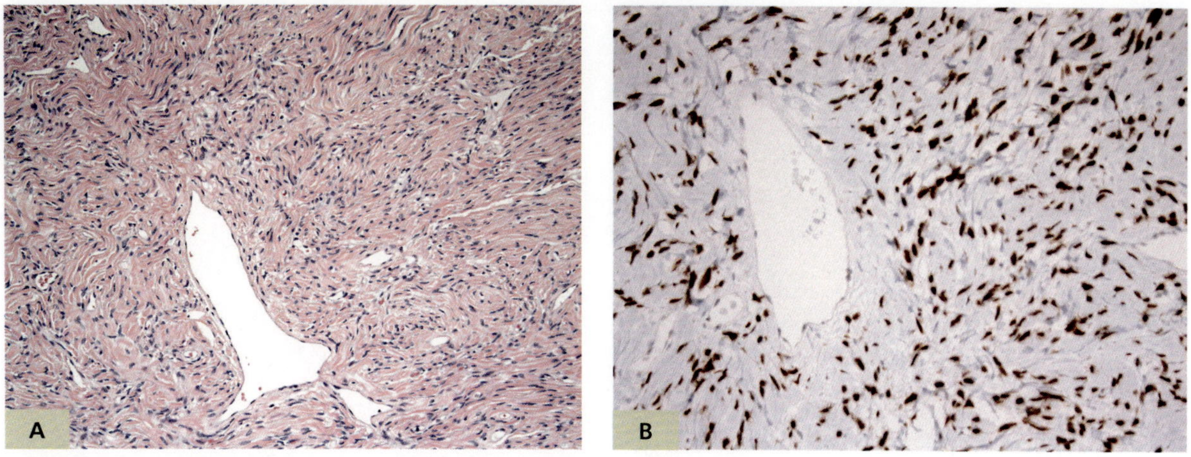

FIGURE 4.17 Solitary fibrous tumor characteristically shows a patternless pattern of spindle cells, varying hypercellular and hypocellular foci, hemangiopericytoma-like vessels, and abundant stromal collagen (A). Nuclear expression of STAT6 is a characteristic and highly specific feature (B).

cellular angiofibroma on morphologic and cytogenetic grounds (213,214,247). This family of tumors bears rearrangements of 13q and 16q. Mammary-type myofibroblastoma is comprised of fascicles of short "stubby" spindled and ovoid myofibroblasts embedded in a collagenous stroma, with frequent wiry collagen fibers (**Figure 4.18A**). Areas of varying cellularity, from paucicellular foci and a more hypercellular component, may be present. Fascicles vary from short to long, and an adipocytic component is frequent. The vessels are typically inconspicuous and thin-walled (in contrast to the thick-walled vessels characteristic of cellular angiofibroma). Mitoses may be present. The myofibroblasts demonstrate positivity for CD34 and desmin, and variable expression of SMA (**Figure 4.18B, C**). Immunohistochemistry for retinoblastoma (Rb) protein, encoded by *RB1* on 13q, can be a useful diagnostic tool for mammary-type myofibroblastoma, cellular angiofibroma, and spindle cell lipoma: secondary to 13q rearrangement, nuclear expression is absent (see Chapter 3; Figure 3.16) (215).

Mammary-type myofibroblastoma may show features suggestive of SFT, which is also positive for CD34. SFT is comprised of ovoid and spindle shaped tumor cells arranged in a patternless architecture and collagenous stroma, with frequent thin-walled hemangiopericytoma-like vessels. The presence of fascicular growth favors mammary-type myofibroblastoma. Immunohistochemistry for STAT6 can reliably identify SFT, which would also have intact Rb expression.

CELLULAR ANGIOFIBROMA

As discussed previously in the section "*Mammary-Type Myofibroblastoma*," cellular angiofibroma shares morphologic and genetic features with spindle cell

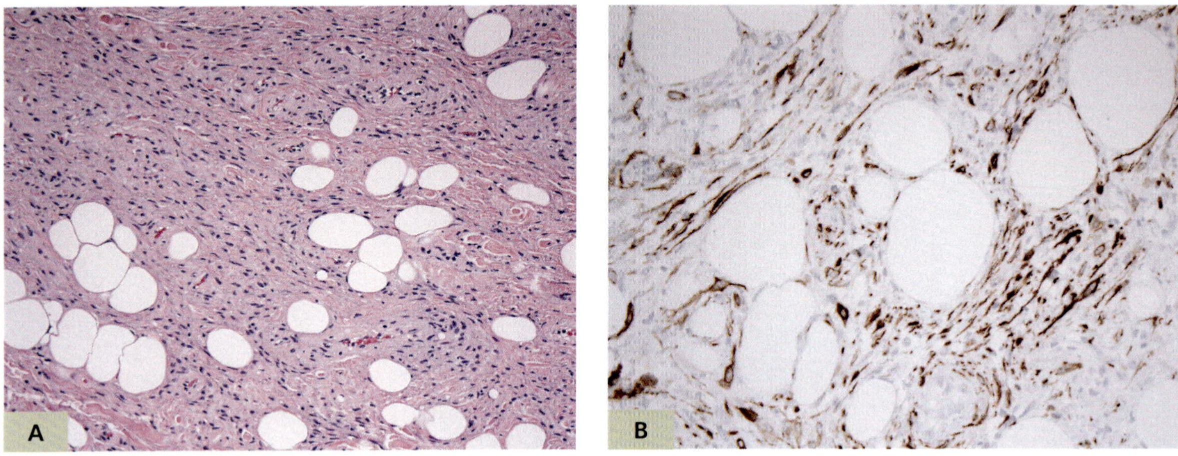

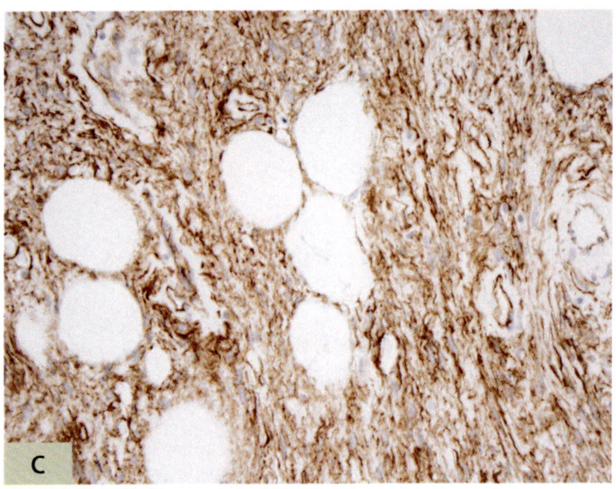

FIGURE 4.18 Mammary-type myofibroblastoma appears as fascicles of short "stubby" spindled and ovoid myofibroblasts embedded in a collagenous stroma, with frequent wiry collagen fibers and an adipocytic component (A). Tumors are positive for desmin (B) and CD34 (C).

lipoma and mammary-type myofibroblastoma. Tumors occur in vulvar, paratesticular, pelvic, and perineal sites in adult patients, and show variable circumscription. Although some tumors are poorly marginated, local recurrence is rare. Similar to mammary-type myofibroblastoma, tumor cells are short, spindled-to-ovoid in shape with nuclei having variably blunt and tapering ends, and arranged in short fascicles (**Figure 4.19**). Wiry collagen within the stroma and between tumor cells is common, as are thick-walled small rounded vessels. Mature adipose tissue may be present (and in some cases, abundant). Cellular angiofibroma is often positive for CD34 and variably positive for desmin and SMA. Secondary to 13q rearrangement, loss of nuclear Rb expression is observed.

The differential diagnosis includes angiomyofibroblastoma; however, angiomyofibroblastoma has thin-walled vessels (**Figure 4.20**) in contrast to the thick-walled, often hyalinized vessels of cellular angiofibroma. Examples of cellular angiofibroma showing a predominance of fascicular growth may

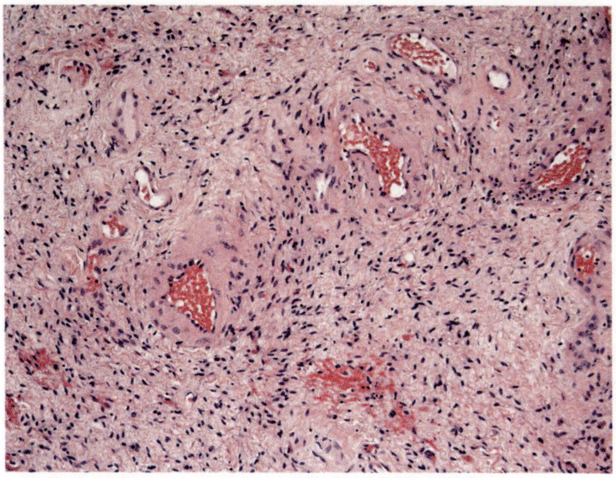

FIGURE 4.19 Cellular angiofibroma is comprised of short spindled-to-ovoid tumor cells arranged in short fascicles, with characteristic small thick-walled rounded vessels.

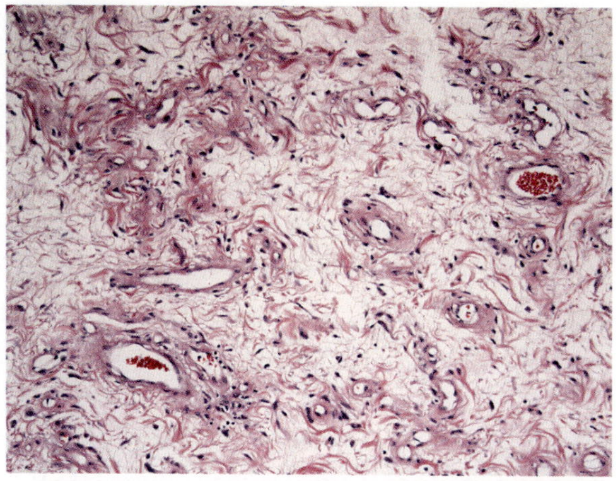

FIGURE 4.20 Angiomyofibroblastoma has ovoid, plump, and stellate tumor cells embedded in a myxoid stroma, with concentric growth around thin-walled capillaries.

mimic smooth muscle neoplasms, which can be excluded by the absence of diffuse desmin, SMA, and caldesmon staining. SFT may occasionally be considered, though cellular angiofibroma bears less resemblance than mammary-type myofibroblastoma.

Most cases of cellular angiofibroma lack significant cytologic atypia, although some cases may show degenerative nuclear atypia, often with stromal edema and hyalinization. The histologic spectrum of cellular angiofibroma is now known to include the rare occurrence of severe cytologic atypia, particularly in vulvovaginal sites (**Figure 4.21**). The presence of severe cytologic atypia is so worrisome that it is often referred to as "sarcomatous transformation." However, the presence of the severe cytologic atypia does not seem to confer any increased tendency for recurrence when compared to conventional tumors (248).

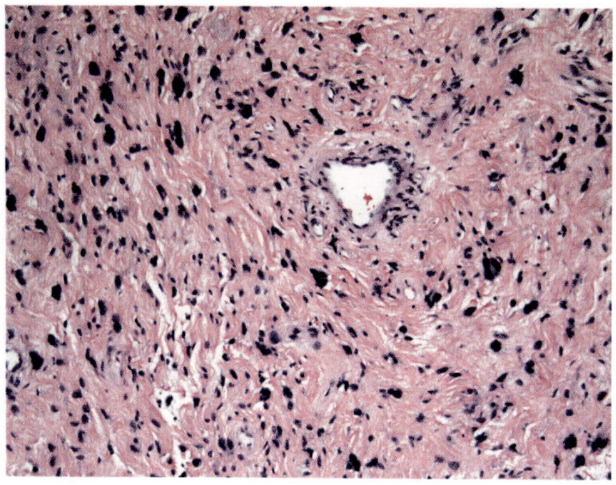

FIGURE 4.21 Cellular angiofibroma rarely shows severe cytologic atypia (or "sarcomatous transformation"), the presence of which does not seem to confer any increased tendency for recurrence.

SOFT TISSUE PERINEURIOMA

Perineuriomas of soft tissue are benign neoplasms that most commonly occur in the extremities of adults. Tumors are well-circumscribed and are more common in superficial sites where they are often smaller in size compared to deep-seated tumors, which can exceed 7.0 cm in size (249). Histologic examination shows spindled perineurial cells arranged in a storiform and whorled architecture (**Figure 4.22A**). Tumor cells are spindled with slender nuclei and long delicate bipolar cytoplasmic processes embedded in a collagenous stroma (**Figure 4.22B**). Cytologic atypia and mitotic activity are typically lacking, though degenerative atypia is sometimes observed. Myxoid stromal changes can occur and sometimes predominate. Immunohistochemistry is positive for epithelial membrane antigen (EMA) and claudin-1, and CD34 staining is seen in over half of cases, which often highlights the characteristic long bipolar cytoplasmic processes (**Figure 4.22C**). Tumors are benign and recurrence is rare.

Soft tissue perineurioma may mimic DFSP, as myxoid and hyalinized examples of DFSP may occur and CD34 positivity is expected. DFSP is typically more cellular and infiltrative in adipose tissue, and tumor cells lack the long delicate processes of perineurial cells.

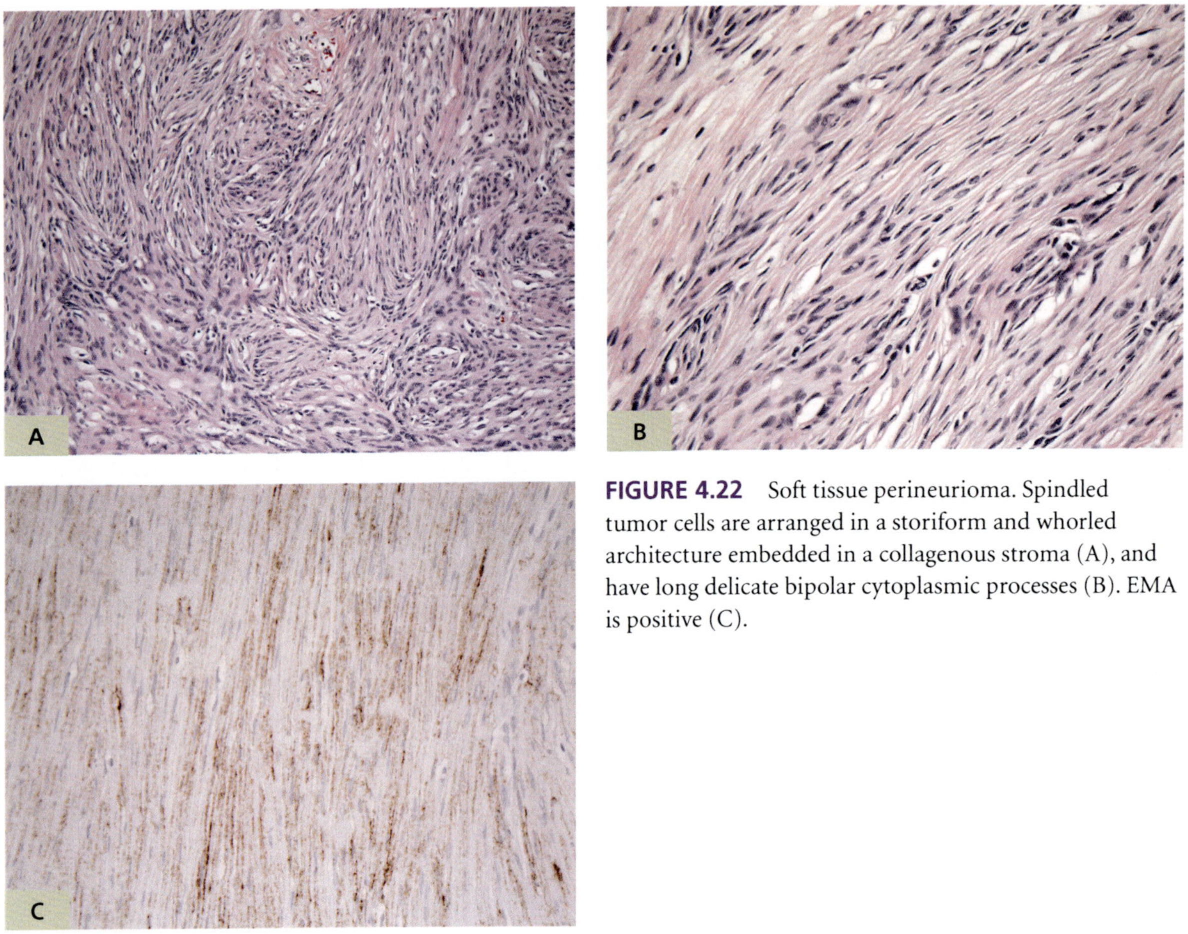

FIGURE 4.22 Soft tissue perineurioma. Spindled tumor cells are arranged in a storiform and whorled architecture embedded in a collagenous stroma (A), and have long delicate bipolar cytoplasmic processes (B). EMA is positive (C).

Especially in examples with myxoid stromal changes, soft tissue perineurioma may closely mimic low-grade fibromyxoid sarcoma (LGFMS), which is also positive for EMA (but not CD34 or claudin-1) and shows a fascicular and whorled growth pattern (**Figure 4.23A, B**). LGFMS is most common in adults between the third and fifth decades, and are more commonly deep-seated tumors in the lower extremity (though in children are more frequently subcutaneous). Histologically, distinction may be difficult as cytologic atypia is mild and mitotic activity is low in LGFMS, and some tumors do not show characteristic features such as abrupt transitions between collagenous and myxoid areas or giant collagenous rosettes. Typically in myxoid foci, thin-walled vessels arranged in arcades can be found in LGFMS and can facilitate distinction. Definitive diagnosis is possible with MUC4 immunohistochemistry, which is a highly sensitive and specific marker for LGFMS (250) (**Figure 4.23C**). Cytogenetic and molecular testing to confirm the translocation t(7;16)(q34;p11) (resulting in *FUS-CREB3L2* fusion) (251) is also diagnostic.

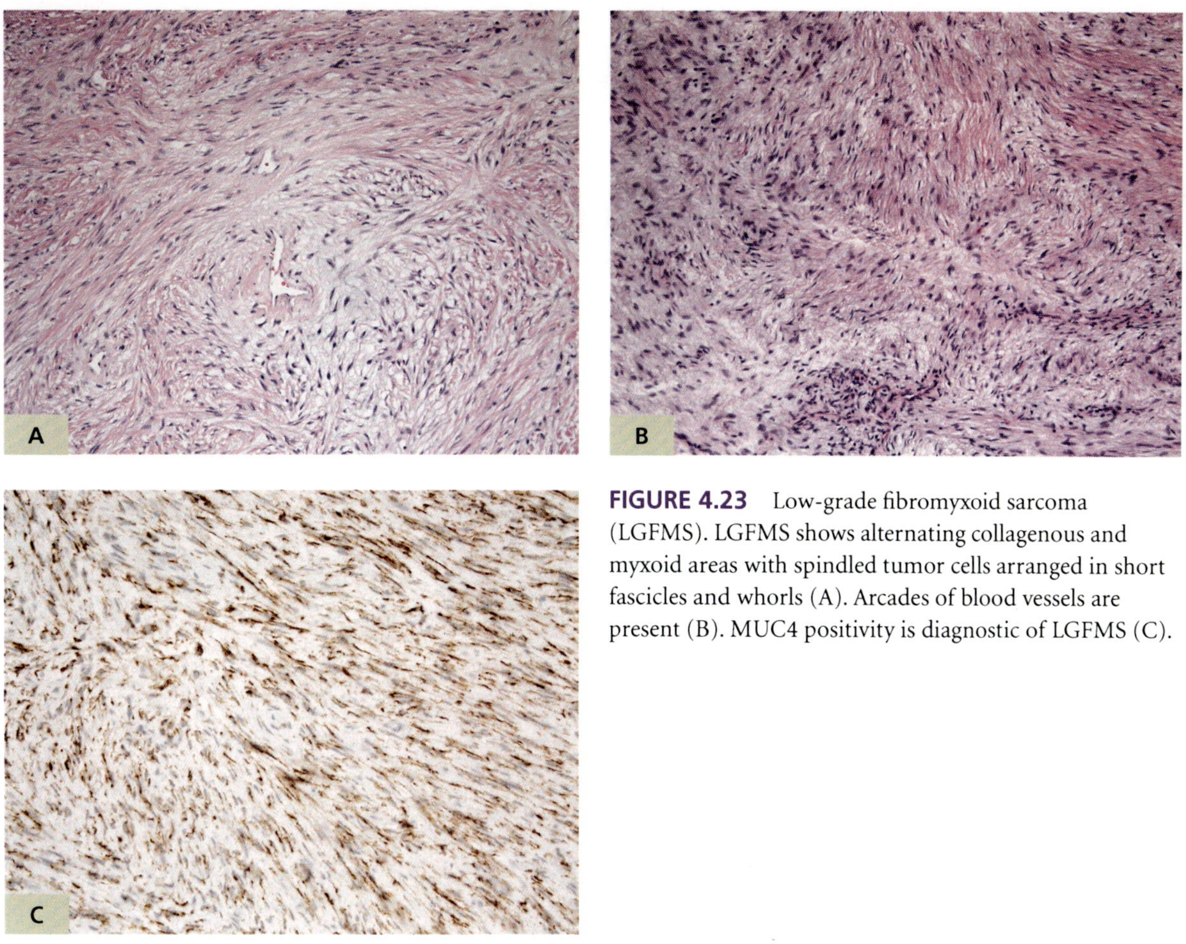

FIGURE 4.23 Low-grade fibromyxoid sarcoma (LGFMS). LGFMS shows alternating collagenous and myxoid areas with spindled tumor cells arranged in short fascicles and whorls (A). Arcades of blood vessels are present (B). MUC4 positivity is diagnostic of LGFMS (C).

The sclerosing variant of perineurioma most commonly occurs in the distal upper extremities. Sclerosing perineurioma is comprised of spindle-to-epithelioid perineurial cells arranged in cords embedded in a dense collagenous stroma (**Figure 4.24**), bearing morphologic resemblance to sclerosing epithelioid fibrosarcoma (SEF) (**Figure 4.25**). SEF is more commonly a deep-seated tumor in the extremities or limb girdles, often exceeding 10 cm in size. A subset of SEF are known to share the same translocation t(7;16)(q33;p11) as LGFMS, and tumors with hybrid features of LGFMS and SEF are recognized (252) (**Figure 4.26**). Most tumors harbor *EWSR1-CREB3L1* fusions (253). MUC4 immunohistochemistry is also positive in up to 90% of SEF and can be a useful diagnostic tool.

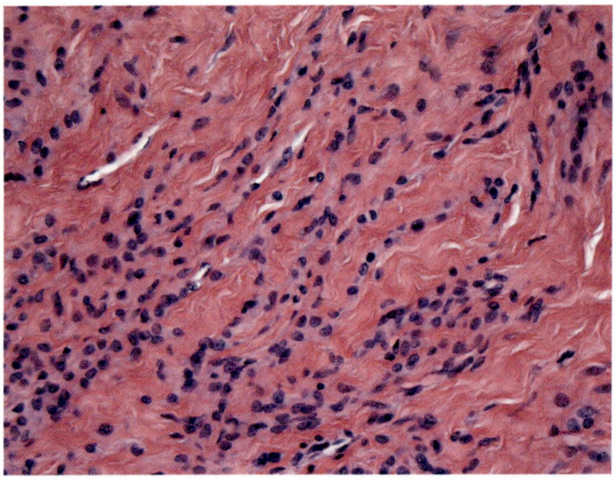

FIGURE 4.24 Sclerosing perineurioma is comprised of spindled-to-epithelioid cells arranged in cords and strands embedded in a dense collagenous stroma.

SUPERFICIAL ANGIOMYXOMA

Superficial angiomyxoma usually arises in adult patients; head and neck, truncal, and vulvovaginal sites are most common. Tumors are small and centered in either the dermis or subcutis. Tumors are multinodular growths of relatively hypocellular myxoid lobules with plump spindled and stellate cells admixed with thin-walled vessels (**Figure 4.27A**). Tumor cells lack cytologic atypia, although occasional mitoses may be seen. A salient characteristic is an inflammatory

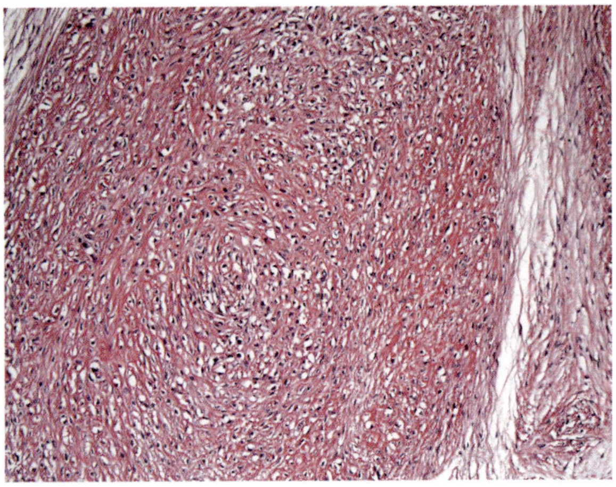

FIGURE 4.25 Sclerosing epithelioid fibrosarcoma. Epithelioid tumor cells are arranged in cords, nests, and small clusters within a dense hyalinized collagenous stroma.

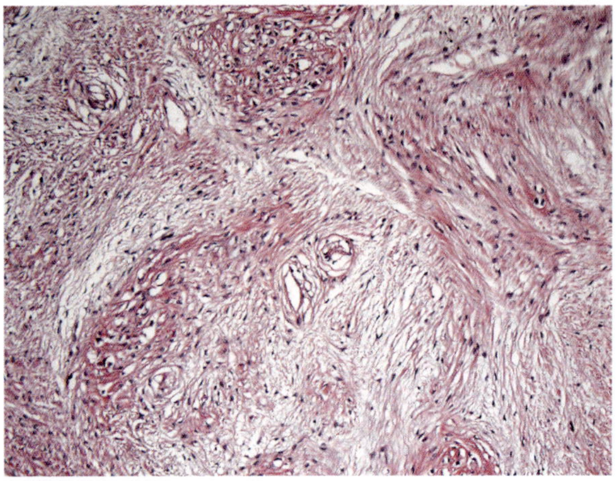

FIGURE 4.26 Some tumors show hybrid features of both low-grade fibromyxoid sarcoma and sclerosing epithelioid fibrosarcoma.

infiltrate with numerous neutrophils in the absence of necrosis or ulceration, observed in 50% of cases (**Figure 4.27B**). Tumors may recur with incomplete excision, but are considered to be benign. However, it should be noted that when superficial angiomyxoma arises in the external ear or breast, or as multicentric lesions at any anatomic site, Carney complex (which includes cardiac myxoma and primary pigmented nodular adrenocortical disease) should be considered.

Superficial angiomyxoma may show features worrisome for myxofibrosarcoma, which is also characterized by multinodular growth and myxoid stroma and may involve dermis and subcutis (**Figure 4.28A**). However, although low-grade myxofibrosarcoma may appear hypocellular with little mitotic activity, appreciable cytologic atypia and hyperchromatic nuclei are present (**Figure 4.28B**).

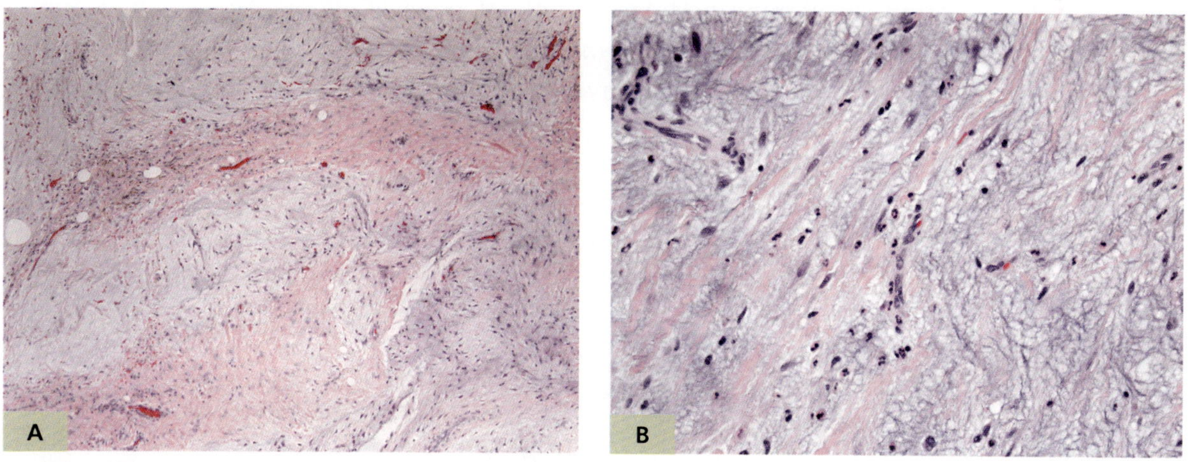

FIGURE 4.27 Superficial angiomyxomas are multinodular (A), comprised of hypocellular myxoid lobules with spindled and stellate cells admixed with thin-walled vessels and variable neutrophils (B).

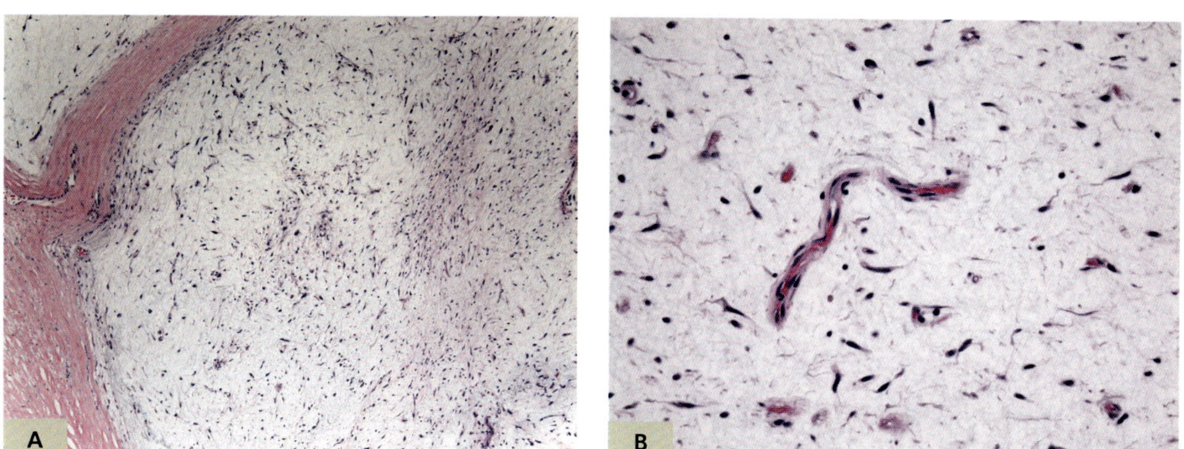

FIGURE 4.28 Myxofibrosarcoma. Low-grade tumors show multinodular growth and are relatively hypocellular with characteristic curvilinear thin-walled vessels (A), but the spindled and stellate tumor cells show cytologic atypia (B).

Long curvilinear thin-walled vessels are a characteristic feature of myxofibrosarcoma, and neutrophils are rare (although a lymphoplasmacytic infiltrate may be seen around vessels). Pseudolipoblasts, or vacuolated tumor cells with abundant intracytoplasmic mucin, are often present. Myxofibrosarcoma is most common in the limbs in a much older, elderly patient population.

INTRAMUSCULAR MYXOMA (INCLUDING CELLULAR MYXOMA)

Intramuscular myxoma is a benign tumor (of uncertain differentiation) that typically presents as a slow-growing intramuscular mass in the limbs (thigh and hip/buttock most commonly) of adults with a female predilection. Tumors are benign and excision is curative. Tumors can grow quite large. Intramuscular myxoma shows multinodular growth of hypocellular and hypovascular myxoid nodules that show entrapment and infiltration of skeletal muscle fibers at the periphery. Within the myxoid nodules are evenly distributed spindle and stellate cells lacking cytologic atypia (**Figure 4.29A, B**).

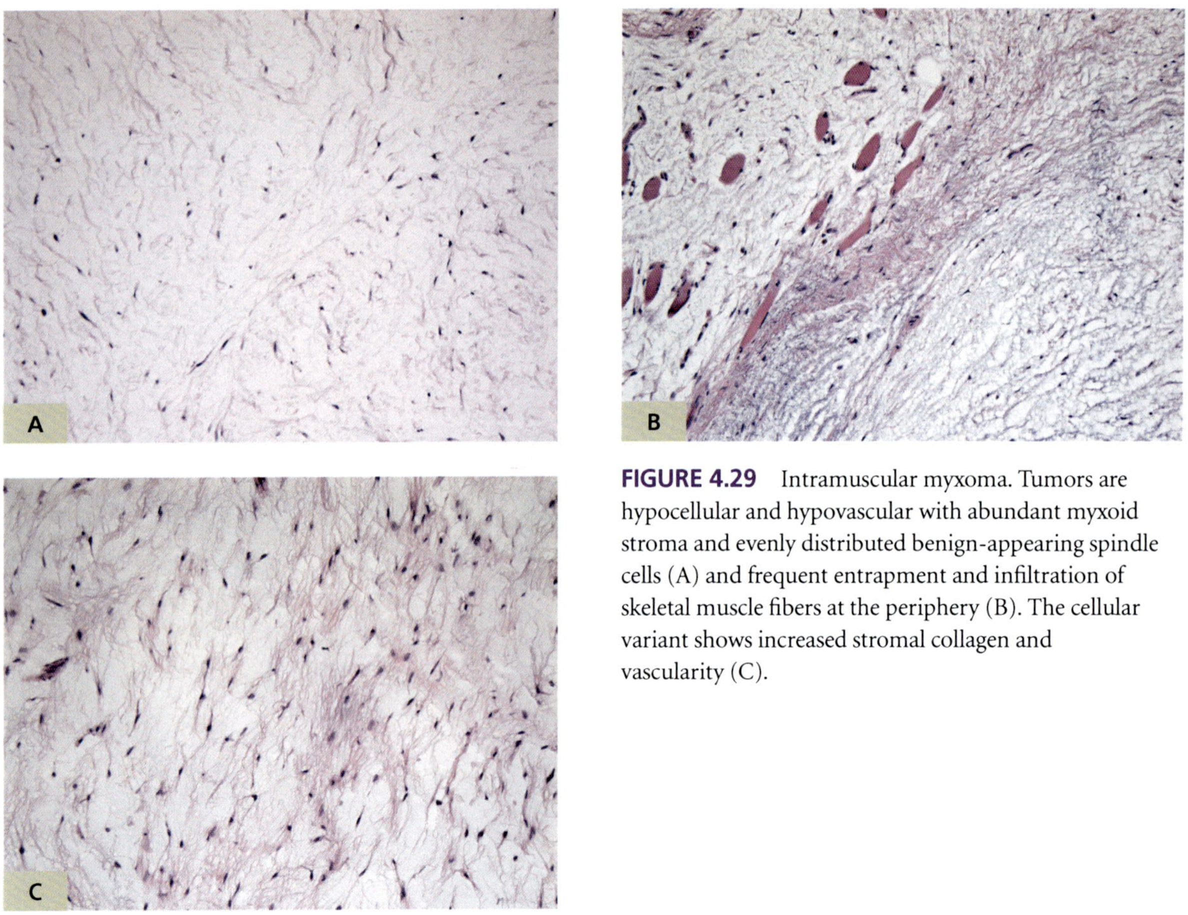

FIGURE 4.29 Intramuscular myxoma. Tumors are hypocellular and hypovascular with abundant myxoid stroma and evenly distributed benign-appearing spindle cells (A) and frequent entrapment and infiltration of skeletal muscle fibers at the periphery (B). The cellular variant shows increased stromal collagen and vascularity (C).

The cellular variant shows increased stromal collagen and vascularity, although mitoses and pleomorphism are still absent (**Figure 4.29C**). *GNAS* point mutations characterize myxomas, although tumors arising near joints (juxta-articular myxomas) lack *GNAS* mutations (254). Notably, Mazabraud syndrome includes multiple intramuscular myxomas along with polyostotic fibrous dysplasia.

Intramuscular myxoma can mimic low-grade myxofibrosarcoma; however, the cytologic atypia, elongated curvilinear vessels, and presence of pseudolipoblasts are diagnostic of myxofibrosarcoma. Cellular myxoma can mimic both soft tissue perineurioma and LGFMS; however, an immunohistochemical panel including EMA, claudin-1, and MUC4 will enable appropriate classification.

SELECTED MIMICS OF PEDIATRIC FIBROBLASTIC/ MYOFIBROBLASTIC NEOPLASMS

FIBROUS HAMARTOMA OF INFANCY

Most cases of fibrous hamartoma of infancy occur within the first 2 years of life, and male infants are more commonly affected. Lesions are most common in the upper extremity and limb girdle, although nearly all anatomic sites have been reported. Lesions are usually slowly growing solitary masses that rarely exceed 5 cm in size. Tumors occur deep dermis and subcutis, and are well-circumscribed but with infiltrative edges. Surgical excision is curative, and recurrence is exceptional.

Four characteristic components comprise fibrous hamartoma of infancy: (a) islands of mature fat; (b) poorly organized collagenous fibrous bands with small vessels and inflammatory cells; (c) a "primitive" population of spindled to stellate cells arranged in nests within a myxoid stroma; and (d) nodules of myofibroblasts arranged in short fascicles (**Figure 4.30A**). When all four characteristic components are present, definitive diagnosis can be made by routine histologic examination. However, the components may be present in variable proportions, and when there is a predominance of the myofibroblastic component (**Figure 4.30B**) the tumor may show morphologic overlap with infantile fibrosarcoma. Infantile fibrosarcoma affects patients during the first year of life, and often presents as a large mass on the extremities that often exceeds the diameter of the affected arm or leg. Lesions are densely cellular, with long cellular fascicles of spindled to ovoid cells (**Figure 4.31A, B**). The clinicopathologic features and thorough tumor sampling will help make the distinction;

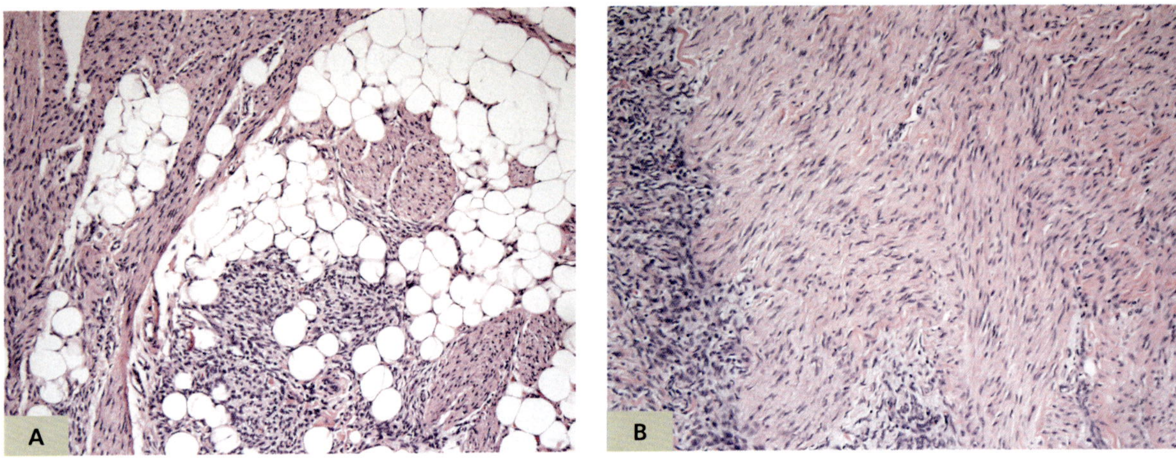

FIGURE 4.30 Fibrous hamartoma of infancy is comprised of islands of mature fat, poorly organized collagenous fibrous bands with small vessels and inflammatory cells, nests of "primitive" spindled to stellate cells within a myxoid stroma, and nodules of myofibroblasts arranged in short fascicles (A). These components may be present in variable proportions, and some examples show a predominance of the myofibroblastic component (B).

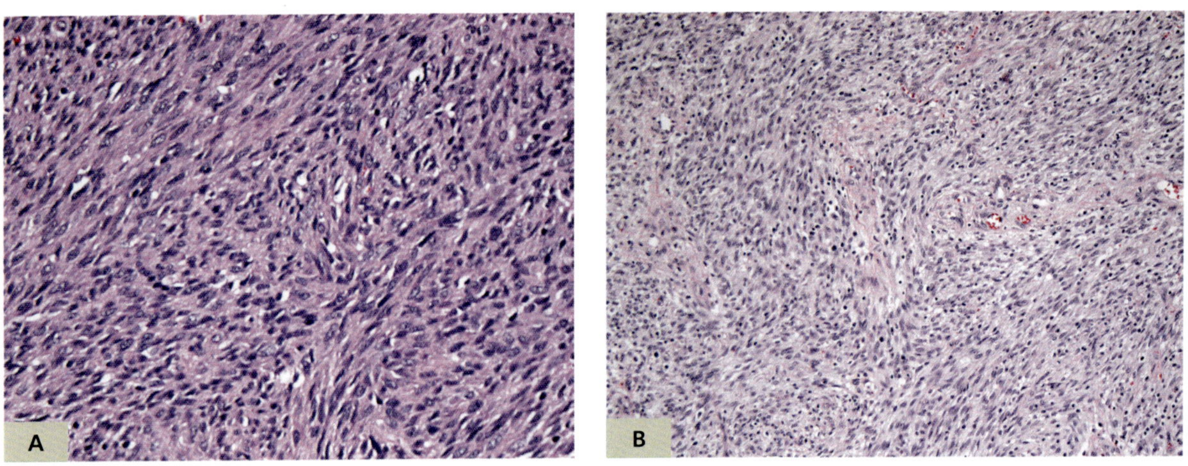

FIGURE 4.31 Infantile fibrosarcoma is comprised of long cellular fascicles of spindled and ovoid tumor cells (A); some tumors have a myoid appearance with palely eosinophilic cytoplasm (B).

furthermore, identification of the translocation t(12;15)(p13;q25), resulting in *ETV6-NRTK3* fusion, is diagnostic of infantile fibrosarcoma (255).

INFANTILE MYOFIBROMATOSIS

Infantile myofibromatosis, a tumor of pericytic differentiation, typically presents before 2 years of age and is congenital in up to a third of cases. Tumors often arise at superficial sites of the head and neck, and a subset of cases can be multicentric. The clinical course is benign, with rare recurrences

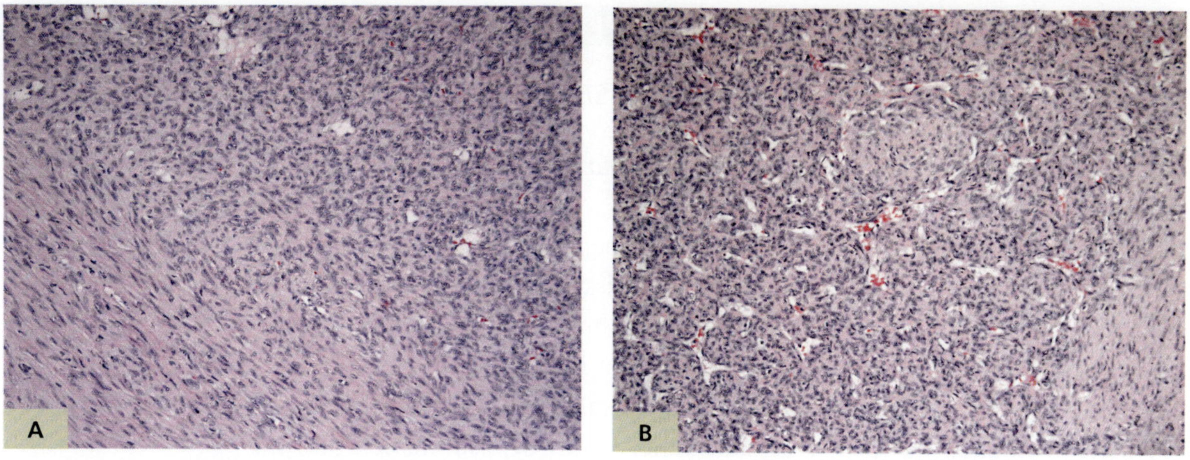

FIGURE 4.32 Infantile myofibroma has a biphasic appearance, with eosinophilic ovoid-to-spindled cells arranged in nodules centrally and more primitive-appearing smaller and rounder cells at the periphery (A). The rounded cell population is often arranged concentrically around hemangiopericytoma-like vessels (B).

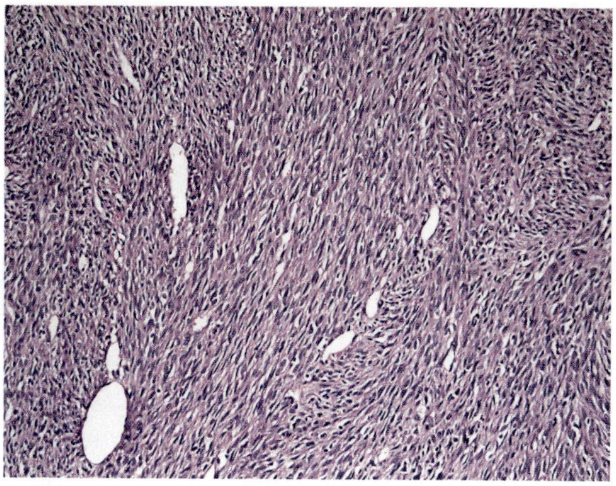

FIGURE 4.33 The fascicular growth of infantile fibrosarcoma often imparts a herringbone-type appearance, and hemangiopericytoma-like vessels are common.

and frequent spontaneous regression of lesions. Tumors are nodular and often show a biphasic appearance, with an eosinophilic ovoid-to-spindle cell component arranged in nodules centrally with abrupt transitions to a more primitive-appearing population of smaller and rounder cells at the periphery (**Figure 4.32A**). Thin-walled slit-like vessels are present at the periphery of nodules, and the rounded cell population is often arranged concentrically around the vessels (**Figure 4.32B**). Hyalinization and chondromyxoid changes to the stroma are common. Lesions that are more cellular in which the characteristic biphasic appearance is not readily apparent may show morphologic overlap with infantile fibrosarcoma. While mitoses and necrosis are common in myofibromatosis, cytologic atypia is absent. The characteristic nodular architecture of infantile myofibromatosis differs from the infiltrative growth of infantile fibrosarcoma. Infantile fibrosarcoma is more densely cellular and fascicular, often forming a herringbone-type appearance (**Figure 4.33**). Although metastasis is rare, up to a half of cases recur. Cytogenetic and molecular testing to identify the characteristic translocation of infantile fibrosarcoma, t(12;15)(p13;q25), is sometimes necessary.

MIMICS OF FIBROHISTIOCYTIC NEOPLASMS

REACTIVE AND INFLAMMATORY PROCESSES

Numerous inflammatory conditions that are characterized by granulomatous inflammation, histiocytes, xanthomatous change, and giant cell reaction can mimic either diffuse or localized tenosynovial giant cell tumors. Tenosynovial giant cell tumors arise in adults in somatic soft tissue sites, most commonly on the hand. The distinction between localized and diffuse types is based on the presence of either circumscribed nodules (localized) or infiltrative margins (diffuse). Tumors are comprised of a mixture of a mononuclear cell population, foamy macrophages, osteoclast-like giant cells, and hemosiderin deposition; components are present in variable proportions in a given tumor (**Figure 4.34**). Characteristic histiocytoid cells with an eccentrically placed nucleus and pale pink cytoplasm with hemosiderin deposition are frequent ("ladybird" cells). Stroma is often hyalinized, and diffuse-type tenosynovial giant cell tumors are multinodular and are occasionally locally aggressive, with a risk of recurrence. Rare cases of sarcomatous progression with recurrence have been reported. Desmin positivity may be seen in the mononuclear cell population, and histiocytic markers (eg, CD163) show multifocal staining. Careful attention for the various cellular components will assist diagnosis. Tenosynovial giant cell tumor is characterized by translocations involving the *CSF1* gene on chromosome 1 (256,257).

Mycobacterial spindle cell pseudotumor is comprised of spindled and epithelioid histiocytes, and can be mass-forming and worrisome for a malignancy (**Figure 4.35A**). The heterogeneous mix of spindled and epithelioid histiocytes and giant cells may mimic tenosynovial giant cell tumor in florid cases. Correlation with clinical history and special stains to identify the presence of acid-fast bacilli will assist in appropriate diagnosis (**Figur 4.35B**).

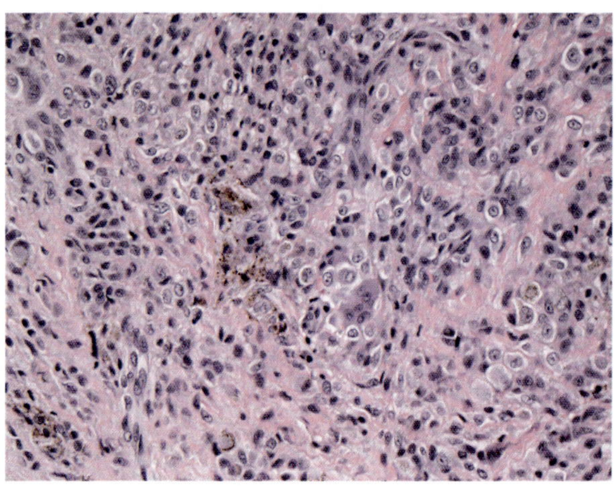

FIGURE 4.34 Tenosynovial giant cell tumors are comprised of a mixture of a mononuclear histiocytoid cell population, osteoclast-like giant cells, and hemosiderin deposition in variable proportions.

Malakoplakia, which is most common in the urinary bladder but may occur at a range of anatomic sites, is a reactive process associated with gram-negative bacterial infection. Lesions are characterized by a proliferation of large epithelioid histiocytes, some with xanthomatous cytoplasm, and occasional giant cell formation, which may mimic tenosynovial giant cell tumors

(**Figure 4.36A**). Diagnosis is facilitated by identification of the characteristic Michaelis–Gutmann bodies by histochemical stains for calcium (von Kossa) and iron (**Figure 4.36B**).

CELLULAR NEUROTHEKEOMA

Cellular neurothekeoma is a benign cutaneous tumor that occurs most commonly on the head and neck and upper extremities in adult patients. Tumors are comprised of nests and lobules of epithelioid and spindled cells separated

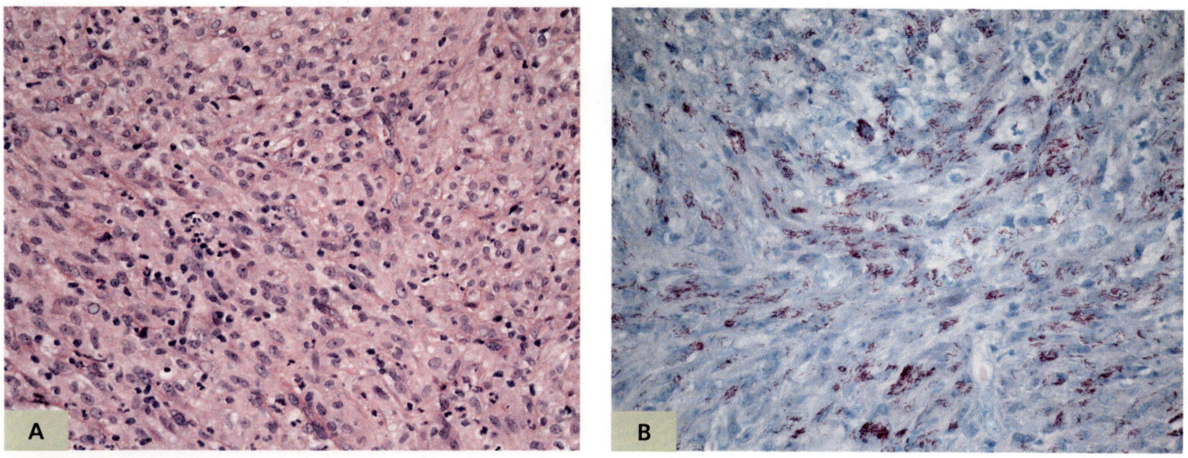

FIGURE 4.35 Mycobacterial spindle cell pseudotumor is comprised of a proliferation of spindled and epithelioid histiocytes (A). Special stain for acid-fast bacilli highlights the causative organisms (B).

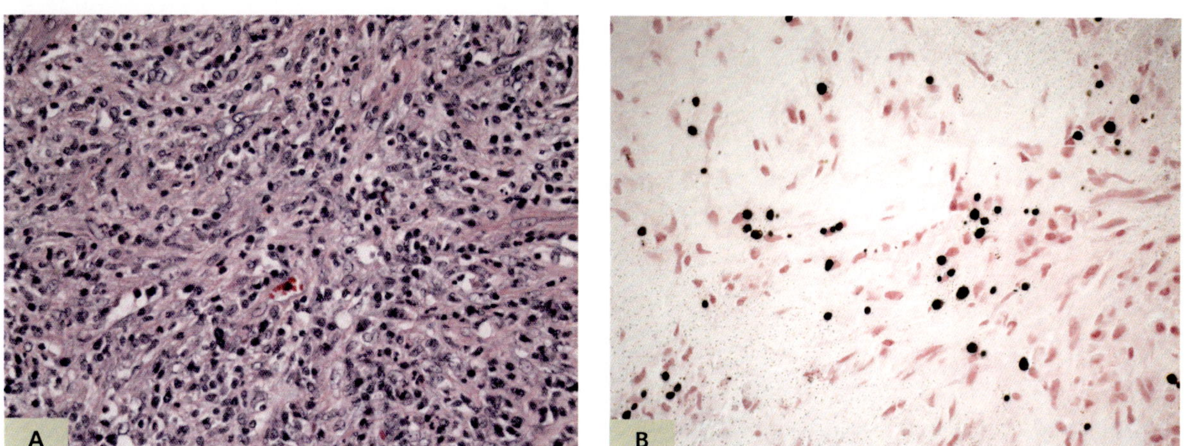

FIGURE 4.36 Malakoplakia is characterized by a proliferation of large epithelioid histiocytes, some with xanthomatous cytoplasm (A). Von Kossa stain (for calcium) identifies the characteristic Michaelis-Gutmann bodies (B).

by hyalinized collagen (**Figure 4.37**). Tumor cells are palely eosinophilic and usually lack significant cytologic atypia. Osteoclast-like giant cells may be present. Lesions may extend into subcutaneous tissue. Immunohistochemical stains for NKI-C3, NSE, and SMA are positive.

Cellular neurothekeoma shows frequent morphologic overlap with plexiform fibrohistiocytic tumor (PFHT) (and some authors believe these are related entities) (258). PFHT occurs in the same anatomic distribution as cellular neurothekeoma, and affects both adults and children. Tumors are comprised of multinodular growth of epithelioid histiocytoid cells, spindled cells, and osteoclast-like giant cells (**Figure 4.38**). Hyalinized and myxoid stroma may be seen. Despite lacking significant cytologic atypia and having low mitotic counts, PFHT is associated with local recurrence (30%) and metastasis (6%; predominantly to lymph nodes) (259, 260). Appropriate classification as PFHT, when possible, is thus important as cellular neurothekeoma rarely recurs. Cellular neurothekeoma rarely shows plexiform growth pattern and lacks histiocytoid nodules, and PFHT tends to be more infiltrative and can involve skeletal muscle.

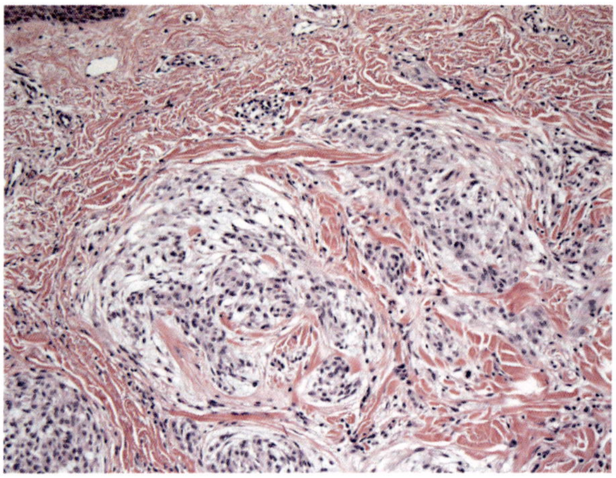

FIGURE 4.37 Cellular neurothekeoma is comprised of nests and lobules of palely eosinophilic epithelioid and spindled cells separated by hyalinized collagen.

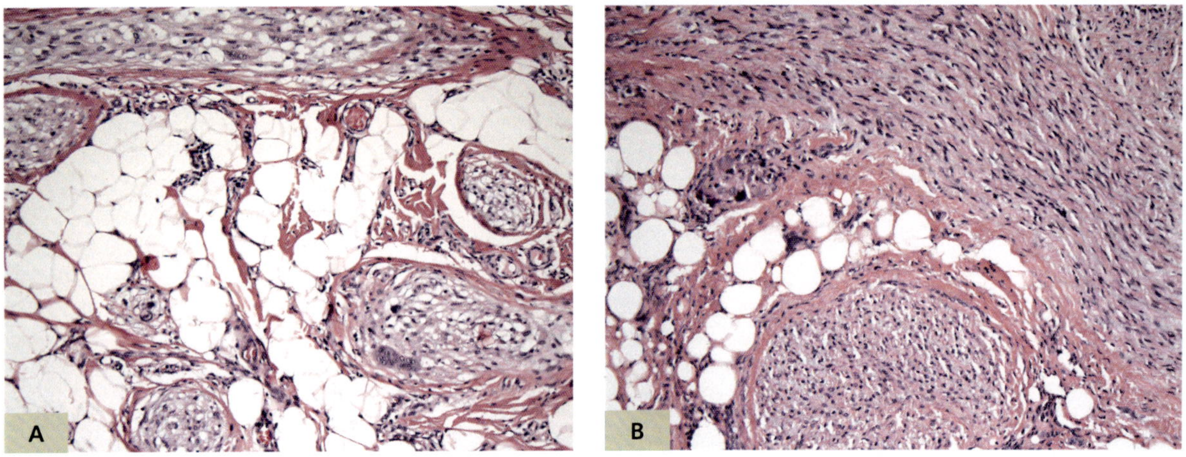

FIGURE 4.38 Plexiform fibrohistiocytic tumor shows multinodular growth of histiocytoid cells and osteoclast-like giant cells, as well as fascicles of spindled myofibroblasts (A). Some tumors show a predominance of the spindled myofibroblastic cells (B).

CELLULAR BENIGN FIBROUS HISTIOCYTOMA

CBFH, discussed previously (see section "*Cellular Benign Fibrous Histiocytoma*" in "*Mimics of Fibroblastic/Myofibroblastic Neoplasms*"), can also mimic giant cell tumor of soft tissue, especially when osteoclast-like giant cells or aneurysmal changes are present (**Figure 4.39**). Giant cell tumor of soft tissue is identical to its counterpart in bone, and has a mononuclear stromal cell component that may be spindled and can show storiform growth (**Figure 4.40**). Osteoclast-like giant cells and foamy cells are distributed throughout. Giant cell tumor of soft tissue differs from CBFH in showing multinodular growth with intervening fibrous septa and frequent peripheral (shell-like) metaplastic bone formation. The peripheral mineralization characteristic of giant cell tumors is sometimes evident on radiographic studies. Giant cell tumor of soft tissue shows recurrence (often greater rates with incomplete resection) and can rarely metastasize.

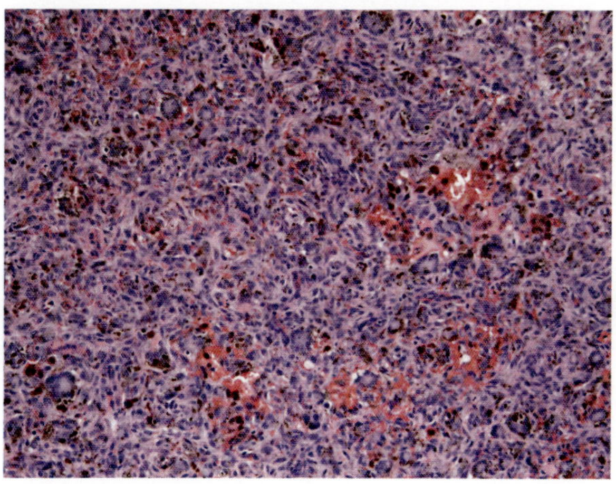

FIGURE 4.39 Some variants of cellular benign fibrous histiocytoma show extensive aneurysmal changes and osteoclast-like giant cells.

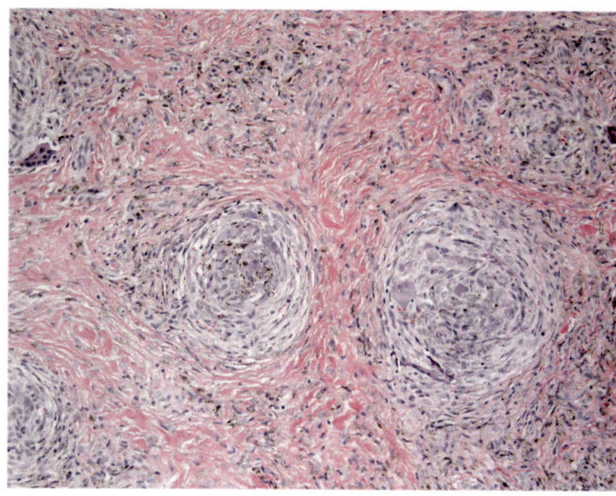

FIGURE 4.40 Giant cell tumor of soft tissue shows a multinodular growth pattern, with nodules of mononuclear cells and osteoclast-like giant cells, separated by fibrous septa. The tumor cells may be spindled and can show storiform growth with admixed foam cells and hemosiderin deposition.

5

Mimics of Smooth Muscle and Skeletal Muscle Neoplasms

Several nonneoplastic lesions and benign neoplasms can mimic smooth muscle and skeletal muscle neoplasms on morphologic grounds. Benign tumors with a smooth muscle component may show overlapping features with leiomyoma or leiomyosarcoma. At soft tissue sites, leiomyosarcoma should be considered more often than leiomyoma (**Figure 5.1**), as benign smooth muscle tumors are very rare in somatic soft tissue and are essentially defined at such locations by an absence of nuclear atypia and mitotic activity. Many benign lesions contain cells that bear resemblance to rhabdomyoblasts, which may lead to consideration of rhabdomyosarcoma or heterologous rhabdomyoblastic differentiation in a malignant germ cell tumor or sarcoma, most commonly malignant peripheral nerve sheath tumor (MPNST) (**Figure 5.2**) or dedifferentiated liposarcoma (DDLPS). Clinicopathologic correlation and adequate sampling will help in these scenarios. While some types of rhabdomyosarcoma are morphologically distinctive and overtly malignant (eg, alveolar and pleomorphic types), the heterogeneity seen in embryonal rhabdomyosarcoma may show morphologic overlap with other lesions containing

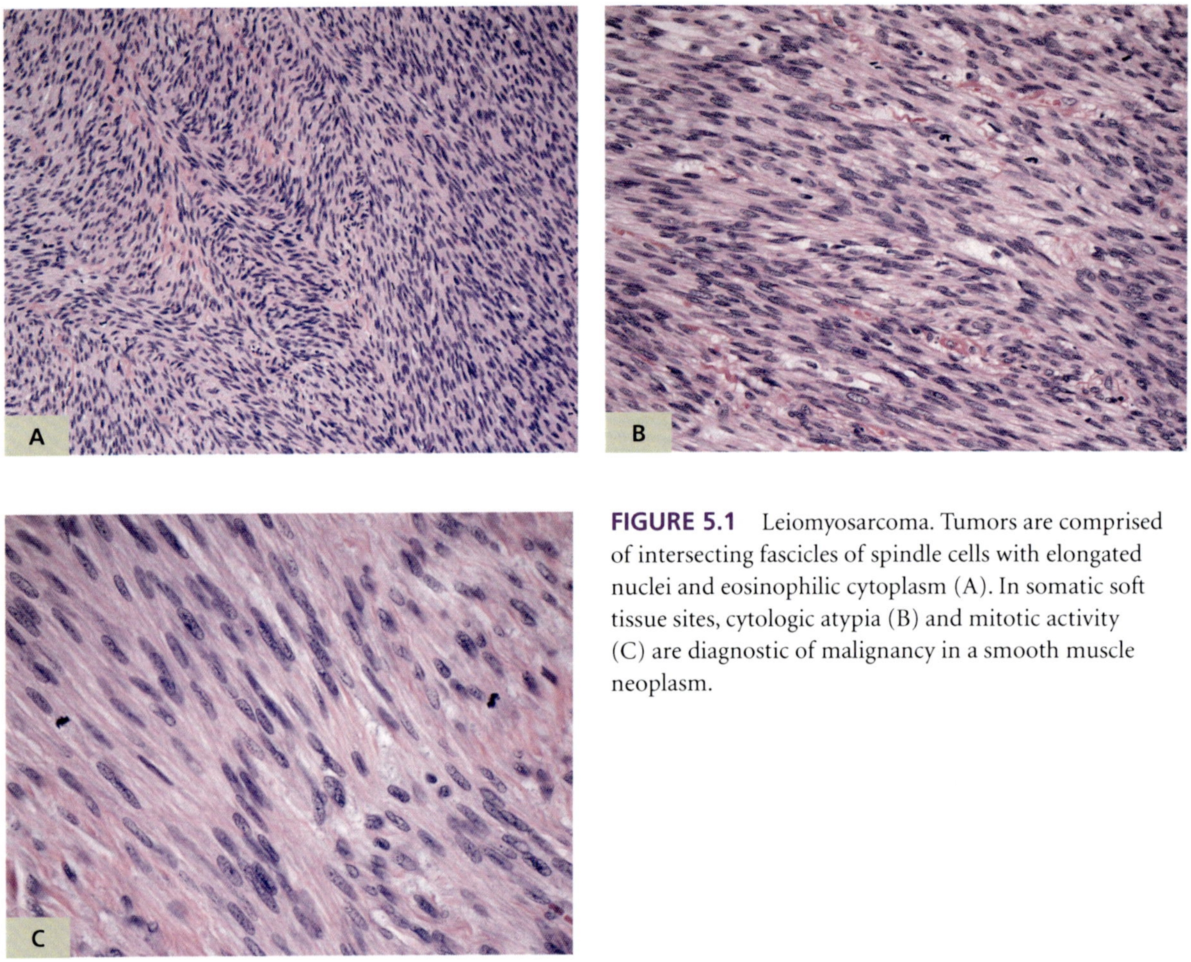

FIGURE 5.1 Leiomyosarcoma. Tumors are comprised of intersecting fascicles of spindle cells with elongated nuclei and eosinophilic cytoplasm (A). In somatic soft tissue sites, cytologic atypia (B) and mitotic activity (C) are diagnostic of malignancy in a smooth muscle neoplasm.

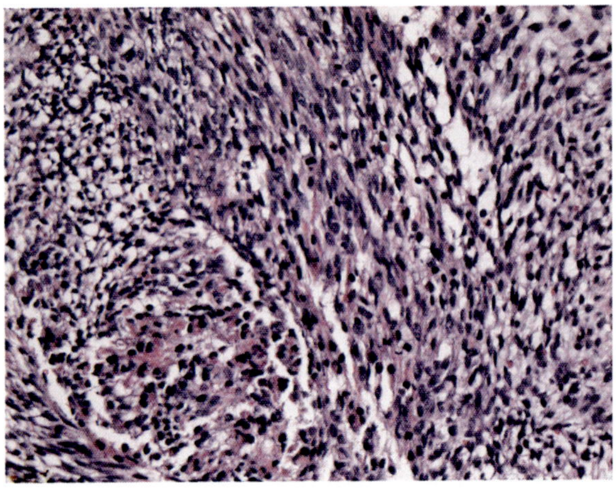

FIGURE 5.2 Malignant peripheral nerve sheath tumor may demonstrate heterologous rhabdomyoblastic differentiation, with foci of rhabdomyoblasts that have eccentric nuclei and abundant brightly eosinophilic cytoplasm.

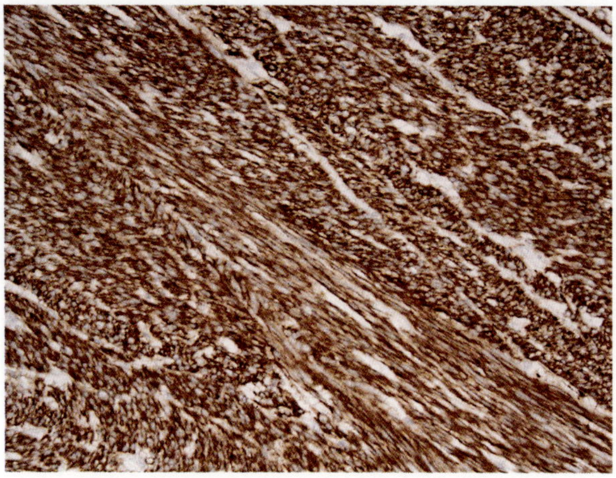

FIGURE 5.3 Smooth muscle differentiation can be supported by diffuse positivity for smooth muscle actin (SMA) (as well as desmin and caldesmon).

rhabdomyoblasts or mimics. Embryonal rhabdomyosarcoma is composed of rhabdomyoblasts in varying stages of differentiation, often associated with hypocellular areas.

Smooth muscle and skeletal muscle differentiation can usually be confirmed by immunohistochemistry. Smooth muscle neoplasms are positive for at least one of the three myogenic markers smooth muscle actin (SMA) (**Figure 5.3**), desmin, and caldesmon. Desmin expression is also characteristic of skeletal muscle differentiation, and rhabdomyoblastic differentiation can be confirmed by immunoreactivity for fast myosin, myogenin, or *MYOD1*.

MIMICS OF SMOOTH MUSCLE NEOPLASMS

MYOPERICYTOMA/MYOFIBROMA

Myofibroma, now classified as a synonym for myopericytoma (261), is a benign perivascular neoplasm that shows a predominance of myoid spindle cells. Tumors arise both in children (including during infancy) and in adults, most commonly on the extremities and head and neck. Lesions are usually superficial and solitary, but can occasionally be multifocal (myofibromatosis), and may be clinically worrisome for sarcoma when presenting as large masses in infants. Histologically, myofibromas are well-circumscribed with a biphasic spindle cell population: eosinophilic spindle cells arranged in bundles or whorls, occasionally bulging into the lumens of dilated, thin-walled blood vessels, and more ovoid, short spindle cells at the periphery of the lesion that grow between prominent slit-like blood vessels (**Figure 5.4**).

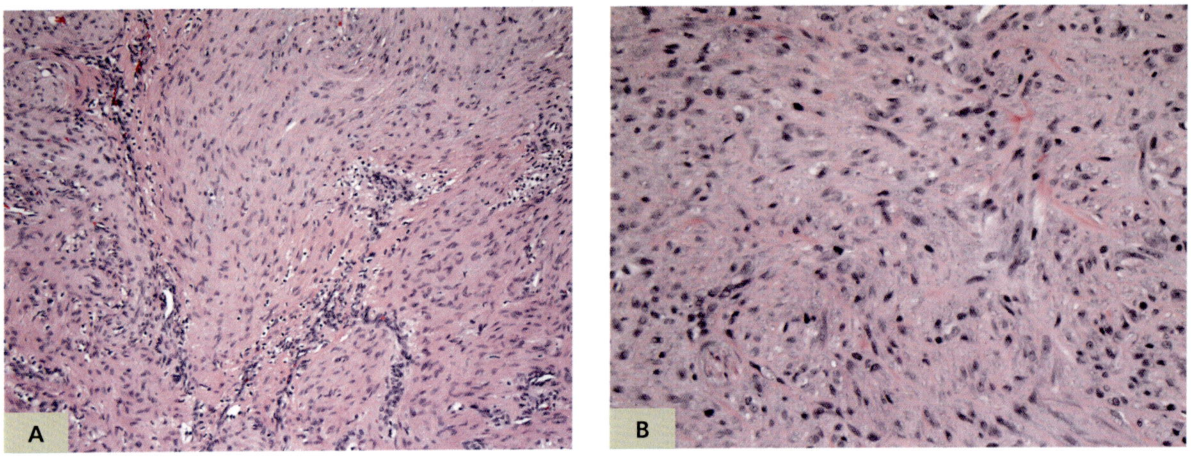

FIGURE 5.4 Myofibroma is typically biphasic, with eosinophilic myoid spindle cells arranged in bundles or whorls and more ovoid, short spindle cells; slit-like compressed vessels and concentric perivascular growth are characteristic features (A). Stromal chondroid or myxoid change is common (B).

Within the nodular areas, the stroma shows frequent chondroid or myxoid change. Because these lesions may show variable mitotic activity and even central necrosis, a diagnosis of leiomyosarcoma may be considered. However, smooth muscle neoplasms have more brightly eosinophilic cytoplasm, show a more uniformly fascicular growth pattern, and lack nuclear atypia and pleomorphism. The chondroid stroma and characteristic vascular pattern are not features of leiomyosarcoma. Immunohistochemistry can also be helpful; although myofibromas share SMA expression with leiomyosarcoma, they are negative for caldesmon and desmin.

PSEUDOSARCOMATOUS MYOFIBROBLASTIC PROLIFERATION

Pseudosarcomatous myofibroblastic proliferation (PMP), previously discussed in Chapter 3 as a mimic of inflammatory myofibroblastic tumor, may also mimic leiomyosarcoma. Tumors can be large (up to 10 cm) and infiltrative, and are composed of a population of spindled-to-stellate myofibroblastic cells arranged in loose fascicles in a myxoid stroma (**Figure 5.5A**). Slit-like vessels and an accompanying sparse lymphocytic infiltrate are common. The fascicular growth of spindled cells and presence of mitotic activity and occasional necrosis observed in PMP may resemble leiomyosarcoma; however, significant nuclear atypia, hyperchromasia, and atypical mitotic figures are absent. PMP shows positivity for SMA and desmin, further contributing to potential confusion with a smooth muscle neoplasm. Cytokeratin may be positive in PMP, but can also be focally present in leiomyosarcoma (in nearly 40% of cases in

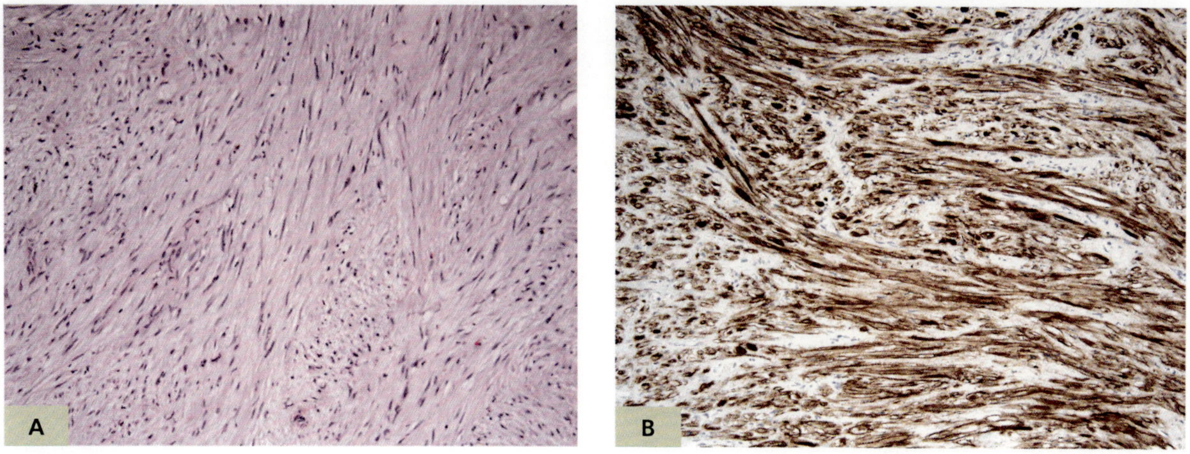

FIGURE 5.5 Pseudosarcomatous myofibroblastic proliferation. Spindled-to-stellate myofibroblastic cells are arranged in loose fascicles in a myxoid stroma (A). ALK overexpression is observed in nearly half of cases, though *ALK* gene rearrangements are usually absent (B).

both tumor types). In half of cases of PMP, *ALK* is overexpressed (but *ALK* gene rearrangements are usually absent) (**Figure 5.5B**); this finding can be a useful diagnostic feature in this distinction, in addition to the absence of true cytologic features of malignancy (238).

Postoperative spindle cell nodule is a synonym for those PMPs that arise following surgery or instrumentation, most often in the urinary bladder. Such lesions are typically small and well-circumscribed, with plump myofibroblastic spindle cells arranged in cellular fascicles, sometimes with frequent mitoses, again resembling leiomyosarcoma. Clinical correlation is informative in these cases. PMP (including postoperative examples) has minimal recurrent potential and no risk of metastasis.

ANGIOLEIOMYOMA

Angioleiomyoma is a benign smooth muscle lesion that arises in association with vessels; it may be subclassified as capillary/solid, venous, or cavernous types (although most authorities do not subclassify these tumors). Tumors occur as painful subcutaneous nodules in the extremities of adults, and rarely recur. Angioleiomyomas are well-circumscribed and occasionally associated with calcifications (**Figure 5.6**). The proliferating smooth muscle cells can show limited mitotic activity, which may raise concern for leiomyosarcoma. The absence of cytologic atypia in angioleiomyoma will help exclude leiomyosarcoma; recognition of the prominent vascular component (and focal perivascular orientation of smooth muscle cells) is critical for appropriate diagnosis.

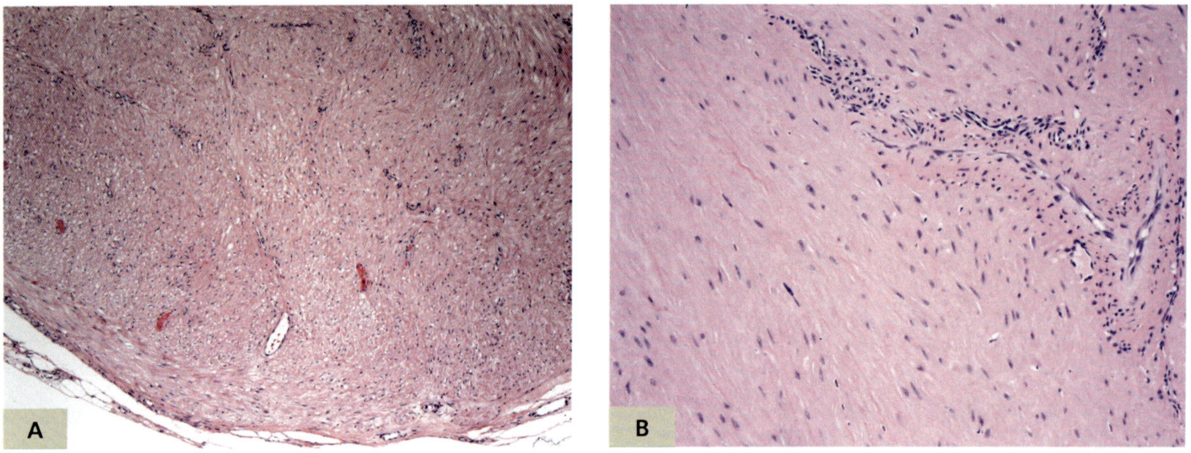

FIGURE 5.6 Angioleiomyoma is a well-circumscribed proliferation of smooth muscle cells associated with prominent blood vessels (often slit-like) (A); the tumor cells can show concentric growth around vessel walls (B).

CELLULAR SCHWANNOMA

The cellular variant of schwannoma, which usually lacks hypocellular (Antoni B) areas and Verocay bodies, can morphologically resemble a smooth muscle neoplasm and therefore be confused with leiomyosarcoma (**Figure 5.7A**). Cellular schwannoma most commonly occurs in the retroperitoneum and posterior mediastinum, but similar to conventional schwannoma, this less common variant can occur at a wide range of anatomic sites. Cellular schwannomas are usually encapsulated and may show a prominent peripheral lymphoid cuff, although in the upper aerodigestive and gastrointestinal tracts, schwannomas are generally unencapsulated (though well-circumscribed) (**Figure 5.7B**). In cellular schwannoma, the spindled tumor cells are arranged in sheets and fascicles and may simulate a smooth muscle neoplasm or even MPNST. Furthermore, degenerative nuclear atypia, low mitotic activity, and focal necrosis can be seen in schwannomas and can also raise concern for malignancy. Features that favor cellular schwannoma are encapsulation or sharp circumscription, thick-walled vessels with hyaline change, and clusters of foamy histiocytes. In comparison to smooth muscle cells, lesional Schwann cells tend to contain more tapering nuclei and paler fibrillary cytoplasm (**Figure 5.7C**). Though mitoses may be present, atypical forms are not seen in a cellular schwannoma. Diffuse immunoreactivity for S-100 protein is diagnostic of schwannoma, and epithelial membrane antigen (EMA) will be positive in the perineurial cells of the capsule, if a capsule is present.

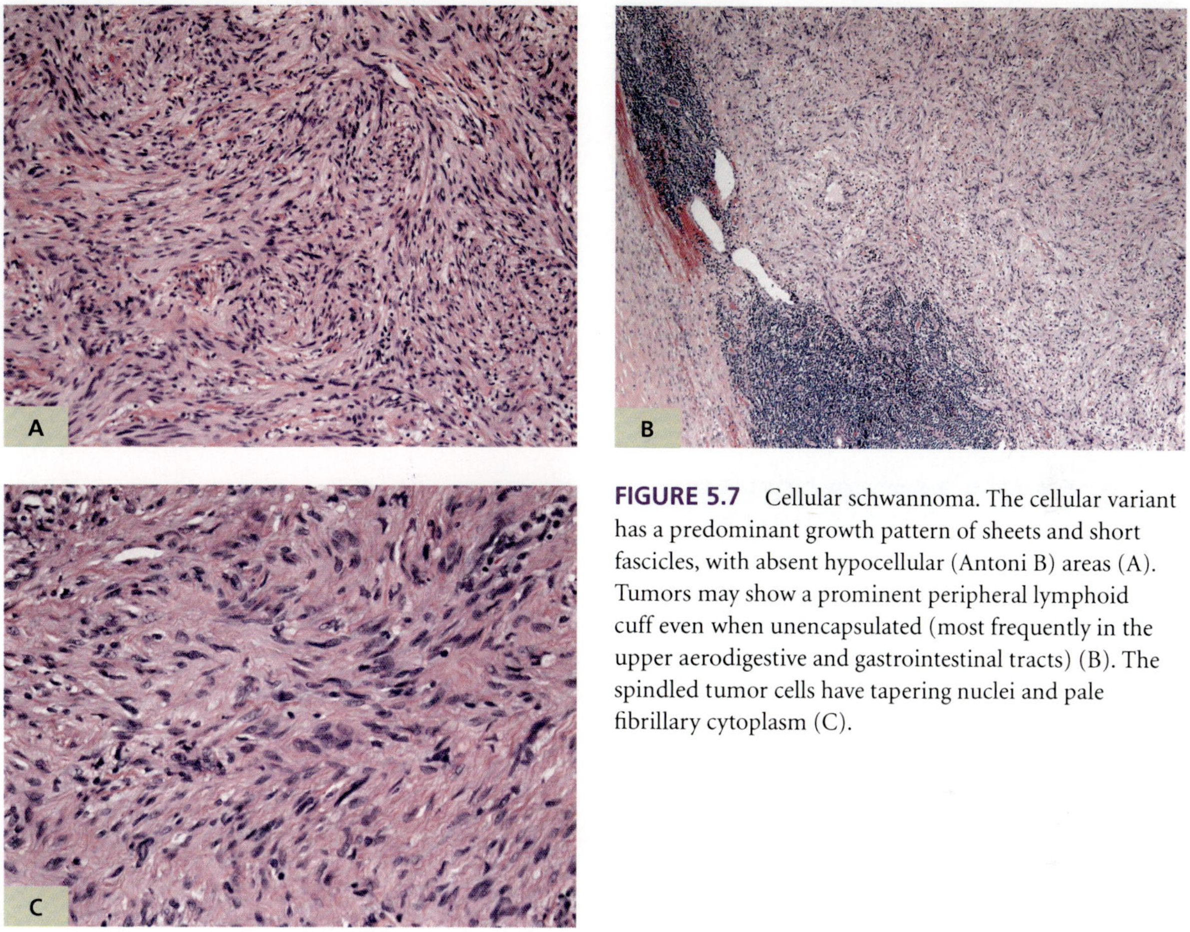

FIGURE 5.7 Cellular schwannoma. The cellular variant has a predominant growth pattern of sheets and short fascicles, with absent hypocellular (Antoni B) areas (A). Tumors may show a prominent peripheral lymphoid cuff even when unencapsulated (most frequently in the upper aerodigestive and gastrointestinal tracts) (B). The spindled tumor cells have tapering nuclei and pale fibrillary cytoplasm (C).

EBV-ASSOCIATED SMOOTH MUSCLE NEOPLASMS

In the immunocompromised setting (usually patients with HIV or who are post-transplant), smooth muscle tumors may arise in association with Epstein–Barr virus (EBV) infection. EBV-associated smooth muscle tumors typically arise at visceral sites and are often multifocal. Lesions are usually recognizable as smooth muscle neoplasms with fascicular growth of eosinophilic spindle cells (although occasional tumors appear more pericytic in appearance with less abundant cytoplasm and focally perivascular growth), and the tumor cells typically lack cytologic atypia but show some degree of mitotic activity (usually three or less per ten high-power field (HPF), but sometimes higher) (262) (**Figure 5.8A, B**). More cellular foci of rounded cells with limited cytoplasm and scattered small lymphocytes are typical features. EBV-associated smooth muscle tumors are positive for SMA, desmin, and caldesmon, as well as EBV-encoded RNA (EBER) by in situ hybridization (**Figure 5.8C**). If the EBV-associated nature of

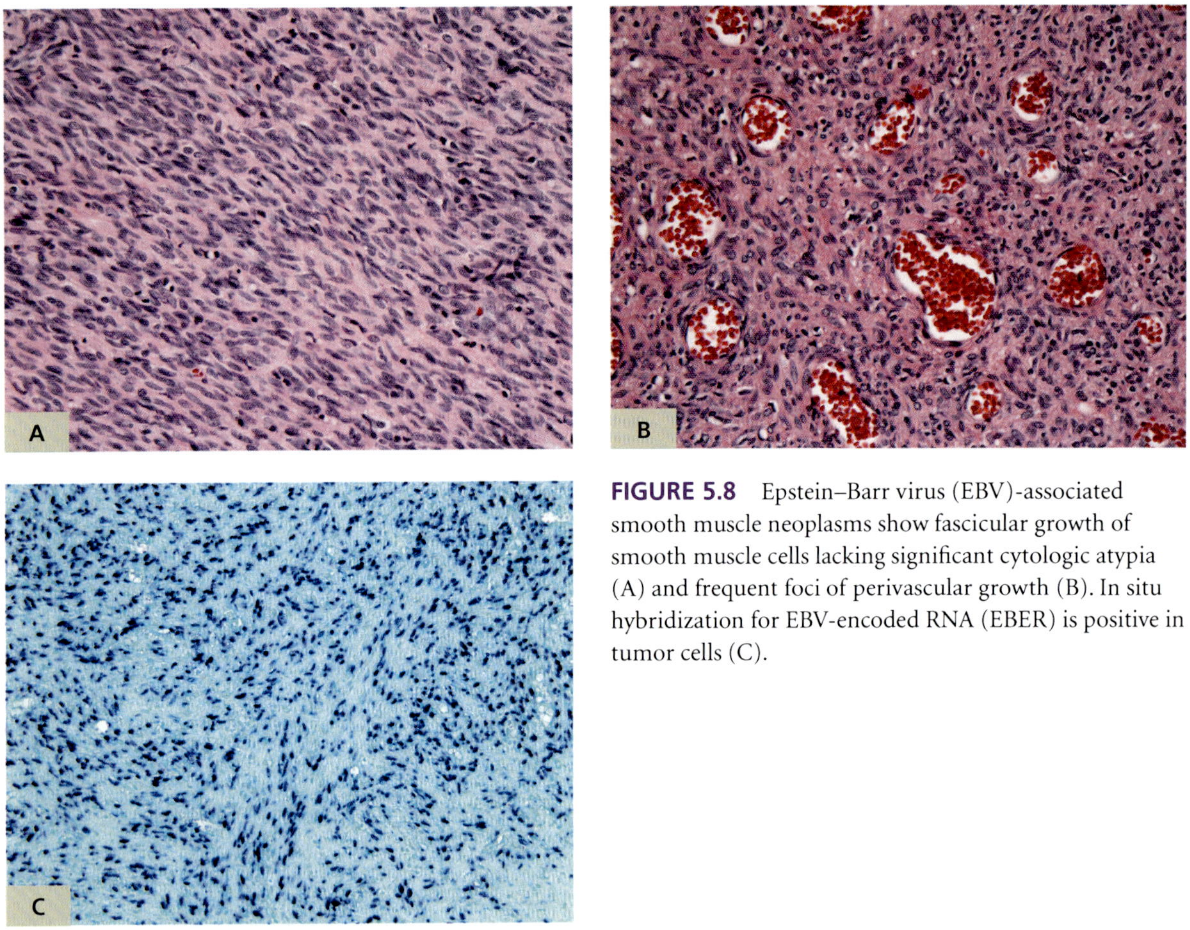

FIGURE 5.8 Epstein–Barr virus (EBV)-associated smooth muscle neoplasms show fascicular growth of smooth muscle cells lacking significant cytologic atypia (A) and frequent foci of perivascular growth (B). In situ hybridization for EBV-encoded RNA (EBER) is positive in tumor cells (C).

the lesion is not recognized, owing to the presence of mitotic activity, leiomyosarcoma may be diagnosed. This distinction is important as EBV-associated smooth muscle tumors have a more favorable prognosis with infrequent metastases and rare mortality in comparison to leiomyosarcoma. Multicentricity of lesions, foci of round cells, and aggregates of lymphocytes favor EBV-associated smooth muscle tumors over conventional leiomyosarcomas.

MIMICS OF SKELETAL MUSCLE NEOPLASMS

CRYSTAL STORING HISTIOCYTOSIS

Most cases of crystal storing histiocytosis arise in the setting of a lymphoproliferative disorder or a plasma cell neoplasm (263,264). Lesions present as either a localized mass or as diffuse disease; lung, skin, kidney, and bone marrow are common sites of involvement (265). Crystal storing histiocytosis is a nonneoplastic

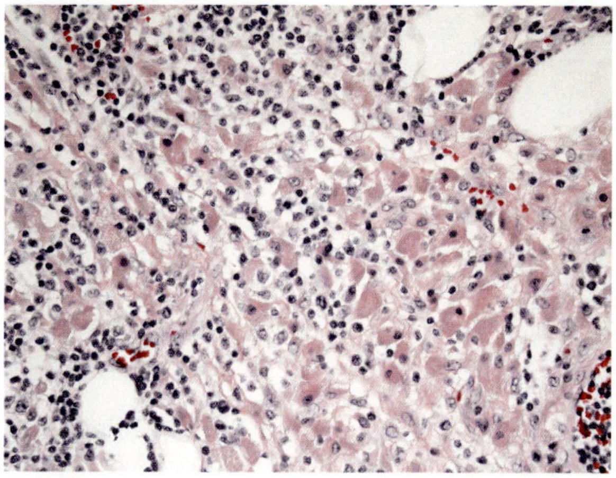

FIGURE 5.9 Crystal-storing histiocytosis is a non-neoplastic proliferation of histiocytes with abundant brightly eosinophilic cytoplasmic inclusions (resulting from ingestion of immunoglobulins).

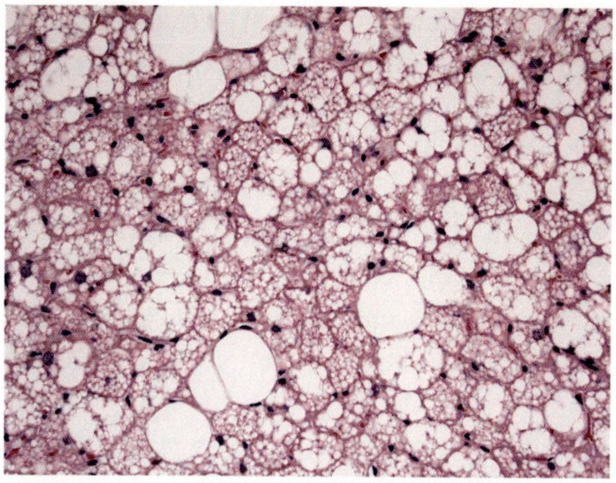

FIGURE 5.10 Hibernoma. The brown fat cells of hibernoma can show a predominance of eosinophilic morphology.

proliferation of histiocytes with abundant brightly eosinophilic cytoplasmic inclusions, resulting from ingestion of immunoglobulins (most commonly kappa light chain) (263) (**Figure 5.9**). The appearance of these histiocytes often mimics mature rhabdomyoblasts, with striated-appearing eosinophilic cytoplasm due to the accumulated crystalline material. A diagnosis of adult-type rhabdomyoma may be considered, and the histiocytes may even be misinterpreted as heterologous rhabdomyoblastic differentiation in a malignant germ cell tumor, MPNST, or DDLPS, depending upon the anatomic location. The absence of a teratomatous or sarcomatous component will exclude these other diagnostic considerations. Immunohistochemistry for histiocyte-specific markers (eg, CD68 or CD163) will confirm the histiocytic nature of the proliferation, and negative staining for desmin and myogenin will exclude myogenic differentiation. Clinical correlation for a history of a monoclonal gammopathy is most helpful in recognition of crystal storing histiocytosis. In some cases, the histiocytic proliferation will be admixed with the lymphoma; appropriate immunohistochemistry can be used to confirm the latter diagnosis. These lesions usually resolve following treatment of the underlying lymphoproliferative disorder or plasma cell neoplasm.

HIBERNOMA

The brown fat cells of hibernoma [a benign adipocytic tumor frequently associated with 11q13 rearrangement (216); initially discussed in Chapter 2] can show a predominance of eosinophilic morphology and mimic adult-type rhabdomyoma (**Figure 5.10**). The anatomic site may be helpful: while both hibernoma and adult-type rhabdomyoma frequently occur in the head and neck, adult-type rhabdomyoma rarely occurs in the extremities where hibernoma is common. Both hibernoma and adult-type rhabdomyoma may show a lobulated architecture; however, in the latter, the tumor cells often show vacuolization ("spider" cells) and contain eosinophilic rod-like inclusions or cross striations (**Figure 5.11**). A component of white fat cells within hibernoma is common, and myogenic markers are negative.

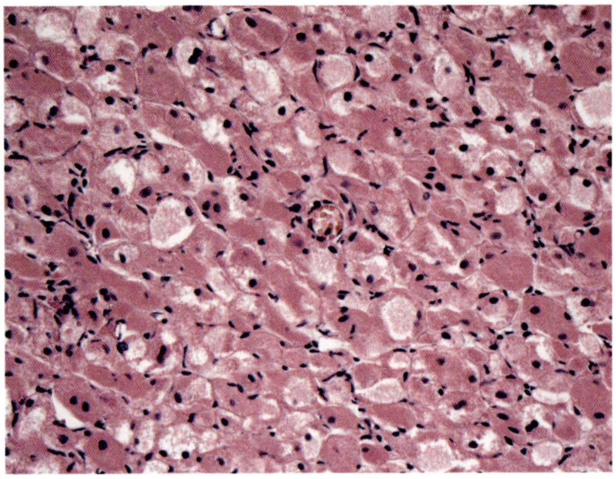

FIGURE 5.11 Adult rhabdomyoma is characterized by large polygonal tumor cells with cytoplasmic vacuolization ("spider" cells), eosinophilic rod-like inclusions, or cross striations.

GRANULAR CELL TUMOR

Granular cell tumor is a benign neoplasm of neuroectodermal differentiation that most frequently arises on the head and neck, but can involve essentially any anatomic site, including visceral organs. Tumors are composed of a round-to-epithelioid cell population containing a round, centrally placed nucleus with indistinct nucleoli, and granular eosinophilic cytoplasm, which may resemble rhabdomyoblasts (**Figure 5.12**). Granular cell tumor shows a predominantly nested and trabecular growth pattern, but infiltrative growth and perineural invasion are often seen at the periphery of these lesions. These features may overlap somewhat with embryonal rhabdomyosarcoma, which is characterized by rhabdomyoblasts in varying stages of differentiation and variable hypocellular regions and stromal hyalinization (**Figure 5.13**). Distinction can be made on morphologic and immunohistochemical grounds. Rhabdomyoblasts contain more brightly eosinophilic cytoplasm than the lesional cells in granular cell tumor, in which the cytoplasm is more uniformly granular, paler, and syncytial in appearance. In subepithelial and submucosal sites, granular cell tumors are often accompanied by overlying pseudoepitheliomatous hyperplasia of squamous epithelium, which may be a helpful diagnostic feature. The immunophenotype of granular cell tumor includes positivity for S-100 protein, NKI-C3, neuron-specific enolase, and CD68; desmin and myogenin are negative. Granular cell tumors are usually benign; recurrence is uncommon after incomplete resection, but metastases are exceptionally rare.

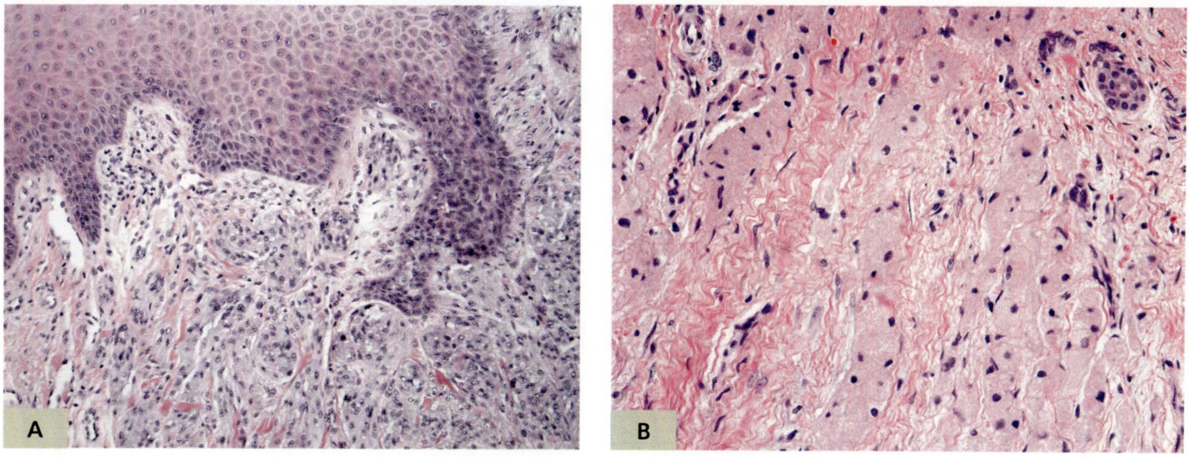

FIGURE 5.12 Granular cell tumor is comprised of round-to-epithelioid tumor cells in a nested or sheet-like growth pattern, which is frequently accompanied by overlying pseudoepitheliomatous hyperplasia of squamous epithelium (A). Tumor cells have a centrally placed round nucleus with indistinct nucleoli and granular eosinophilic cytoplasm (B).

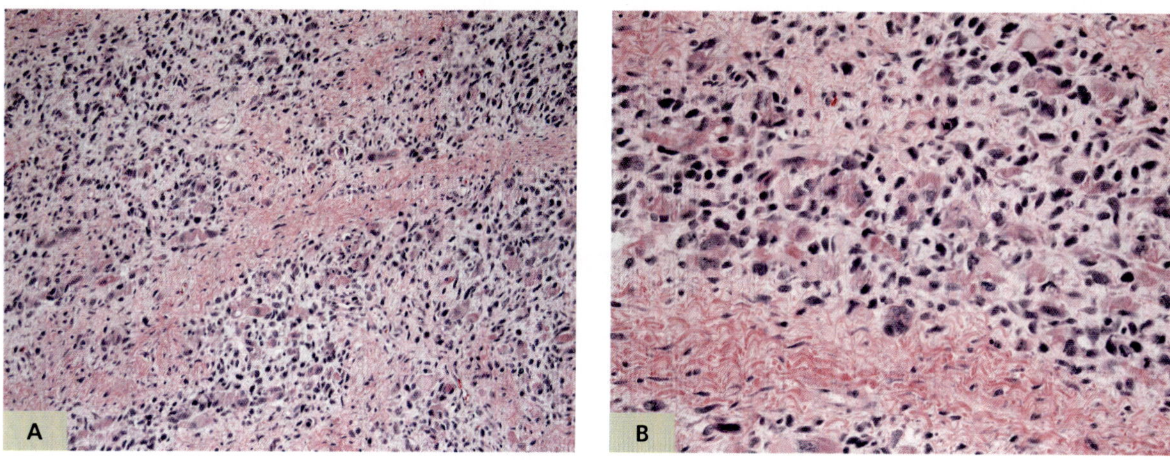

FIGURE 5.13 Embryonal rhabdomyosarcoma contains rhabdomyoblasts in varying stages of differentiation with variable hypocellular regions, myxoid foci, and stromal hyalinization (A). The rhabdomyoblasts have cytologically atypical nuclei and range in morphology from primitive-appearing stellate cells to larger polygonal, tadpole and spider cells with brightly eosinophilic cytoplasm (B).

PROLIFERATIVE FASCIITIS/PROLIFERATIVE MYOSITIS

Discussed in Chapter 3, the self-limited benign lesions proliferative fasciitis and proliferative myositis may exhibit overlapping histologic features with either rhabdomyoma or even embryonal rhabdomyosarcoma, especially in lesions in which the ganglion cell-like component predominates. The presence of mitoses and characteristic infiltrative growth of proliferative fasciitis and myositis may also seem worrisome as features of malignancy. The ganglion-like cells

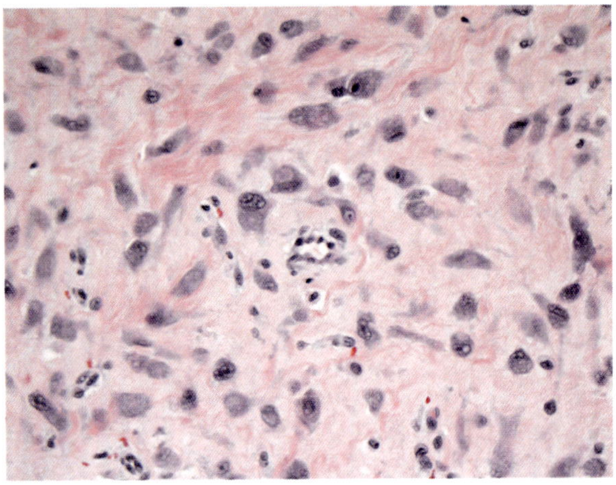

FIGURE 5.14 Proliferative fasciitis has a ganglion cell-like component with abundant amphophilic cytoplasm.

may resemble rhabdomyoblasts, but tend to be basophilic rather than brightly eosinophilic (**Figure 5.14**). Significant cytologic atypia is absent. While desmin reactivity may be focal in proliferative fasciitis and proliferative myositis, diffuse staining is typically not observed and myogenin is negative.

FETAL RHABDOMYOMA

Fetal rhabdomyomas typically present in the head and neck region of infants and young children, and are well-circumscribed and occasionally polypoid masses. Tumors have a myxoid stroma in which eosinophilic spindle cells with a range of morphologic appearances are embedded. The strap-like rhabdomyoblasts show a range of maturation, including immature cells loosely arranged singly or in irregular bundles, fascicular growth of spindle cells, and rounder rhabdomyoblasts (**Figure 5.15**). The chief consideration is distinction from the embryonal and spindle cell subtypes of rhabdomyosarcoma. Embryonal rhabdomyosarcoma is also composed of rhabdomyoblasts in varying stages of differentiation, as well as hypocellular regions and foci of stromal hyalinization (Figure 5.13), whereas spindle cell rhabdomyosarcoma is characterized by a fascicular and storiform growth pattern of uniform spindle cells (**Figure 5.16**). Fetal rhabdomyoma is well-circumscribed, while rhabdomyosarcomas are frequently infiltrative. Rhabdomyosarcoma should be considered if there are any histologic features worrisome for malignancy, specifically mitotic figures, atypical mitoses, cytologic atypia, and necrosis. Recurrent *NCOA2* gene rearrangements and mutations in *MYOD1* have been described in congenital/infantile and pediatric and adult spindle cell/sclerosing rhabdomyosarcoma, respectively (266,267). Postchemotherapy, rhabdomyosarcoma may show cytodifferentiation and lack overtly malignant features; correlation with clinical history will avoid this diagnostic pitfall.

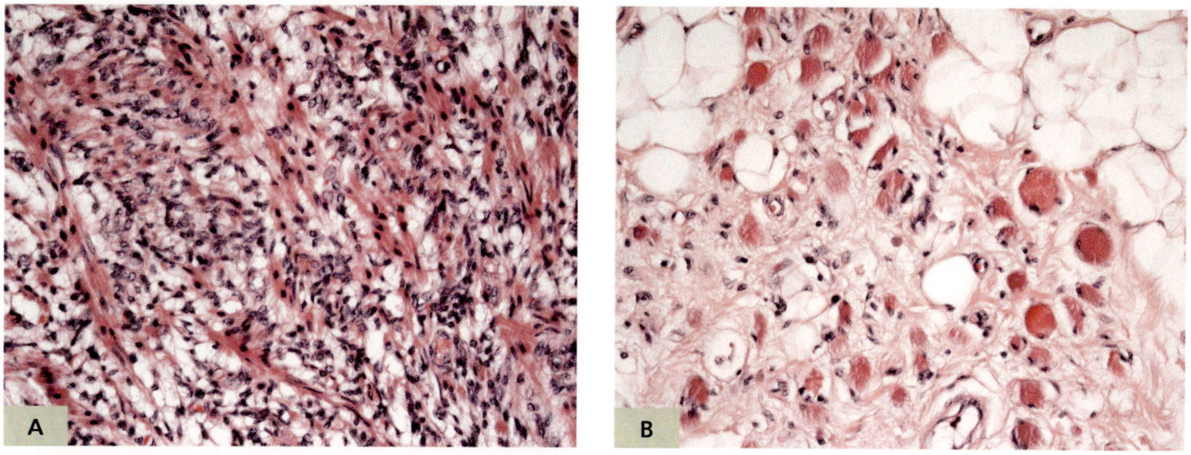

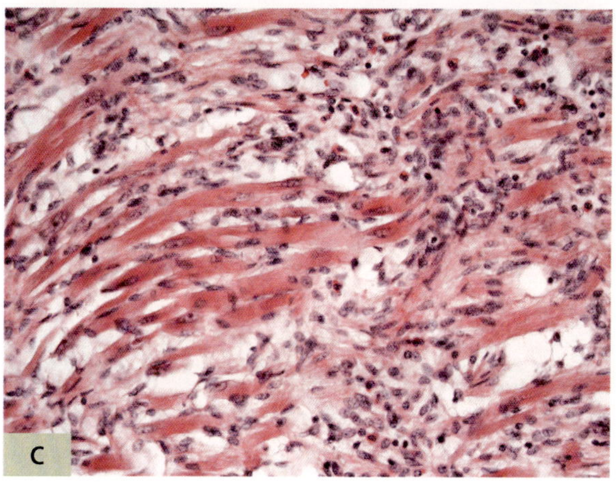

FIGURE 5.15 Fetal rhabdomyoma shows a range of maturation of immature skeletal muscle cells, with strap-like rhabdomyoblasts (A) and rounder rhabdomyoblasts (B), arranged singly or in loose bundles and fascicles (C) within a myxoid stroma.

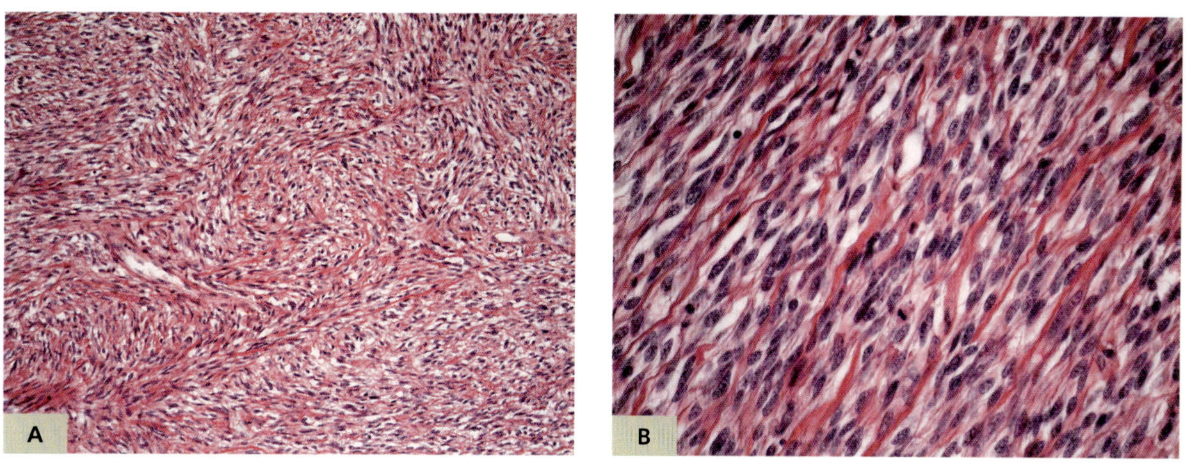

FIGURE 5.16 Spindle cell rhabdomyosarcoma shows a fascicular and storiform growth pattern of relatively uniform spindle cells (A) with cytologic atypia and mitotic activity (B).

6 Mimics of Vascular Neoplasms

- INTRAVASCULAR PAPILLARY ENDOTHELIAL HYPERPLASIA
- REACTIVE ANGIOENDOTHELIOMATOSIS
- EPITHELIOID ANGIOMATOUS NODULE
- BACILLARY ANGIOMATOSIS
- SYMPLASTIC HEMANGIOMA
- MICROVENULAR HEMANGIOMA
- HOBNAIL HEMANGIOMA
- PSEUDOANGIOMATOUS STROMAL HYPERPLASIA
- PERILOBULAR HEMANGIOMA
- ANASTOMOSING HEMANGIOMA OF THE GENITOURINARY TRACT
- VASCULAR TRANSFORMATION OF LYMPH NODE SINUSES
- SPINDLE CELL HEMANGIOMA
- EPITHELIOID HEMANGIOMA OF SOFT TISSUE AND BONE
- SPLENIC HEMANGIOMA AND LITTORAL CELL ANGIOMA
- ATYPICAL POSTRADIATION VASCULAR PROLIFERATION
- KAPOSI SARCOMA

There are many diagnostic challenges in vascular neoplasms, particularly because both benign and malignant lesions can show architectural heterogeneity. Many vascular lesions are superficial; patients frequently undergo shave or core needle biopsies in which architectural features cannot be fully assessed. Most benign vascular proliferations show a lobular growth pattern, lack infiltrative growth and significant endothelial atypia, and exhibit intact microvascular architecture with pericytes around small vessels.

Immunohistochemistry for ERG, CD31, and CD34 can be useful in confirming endothelial differentiation. Smooth muscle actin (SMA) is positive in pericytes, which can be used in combination with endothelial markers to assess whether a lesion has an intact pericytic layer around vessels (which can be helpful in areas of seemingly solid growth of proliferating vessels). Despite the fact that many vascular neoplasms are now known to be characterized by recurrent molecular alterations, few entity-specific immunohistochemical markers currently exist.

Angiosarcoma can show a wide range of morphologic appearances, ranging from low-grade malignancies comprised of only subtly dissecting vascular channels lined by atypical endothelial cells, to high grade lesions with solid growth of spindled or epithelioid tumor cells (**Figure 6.1**). However, the histologic grade of angiosarcoma is not associated with biologic behavior (268), underscoring the importance of the distinction between a morphologically low-grade angiosarcoma and a benign mimicker.

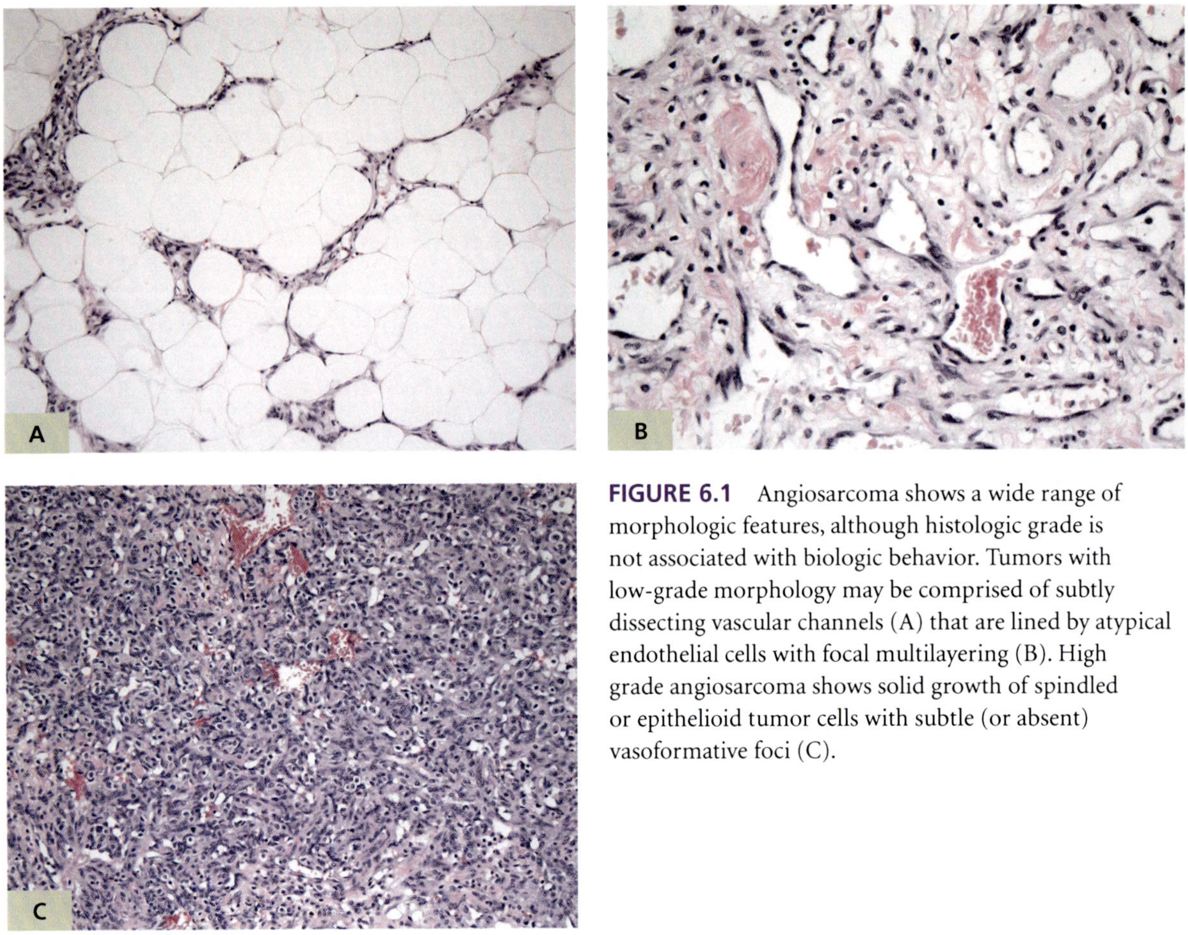

FIGURE 6.1 Angiosarcoma shows a wide range of morphologic features, although histologic grade is not associated with biologic behavior. Tumors with low-grade morphology may be comprised of subtly dissecting vascular channels (A) that are lined by atypical endothelial cells with focal multilayering (B). High grade angiosarcoma shows solid growth of spindled or epithelioid tumor cells with subtle (or absent) vasoformative foci (C).

INTRAVASCULAR PAPILLARY ENDOTHELIAL HYPERPLASIA

Intravascular papillary endothelial hyperplasia (also known as Masson's tumor) is a reactive process that may develop within a pre-existing blood vessel, a pre-existing vascular lesion (most commonly hemangioma), or a hematoma. It is considered an unusual form of organizing thrombus, in which the dilated vascular space or hematoma is filled by papillary structures containing either fibrin or acellular collagenous cores (**Figure 6.2**). Each papilla is surrounded by a single layer of benign-appearing endothelial cells. Lesions are usually well-circumscribed, except for those arising within a hemangioma, which may initially appear to be comprised of infiltrating vascular channels. Association with a vein wall is usually evident with thorough sampling and histologic examination. Some cases of intravascular papillary endothelial hyperplasia may mimic the infiltrative and dissecting growth pattern of a well-differentiated angiosarcoma, but can be distinguished by the lack of cytologic atypia, mitotic activity, endothelial multilayering, and true dissecting growth. Evidence of an adjacent organizing thrombus may be present, which is a helpful diagnostic clue.

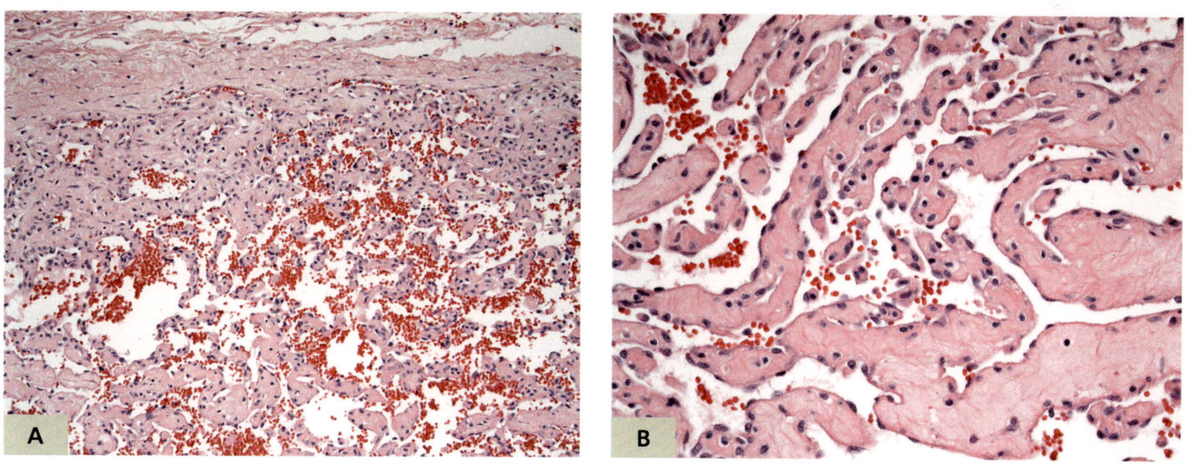

FIGURE 6.2 Intravascular papillary endothelial hyperplasia (Masson's tumor) is considered an unusual form of organizing thrombus, in which a dilated vascular space or hematoma is filled by papillary structures containing either fibrin or acellular collagenous cores (A). Papillae are surrounded by a single layer of benign-appearing endothelial cells (B).

REACTIVE ANGIOENDOTHELIOMATOSIS

Reactive angioendotheliomatosis (RAE) has a characteristic presentation of multifocal plaques, papules, nodules, and ecchymoses covering the chest, trunk, limbs, and/or face, which is often clinically worrisome for angiosarcoma. The majority of affected patients have coexistent systemic diseases, most commonly renal disease, cardiovascular disease, or immunosuppression; RAE is considered to be reactive in nature (269). RAE is a dermal proliferation of tightly packed capillaries varying in size, either in a lobular or diffuse growth pattern (**Figure 6.3A, B**). Occasional cases show a somewhat infiltrative growth pattern

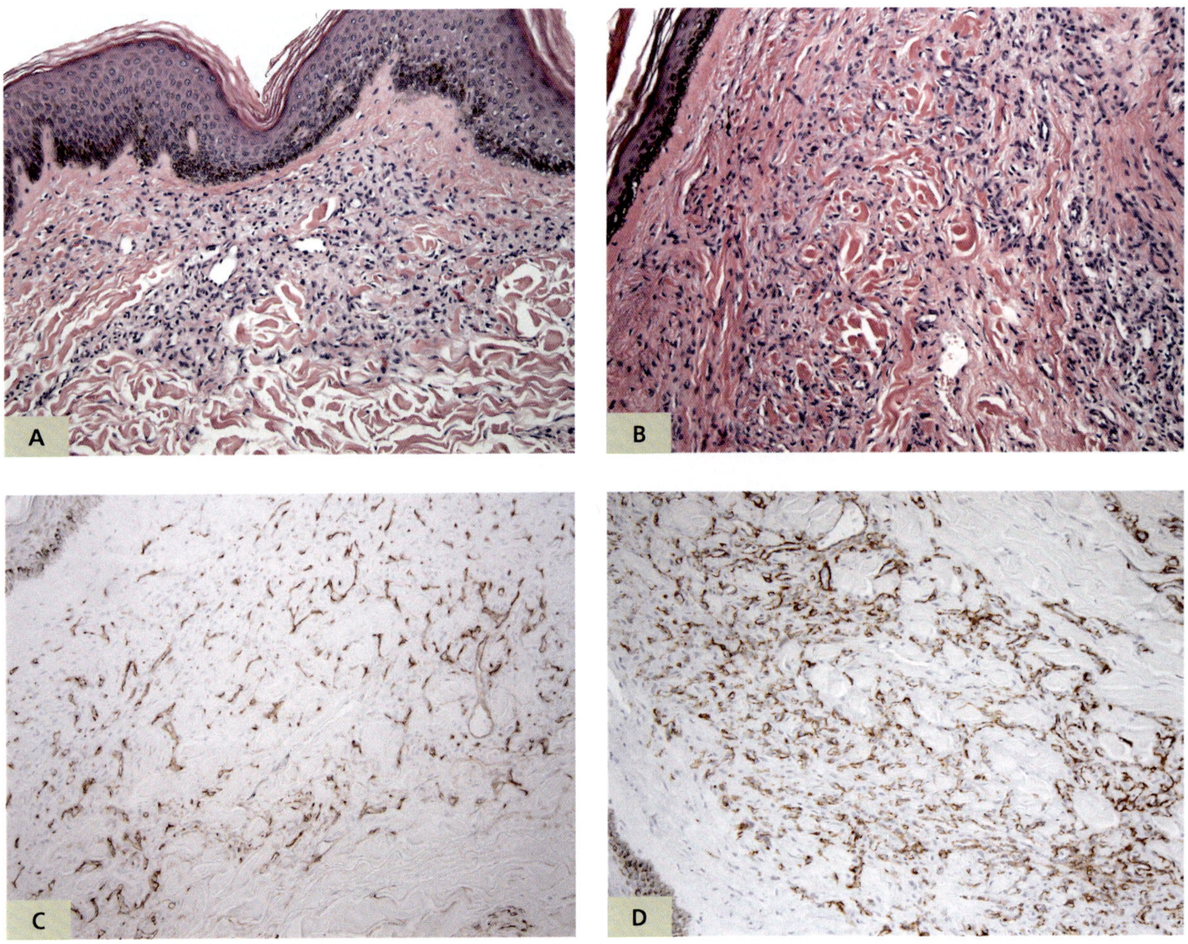

FIGURE 6.3 Reactive angioendotheliomatosis is a dermal proliferation of tightly packed capillaries varying in size, either in a lobular or diffuse growth pattern (A). Some cases may show a somewhat infiltrative growth pattern through dermal collagen (B). The capillary architecture can be highlighted by immunohistochemical positivity for CD34 in lining endothelial cells (C) and SMA staining in pericytes that surround vascular spaces (D).

through dermal collagen or focal extension into subcutis. Fibrin microthrombi are common in RAE, and the adjacent dermis can show red blood cell extravasation, chronic inflammation, or a reactive proliferation of myofibroblasts. Angiosarcoma can be excluded on the basis of absent endothelial atypia or multilayering. Immunohistochemistry for endothelial and pericytic markers will confirm the proliferation of tightly packed intact capillaries and an absence of solid growth (**Figure 6.3C, D**). The clinical course of RAE is mixed, with resolution in some patients and disease persistence or progression (as development of additional lesions) in others (269).

EPITHELIOID ANGIOMATOUS NODULE

Epithelioid angiomatous nodule is a benign vascular proliferation that affects adult patients most frequently on the trunk as single lesions. Lesions present with a short duration, and have no risk of recurrence or metastasis (270,271). On histologic section, epithelioid angiomatous nodule appears as a well-circumscribed dermal nodule with a solid proliferation of epithelioid endothelial cells containing abundant pale pink cytoplasm and occasional intracytoplasmic vacuoles (**Figure 6.4**). Given the absence of vascular channel formation and epithelioid cytomorphology, the findings may raise suspicion for epithelioid angiosarcoma (although the lesions are most commonly confused with epithelioid hemangioma; see section "*Epithelioid Hemangioma of Soft Tissue and Bone*"). However, epithelioid angiomatous nodule is well-circumscribed and lacks cytologic atypia and significant mitotic activity.

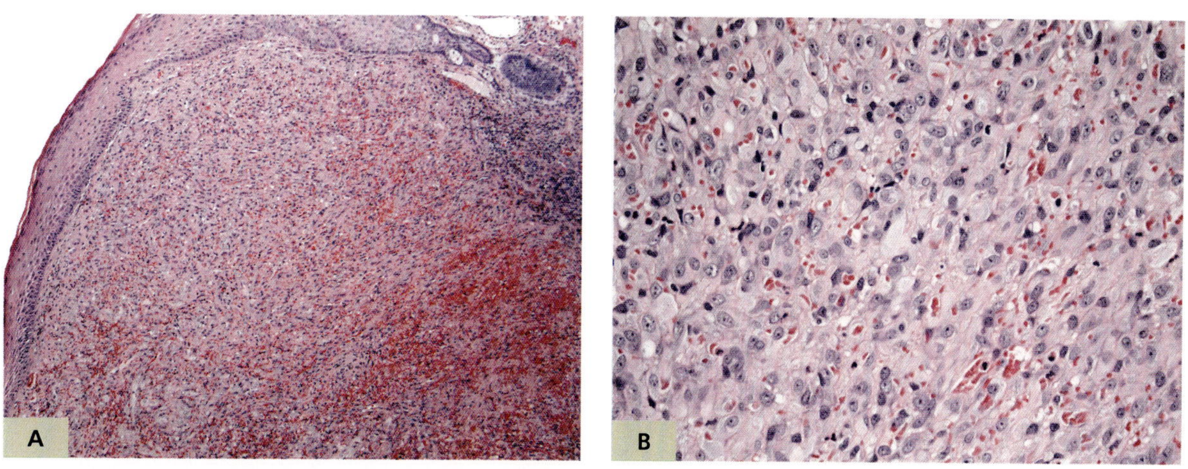

FIGURE 6.4 Epithelioid angiomatous nodule is a well-circumscribed dermal nodule with a solid proliferation of epithelioid endothelial cells (A) that contain abundant pale pink cytoplasm and occasional intracytoplasmic vacuoles, and lack significant cytologic atypia (B).

BACILLARY ANGIOMATOSIS

Most cases of bacillary angiomatosis can be readily recognized by clinical correlation and the presence of the causative basophilic bacterial forms, most commonly the rickettsia *Bartonella* species. The gram-negative bacilli are frequently conspicuous on hematoxylin-and-eosin (H&E) stain. Bacillary angiomatosis presents as multifocal cutaneous lesions comprised of well-demarcated proliferations of capillaries, often in a lobular architecture (**Figure 6.5A, B**). The differential diagnosis includes epithelioid hemangioma (see section "*Epithelioid Hemangioma of Soft Tissue and Bone*"), nodular Kaposi sarcoma (KS) (see section "*Kaposi Sarcoma*"), and epithelioid angiosarcoma. Bacillary angiomatosis is comprised of proliferating microvessels, and the endothelial cells may be epithelioid but lack cytologic atypia. A prominent infiltrate of neutrophils is usually present, which is a helpful diagnostic feature. In addition to Gram stain, a Warthin–Starry (**Figure 6.5C**) or Steiner stain will also highlight the causative organisms.

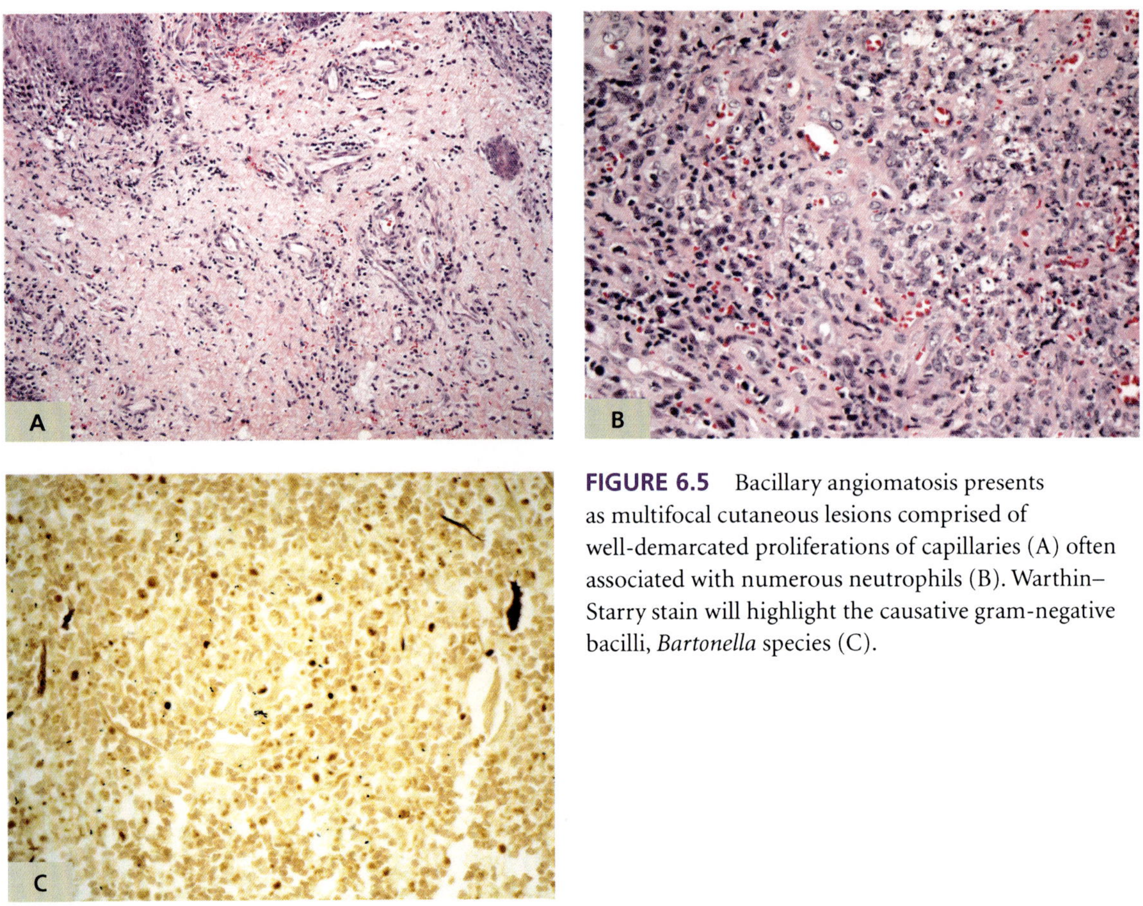

FIGURE 6.5 Bacillary angiomatosis presents as multifocal cutaneous lesions comprised of well-demarcated proliferations of capillaries (A) often associated with numerous neutrophils (B). Warthin–Starry stain will highlight the causative gram-negative bacilli, *Bartonella* species (C).

SYMPLASTIC HEMANGIOMA

Pre-existing dermal hemangiomas can undergo degenerative changes, resulting in atypical stromal or smooth muscle cells in the vessel walls (**Figure 6.6**). The atypical cells can be enlarged, hyperchromatic, and multinucleated; rare mitotic activity can be seen. These features may raise the possibility of angiosarcoma. However, careful examination for a benign-appearing endothelial cell population lacking atypia and multilayering, and confinement of the atypical cells to the vessel walls will support the diagnosis of symplastic hemangioma.

MICROVENULAR HEMANGIOMA

Microvenular hemangioma, which commonly occurs in middle-aged adults on the extremities, is a benign entity that may be histologically worrisome for angiosarcoma. Lesions are comprised of a dermal proliferation of venules that dissect through dermal collagen; on low power the vessels appear to run alternately parallel and perpendicular to the epidermis (**Figure 6.7A**). Despite the dissecting growth pattern, the veins lack endothelial atypia and multilayering, and each vessel has an intact layer of pericytes. Microvenular hemangiomas show

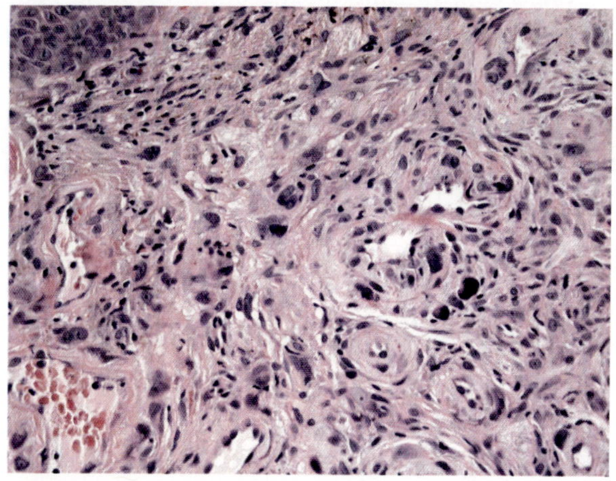

FIGURE 6.6 Symplastic hemangioma represents degenerative changes in pre-existing hemangiomas, resulting in atypical cells confined to the vessel walls.

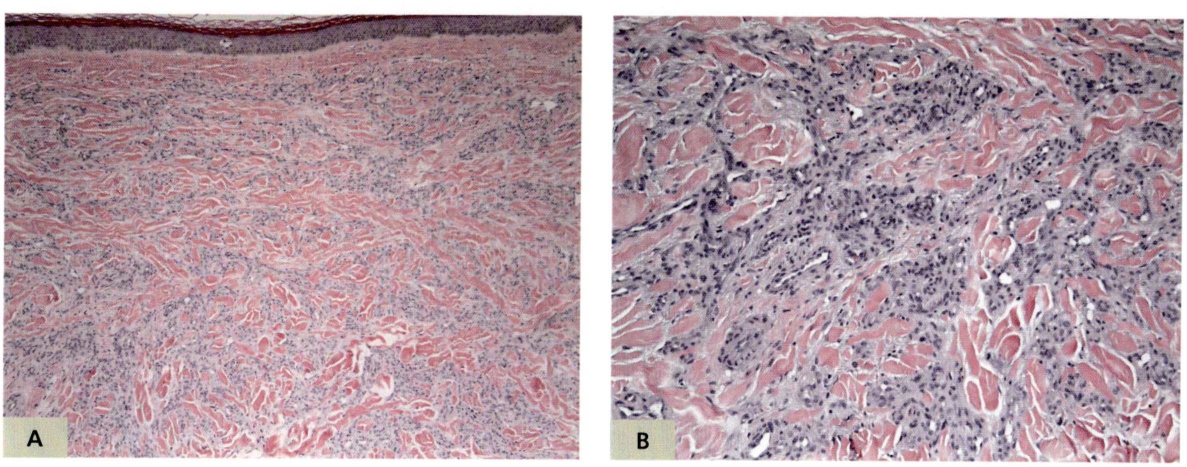

FIGURE 6.7 Microvenular hemangioma is a dermal proliferation of venules that dissect through dermal collagen and appear to run alternately parallel and perpendicular to the epidermis (A). Lesions show "maturation" of vessels, with veins having open lumina at the superficial aspect and becoming progressively more slit-like toward the deeper dermis (B).

a "maturation" of vessels toward the deeper dermis, with veins having open lumina at the superficial end and becoming progressively more slit-like at the deeper aspect (**Figure 6.7B**), which facilitates diagnosis.

HOBNAIL HEMANGIOMA

Also known as targetoid hemosiderotic hemangioma, hobnail hemangioma has a distinct clinical appearance of a target-like erythematous lesion with a darker, elevated central zone on the limbs or back. Histologically, these dermal-based lesions may appear worrisome given the characteristic irregular shapes of the dissecting vessels lined by "hobnail" endothelial cells, which protrude into the lumen and have mild nuclear hyperchromasia (**Figure 6.8A**). Papillary tufting of endothelial cells into the lumen can be seen, but are more prominent in the superficial area of the lesion. Hobnail hemangioma shows a characteristic maturation toward its deeper aspect, with vessels appearing more slit-like with flattened endothelial cells (**Figure 6.8B**). Lesions are benign and resection is curative.

Hobnail hemangioma may mimic three vascular neoplasms: papillary intralymphatic angioendothelioma (PILA; also known as Dabska tumor), retiform hemangioendothelioma, and angiosarcoma. PILA occurs in pediatric patients, and differs by showing extension into subcutaneous tissue and having a better developed papillary component with fibrous cores (**Figure 6.9**). It is considered by some authors to represent the childhood counterpart of

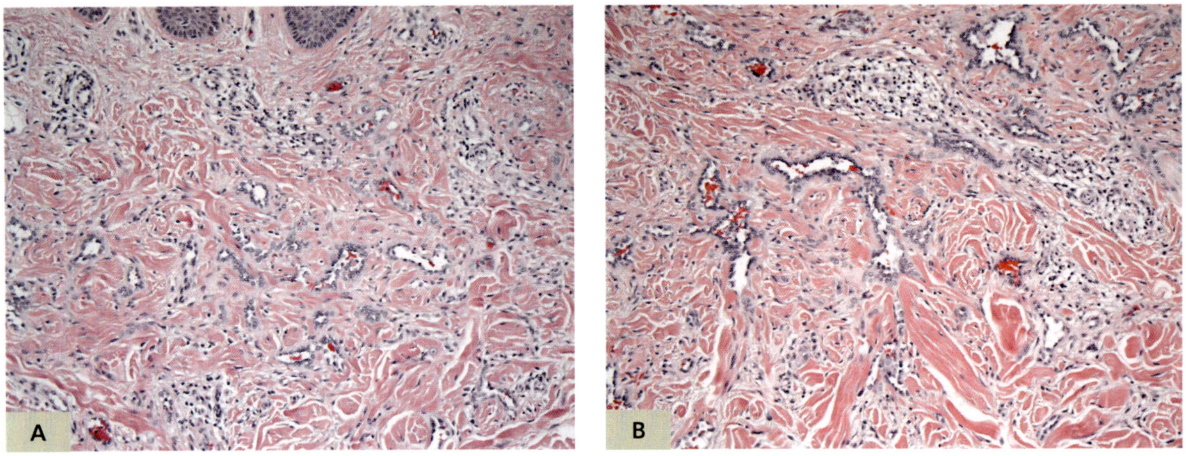

FIGURE 6.8 Hobnail hemangiomas are dermal-based lesions comprised of irregularly shaped dissecting vessels lined by protuberant "hobnail" endothelial cells (A). Tumors show a characteristic maturation with depth, where vessels appearing more slit-like with flattened endothelial cells (B).

retiform hemangioendothelioma. Retiform hemangioendothelioma shows a high recurrence rate. In contrast to hobnail hemangioma, retiform hemangioendothelioma shows a more complex architecture with infiltrative growth (often involving subcutis) of anastomosing dilated vessels lined by plump and atypical endothelial cells; foci of solid growth of endothelial cells can be seen (**Figure 6.10**). Hobnail hemangioma lacks the endothelial multilayering, cytologic atypia, and anastomosing architecture characteristic of angiosarcoma.

In lesions that arise in the postradiation setting (ie, following breast surgery and adjuvant radiation), atypical postradiation vascular proliferation (APRVP) should be favored. APRVP is typically confined to the dermis but shows more irregular borders and lacks maturation (see section "*Atypical Postradiation Vascular Proliferation*"). Chronic inflammation and papillary projections are not features of APRVP.

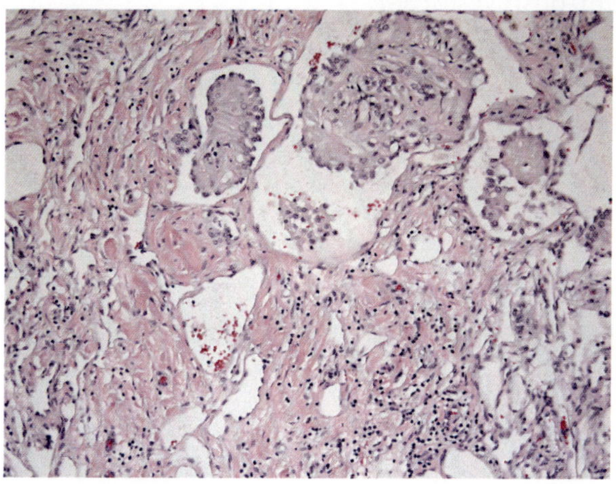

FIGURE 6.9 Papillary intralymphatic angioendothelioma shows lymphatic channels lined by protuberant endothelial cells with intraluminal papillary tufts having hyaline cores.

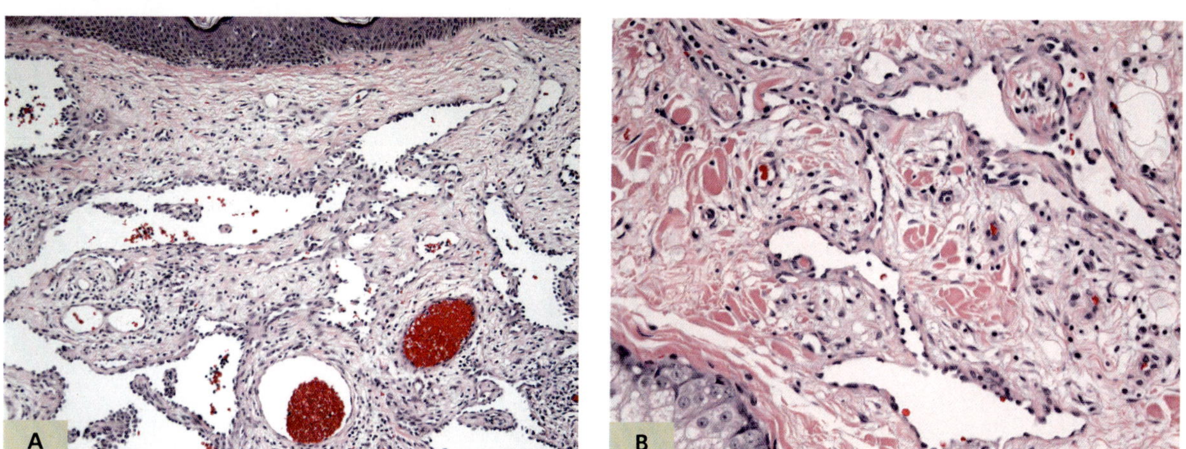

FIGURE 6.10 Retiform hemangioendothelioma shows a complex infiltrative growth pattern of dilated vessels lined by plump and atypical endothelial cells (A); vessels have a characteristic anastomosing and arborizing architecture, and stromal lymphocytes are common (B).

PSEUDOANGIOMATOUS STROMAL HYPERPLASIA

Pseudoangiomatous stromal hyperplasia (PASH) may present as a palpable or mammographic mass in the breast, and especially on biopsy may be mistaken for angiosarcoma. PASH is a benign myofibroblastic lesion, in which myofibroblasts are embedded in a hyalinized and collagenous stroma. The stroma has an anastomosing quality in which there are abundant clefts and slit-like spaces; the myofibroblasts are situated at the edge of the clefts, which imparts a pseudovascular pattern (**Figure 6.11A, B**). The "lining" layer is discontiguous, in contrast to true endothelial lining of lymphovascular spaces. Occasionally, the myofibroblasts are more proliferative (*fascicular PASH*) (**Figure 6.11C**), which may also be worrisome for a vascular malignancy. The myofibroblasts lack cytologic atypia, and are negative for endothelial markers but positive for CD34 with variable reactivity for SMA and desmin. Surgical resection is curative.

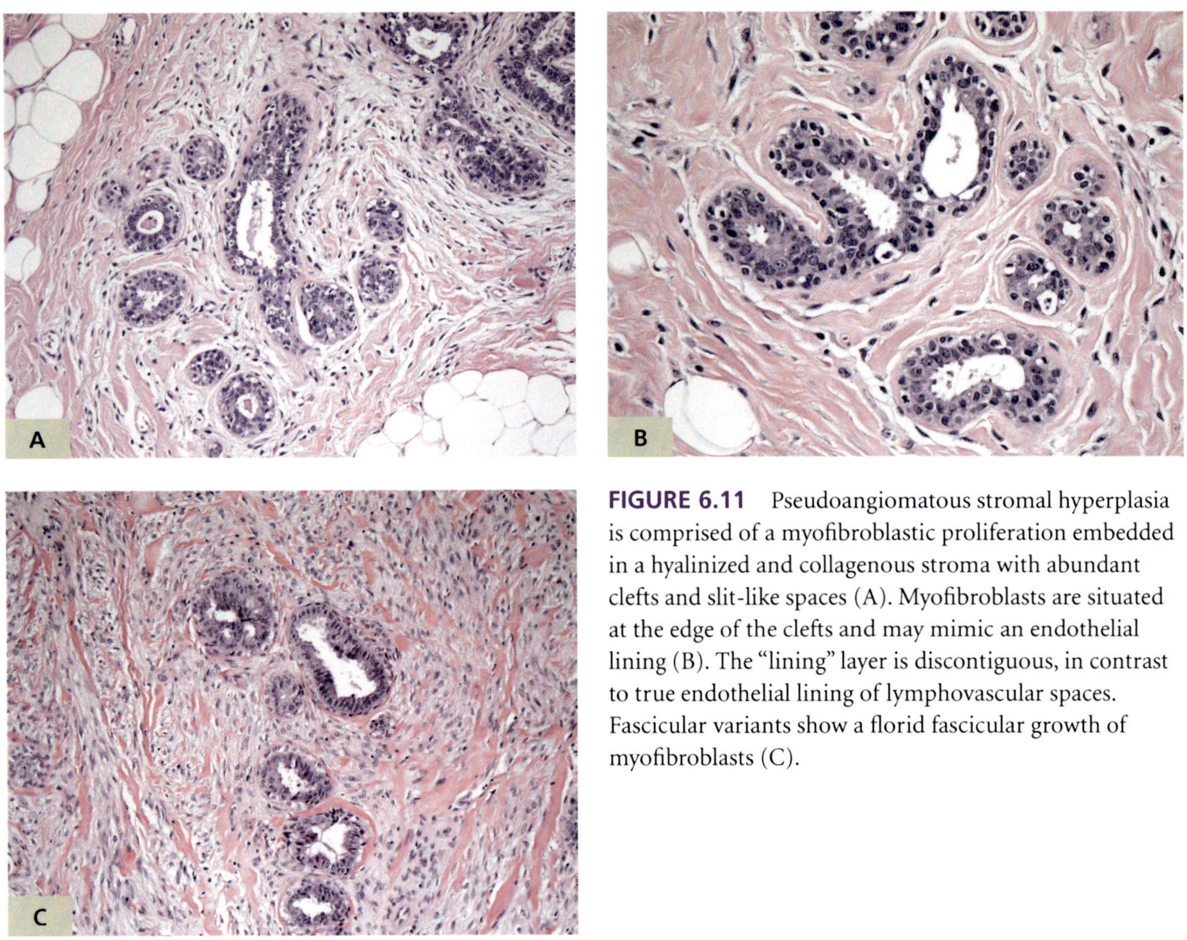

FIGURE 6.11 Pseudoangiomatous stromal hyperplasia is comprised of a myofibroblastic proliferation embedded in a hyalinized and collagenous stroma with abundant clefts and slit-like spaces (A). Myofibroblasts are situated at the edge of the clefts and may mimic an endothelial lining (B). The "lining" layer is discontiguous, in contrast to true endothelial lining of lymphovascular spaces. Fascicular variants show a florid fascicular growth of myofibroblasts (C).

PERILOBULAR HEMANGIOMA

Perilobular hemangiomas in the breast can be challenging, particularly in small biopsies. These are usually incidental findings. Lesions are well-circumscribed, but may appear infiltrative as they can involve the intra- and interlobular stroma and seemingly dissect between ductules within a lobule (**Figure 6.12**) (272). Vessels are well-developed (which can be highlighted using endothelial and pericytic markers) and lined by flattened, benign-appearing endothelial cells. They can be distinguished from morphologically low-grade angiosarcomas by the lack of anastomosing architecture and cytologic atypia.

ANASTOMOSING HEMANGIOMA OF THE GENITOURINARY TRACT

Anastomosing hemangioma of the genitourinary tract most frequently arises in the kidney, although cases have been described in the ovary and testis (273,274). Lesions are well-circumscribed, show a lobular architecture, and are frequently associated with a muscular vessel. They are comprised of anastomosing small vessels lined by spindled-to-epithelioid endothelial cells lacking significant cytologic atypia and multilayering (**Figure 6.13**). Microthrombi are

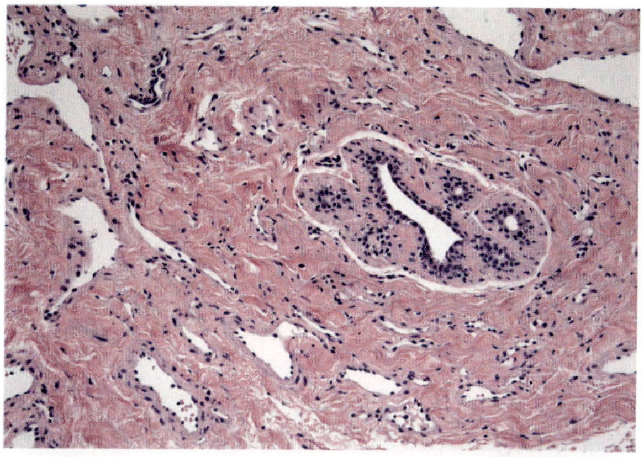

FIGURE 6.12 Perilobular hemangiomas are overall well-circumscribed, but may appear infiltrative within the lesion with involvement of intra- and interlobular stroma and dissection around lobules.

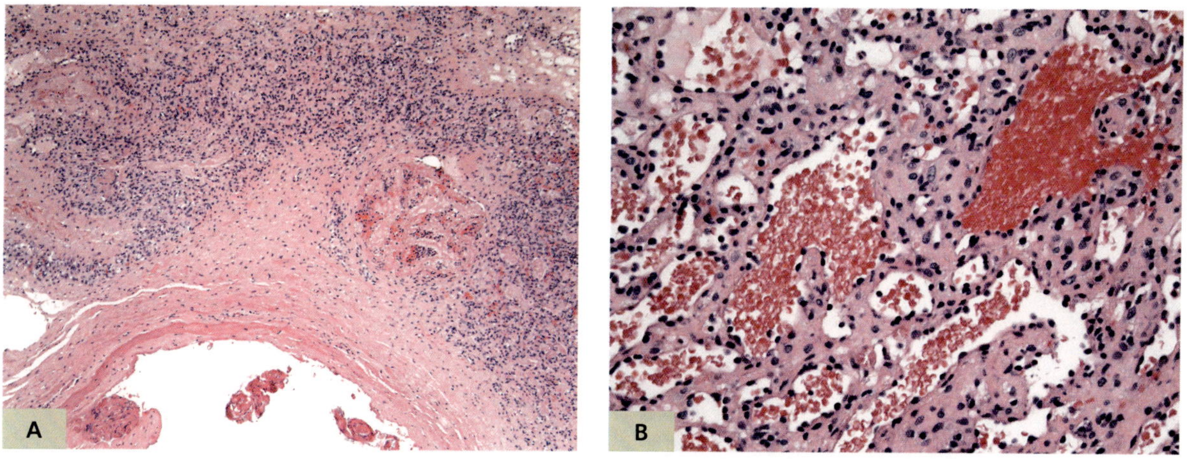

FIGURE 6.13 Anastomosing hemangiomas are frequently associated with a muscular vessel, and show a lobular configuration of anastomosing small vessels (A) which are lined by spindled-to-epithelioid endothelial cells lacking significant cytologic atypia and multilayering (B).

frequently present, and a subset has been described to show extramedullary hematopoiesis (273,274). Lesions are benign and should be distinguished from angiosarcoma despite the anastomosing vascular pattern. Attention to the lesional circumscription and presence of a "feeder" vessel will help identify anastomosing hemangioma. The clinicopathologic spectrum of anastomosing hemangioma appears to be expanding, as similar lesions are now recognized in the liver and gastrointestinal tract (275).

VASCULAR TRANSFORMATION OF LYMPH NODE SINUSES

Vascular transformation of sinuses is a reactive process, possibly associated with lymphatic vessel obstruction. Vascular transformation of sinuses may present as lymphadenopathy but is more often observed as an incidental finding. Involved lymph nodes show a proliferation of anastomosing small vessels in a strictly sinusoidal distribution (**Figure 6.14**). The vessels tend to be better formed at the periphery, and lumina are better seen under the capsule. Extravasation of red blood cells and adjacent stromal sclerosis are common features. Vascular transformation of the sinuses may be mistaken for KS; however, KS shows a multinodular growth within the lymph node parenchyma and characteristically spares the sinuses (**Figure 6.15A**). Early KS is typically confined to the capsular region, which is rare for vascular transformation of lymph node sinuses. The endothelial cells in KS are spindled and show a more fascicular growth pattern, are less vasoformative, and contain at least focal cytoplasmic eosinophilic hyaline globules (**Figure 6.15B**). Pericytes are absent given the lack of vascular channel formation. Immunohistochemistry for human herpesvirus-8 (HHV-8) is positive in KS (**Figure 6.15C**).

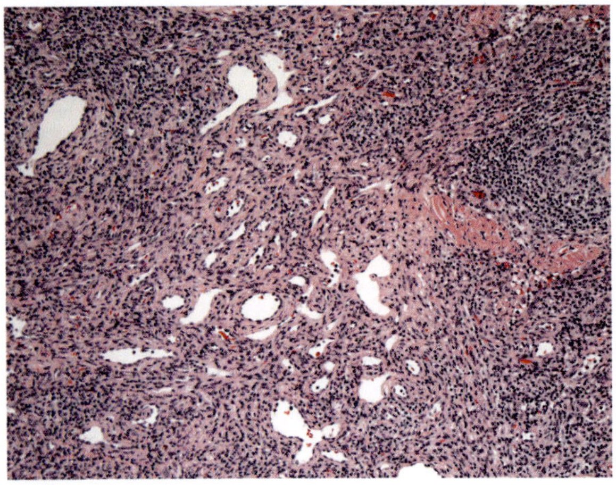

FIGURE 6.14 Vascular transformation of sinuses is a proliferation of anastomosing small vessels in a sinusoidal distribution in a lymph node.

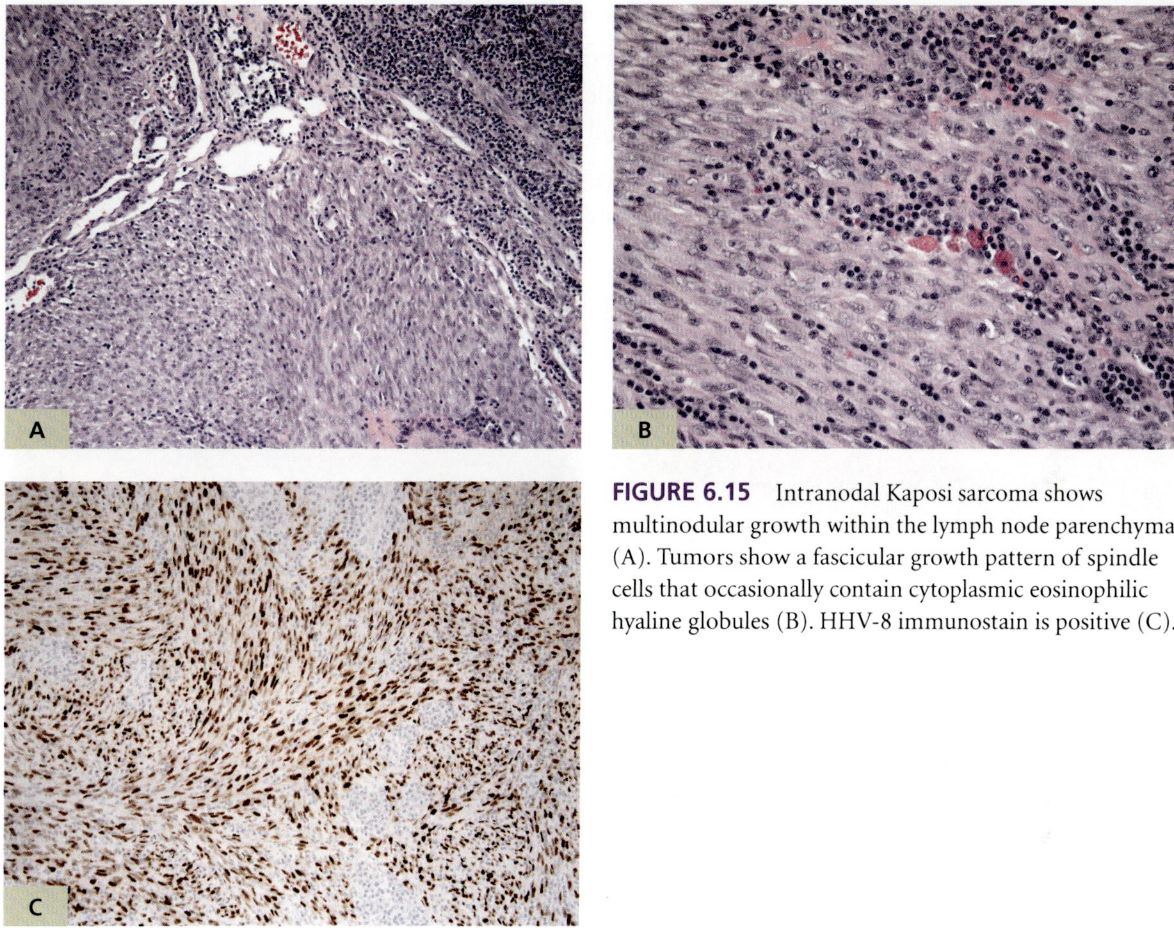

FIGURE 6.15 Intranodal Kaposi sarcoma shows multinodular growth within the lymph node parenchyma (A). Tumors show a fascicular growth pattern of spindle cells that occasionally contain cytoplasmic eosinophilic hyaline globules (B). HHV-8 immunostain is positive (C).

SPINDLE CELL HEMANGIOMA

Spindle cell hemangioma most commonly occurs in young adults on the distal extremities. Most lesions are small, slow growing, and frequently multiple. Lesions are centered in the dermis and subcutis, and comprised of a uniform population of spindled endothelial cells lining vessels and aggregating in clusters. Fibrous septa are frequent. Mitotic activity and nuclear atypia are absent. Some of the vessels are dilated cavernous veins, often associated with phleboliths. While lesions are predominantly vasoformative, with the cavernous-type spaces and slit-like vessels, there are also more solid-appearing foci with clusters of vacuolated endothelial cells with clear cytoplasm (**Figure 6.16**). Spindle cell hemangioma may show overlapping morphologic features with nodular KS. However, KS lacks foci of vacuolated cells and cavernous venous spaces. At least rare foci of intracytoplasmic and extracellular pink hyaline globules are seen in KS (**Figure 6.17**), and immunohistochemistry for HHV-8 is positive in all cases.

Clinical correlation may be helpful, as spindle cell hemangioma may be a manifestation of Maffucci syndrome. Spindle cell hemangioma is considered to be a benign neoplasm despite affected patients developing multiple lesions. Spindle cell hemangiomas have recently been shown to harbor *IDH1* and *IDH2* mutations (276,277).

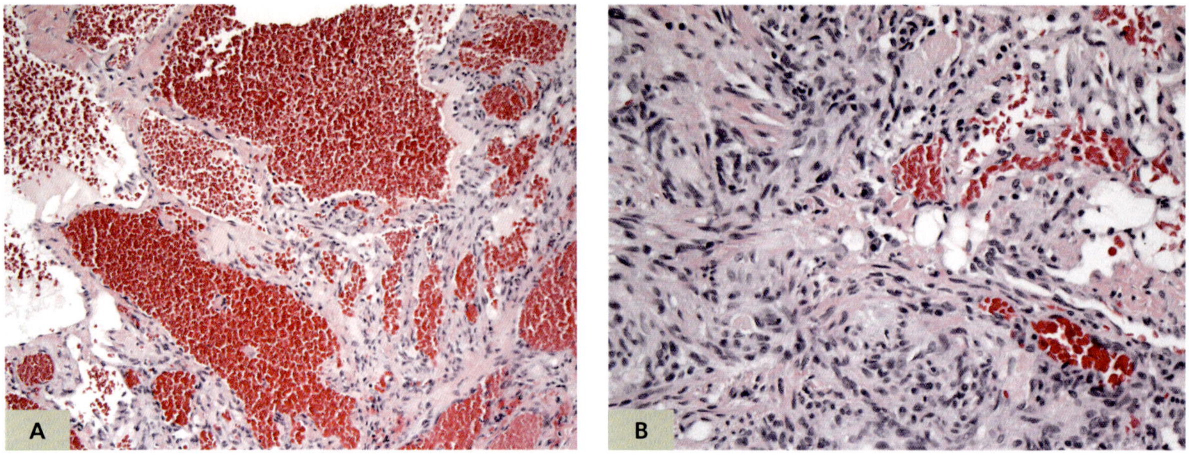

FIGURE 6.16 Spindle cell hemangioma is comprised of a uniform population of spindle cells adjacent to cavernous-type spaces and slit-like vessels (A). Solid-appearing foci with clusters of vacuolated epithelioid endothelial cells with clear cytoplasm are present (B).

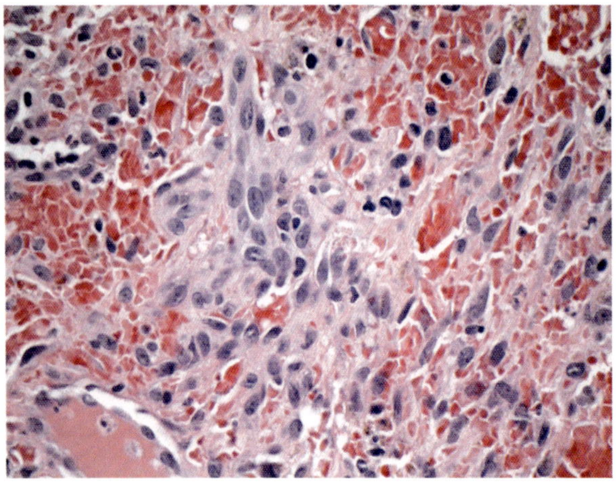

FIGURE 6.17 Kaposi sarcoma has fascicular spindle cells and at least rare foci of intracytoplasmic and extracellular pink hyaline globules.

EPITHELIOID HEMANGIOMA OF SOFT TISSUE AND BONE

Epithelioid hemangioma typically presents in the head and neck region of adults; periauricular sites are most common. Epithelioid hemangioma has also been known as angiolymphoid hyperplasia with eosinophilia, and historically was considered synonymous with Kimura disease (though now they are recognized as separate clinicopathologic entities). Lesions are well-circumscribed with a lobular arrangement of proliferating capillaries, most frequently situated in the dermis. The small-to-medium-sized vessels are lined by plump epithelioid endothelial cells with abundant pale pink cytoplasm and occasional intracytoplasmic vacuoles (**Figure 6.18**). The endothelial cells lack significant cytologic atypia and mitoses are rare. The endothelial cells can hobnail or protrude into the vascular lumina, and areas of seemingly solid growth can be seen (often secondary to the plump epithelioid cells obscuring the vascular lumen). An inflammatory infiltrate of lymphocytes, eosinophils, mast cells, and plasma cells is often present at the periphery of and within the lesion. Immunohistochemistry for endothelial and pericytic markers can be helpful in highlighting the predominance of well-formed vessels in the tumor.

Epithelioid hemangioendothelioma (EHE) and epithelioid angiosarcoma are important exclusions. EHE is not vasoformative; tumor cells are arranged in a cordlike growth pattern embedded in a myxohyaline stroma (**Figure 6.19**).

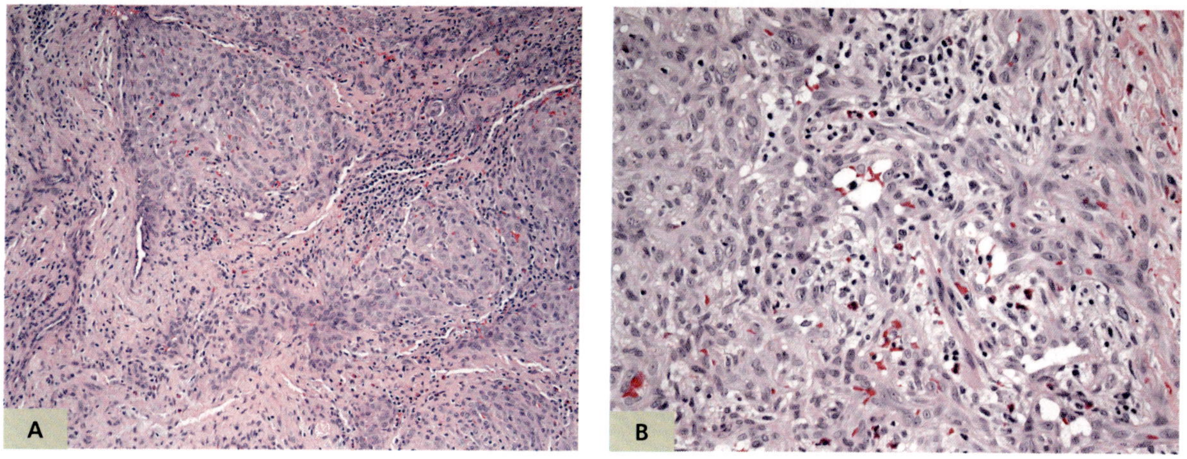

FIGURE 6.18 Epithelioid hemangioma. Lesions are well-circumscribed with a lobular arrangement of proliferating capillaries (A). Vessels are lined by plump epithelioid endothelial cells with abundant pale pink cytoplasm and occasional intracytoplasmic vacuoles; eosinophils are common (B).

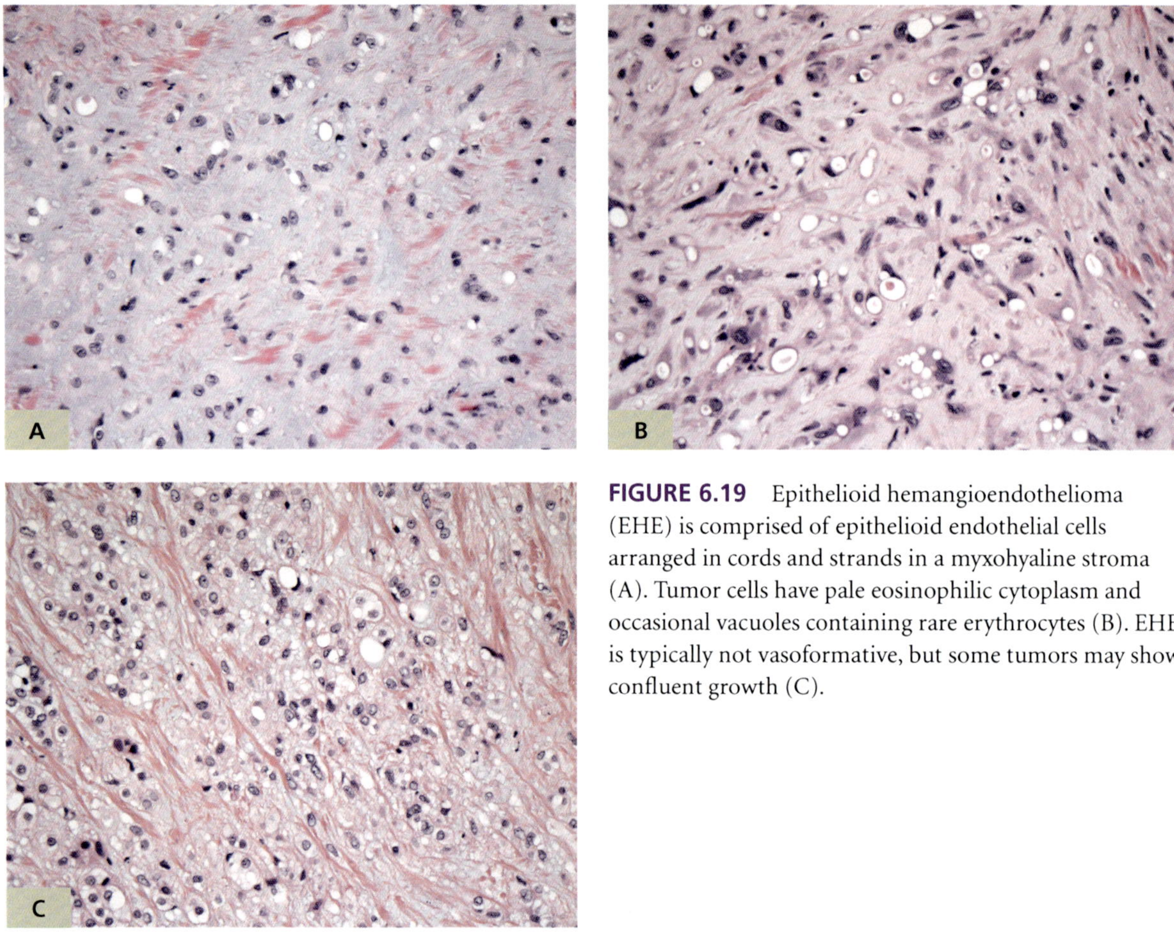

FIGURE 6.19 Epithelioid hemangioendothelioma (EHE) is comprised of epithelioid endothelial cells arranged in cords and strands in a myxohyaline stroma (A). Tumor cells have pale eosinophilic cytoplasm and occasional vacuoles containing rare erythrocytes (B). EHE is typically not vasoformative, but some tumors may show confluent growth (C).

Furthermore, EHE is characterized by a t(1;3)(p36;q23-25) translocation resulting in *CAMTA1-WWTR1* fusion (278); a subset of EHE showing more vasoformative morphology have *YAP1-TFE3* fusion; this group of tumors is positive for TFE3 by immunohistochemistry(279). Epithelioid angiosarcoma is rarely vasoformative with more frequent solid and infiltrative growth, and has cytologic features of malignancy (atypia, mitotic activity, and atypical mitoses) (**Figure 6.20**).

Epithelioid hemangiomas in deep soft tissue and bone are often characterized by more solid growth and increased cytologic atypia (which is still mild) (**Figure 6.21**). A subtype of epithelioid hemangiomas is now known to harbor a *ZPF36-FOSB* fusion, most frequently in penile locations (280).

Epithelioid hemangioma of bone may be worrisome for angiosarcoma, especially because lesions are locally aggressive; complete resection (sometimes followed by radiation therapy) is required for clinical management. Tumors fill the marrow space and are comprised of a multilobular arrangement of small vessel proliferation and more cellular central foci with vasoformative and solid architecture (**Figure 6.22**). The lining endothelial cells are epithelioid and eosinophilic, with occasional vacuolization. Significant cytology atypia is absent, which distinguishes epithelioid hemangioma from angiosarcoma.

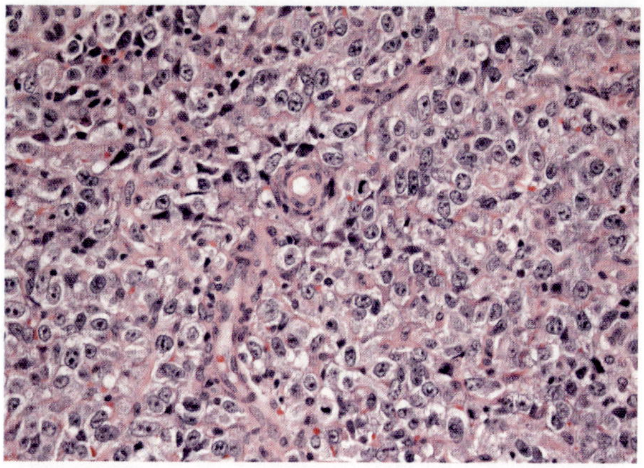

FIGURE 6.20 Epithelioid angiosarcoma is characterized by solid growth of cytologically malignant epithelioid cells and frequent mitotic activity.

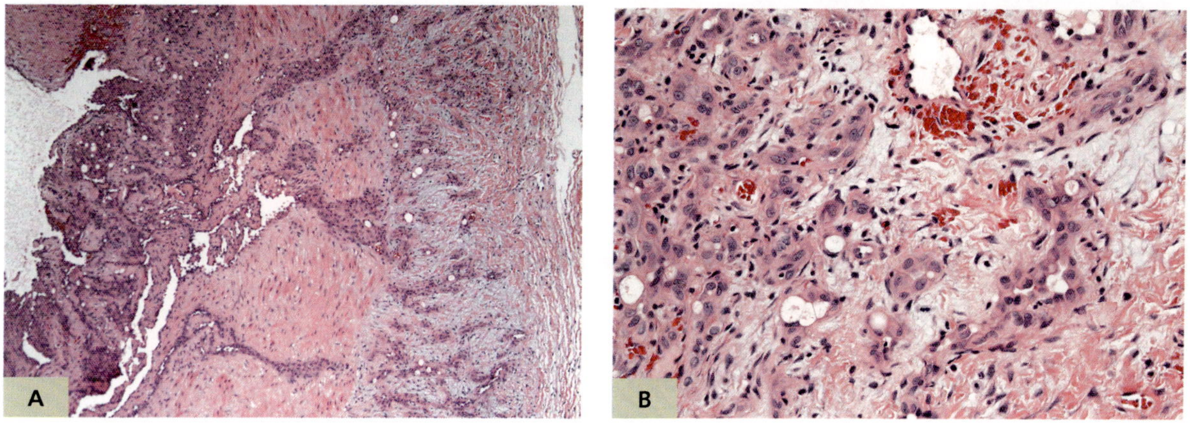

FIGURE 6.21 Epithelioid hemangioma in deep soft tissue arising from a vessel wall with vasoformative foci (A). Tumors typically show more solid growth and increased cytologic atypia compared to superficial examples (B).

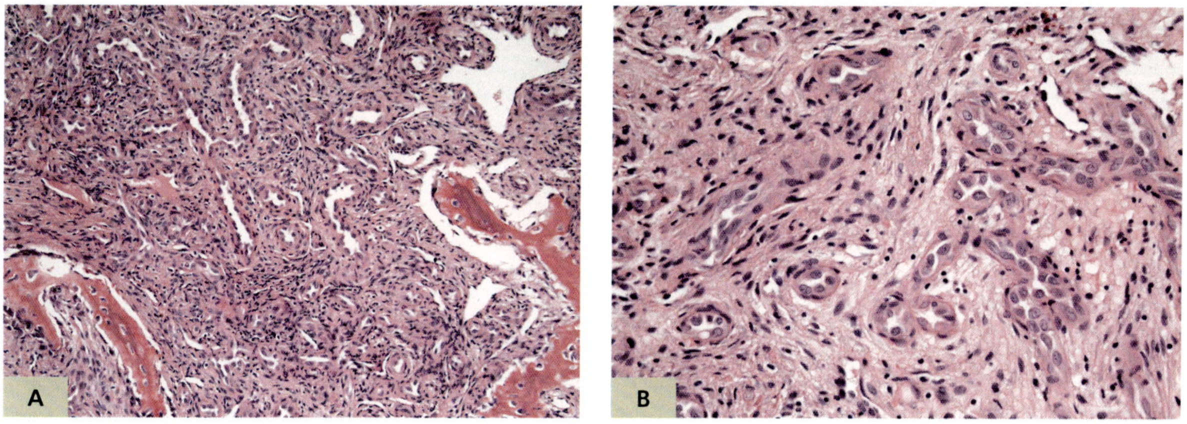

FIGURE 6.22 Epithelioid hemangioma of bone appears as a multilobular small vessel proliferation that fills the marrow space (A). The lining endothelial cells are epithelioid and eosinophilic, with occasional cytoplasmic vacuolization (B).

SPLENIC HEMANGIOMA AND LITTORAL CELL ANGIOMA

Benign vascular lesions of the spleen are typically well-circumscribed and should be distinguished from primary angiosarcoma of the spleen. Hemangioma and littoral cell angioma are often incidental findings, though patients can occasionally present with splenomegaly or rupture. Both splenic hemangioma (**Figure 6.23**) and littoral cell angioma are well-circumscribed lesions within the spleen; angiosarcomas show more infiltrative growth into adjacent splenic parenchyma and more complex vasoformative architecture (**Figure 6.24**).

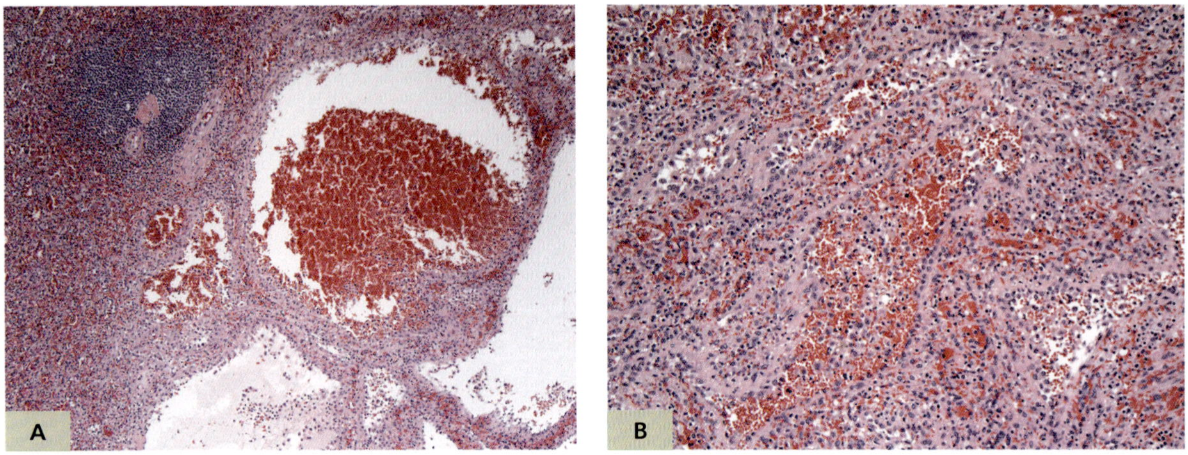

FIGURE 6.23 Splenic hemangiomas are well-circumscribed lesions (A) and the lining endothelial cells lack cytologic atypia and multilayering (B).

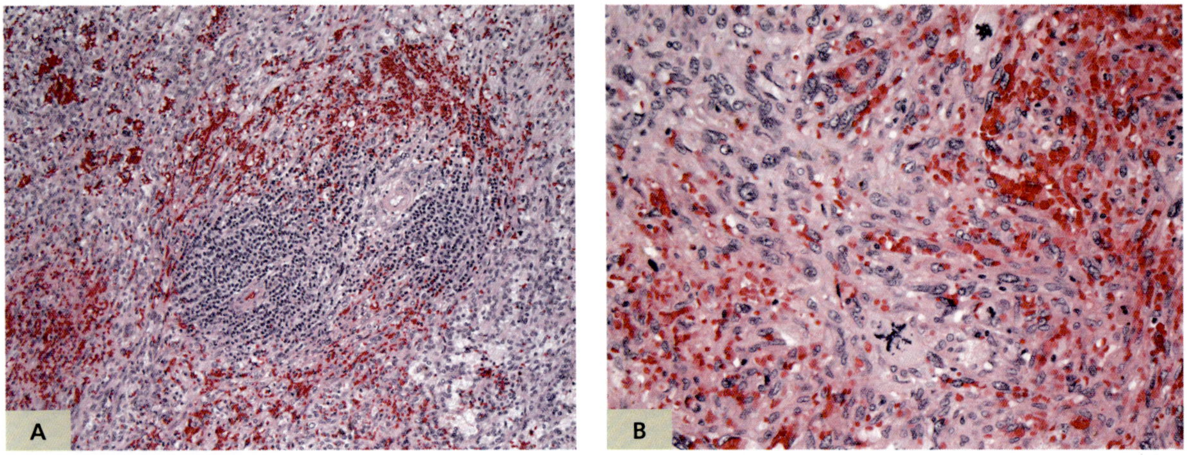

FIGURE 6.24 Splenic angiosarcoma shows infiltrative growth into adjacent splenic parenchyma and a more complex vasoformative architecture (A), and exhibits cytologic atypia and frequent mitotic activity (including atypical forms) (B).

Hemangiomas lack endothelial cytologic atypia and multilayering, and the use of endothelial and pericytic immunohistochemical markers will highlight the microvascular architectural pattern.

Littoral cell angioma is a benign splenic lesion in which the anastomosing vessels are lined by plump palely eosinophilic, often vacuolated, cells showing littoral cell differentiation (**Figure 6.25A**). The endothelial cells have ovoid indented nuclei, with intracytoplasmic hyaline globules. Exfoliation of these endothelial cells into the vascular lumina is common. Littoral cell angioma has a specialized immunophenotype including positivity for CD31, CD163, and CD21 (**Figure 6.25B, C**). Interestingly, CD34 and CD8 are negative (which are both positive in the sinus-lining cells in the spleen).

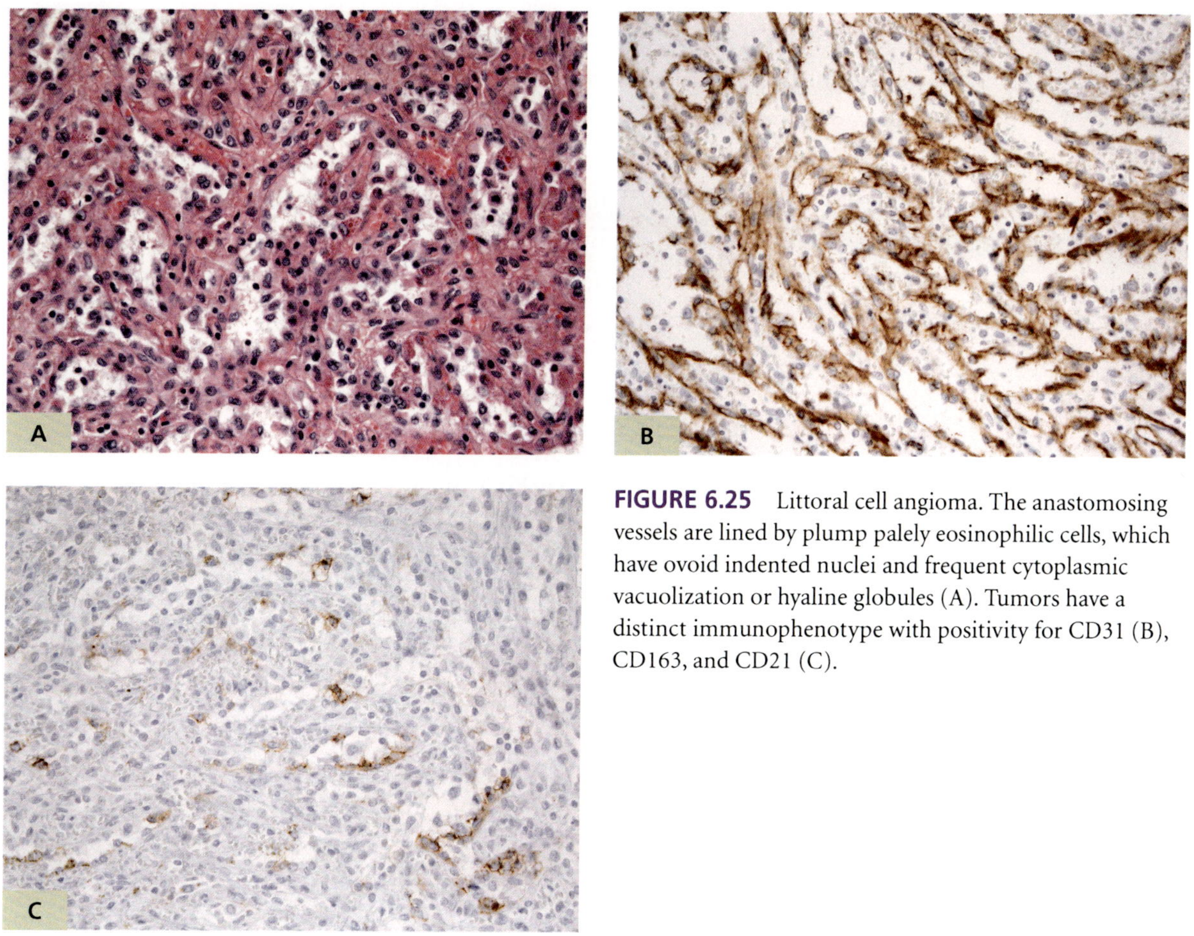

FIGURE 6.25 Littoral cell angioma. The anastomosing vessels are lined by plump palely eosinophilic cells, which have ovoid indented nuclei and frequent cytoplasmic vacuolization or hyaline globules (A). Tumors have a distinct immunophenotype with positivity for CD31 (B), CD163, and CD21 (C).

ATYPICAL POSTRADIATION VASCULAR PROLIFERATION

Patients who have undergone radiation therapy, most commonly for breast carcinoma, may develop cutaneous APRVP in the field of radiation that can clinically or histologically mimic low-grade angiosarcoma (281). Although the time lapse between radiation and development of disease is usually shorter for APRVP (less than five years) in comparison to angiosarcoma (mean, five–seven years), the clinical presentation is not always discriminatory as both may present as multiple macules and papules that vary in color from red to skin-colored, although postradiation angiosarcoma often presents as large ecchymotic or nodular lesions. Despite some studies that suggest that a subset of APRVP may be a precursor to radiation-associated angiosarcoma (281,282), many authors believe that APRVP is a benign process (283). Nonetheless, some lesions may exhibit an architectural growth pattern that mimics low-grade angiosarcoma. APRVP is usually well-circumscribed, with vascular spaces lined by endothelial cells ranging from flattened to hobnail, with mild atypia (**Figure 6.26**). However, frank pleomorphism and multilayering are absent, as are mitotic figures; if any of these features are present, angiosarcoma should be considered, as well as dissecting growth extending beyond the dermis (**Figure 6.27A, B**). Recently, it has been shown that radiation-associated angiosarcoma (and a subset of primary angiosarcomas) are characterized by amplification of 8q24, the *MYC* locus (284,285); immunohistochemistry showing MYC overexpression can distinguish APRVP from a low-grade angiosarcoma (**Figure 6.27C**).

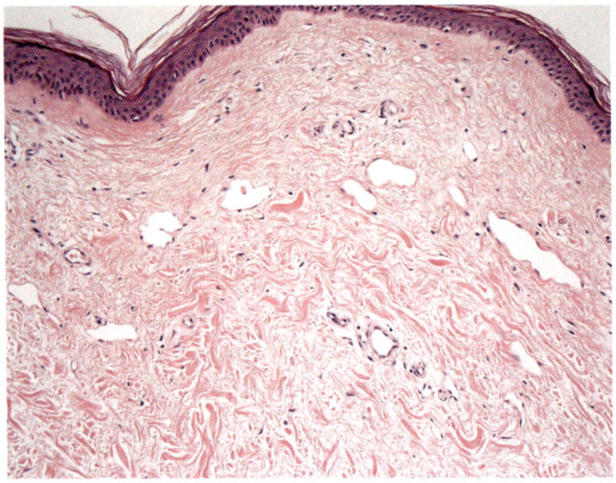

FIGURE 6.26 Atypical postradiation vascular proliferation is comprised of vascular spaces lined by endothelial cells ranging from flattened to hobnail that exhibit mild atypia, but frank pleomorphism, mitotic activity, and endothelial multilayering are absent.

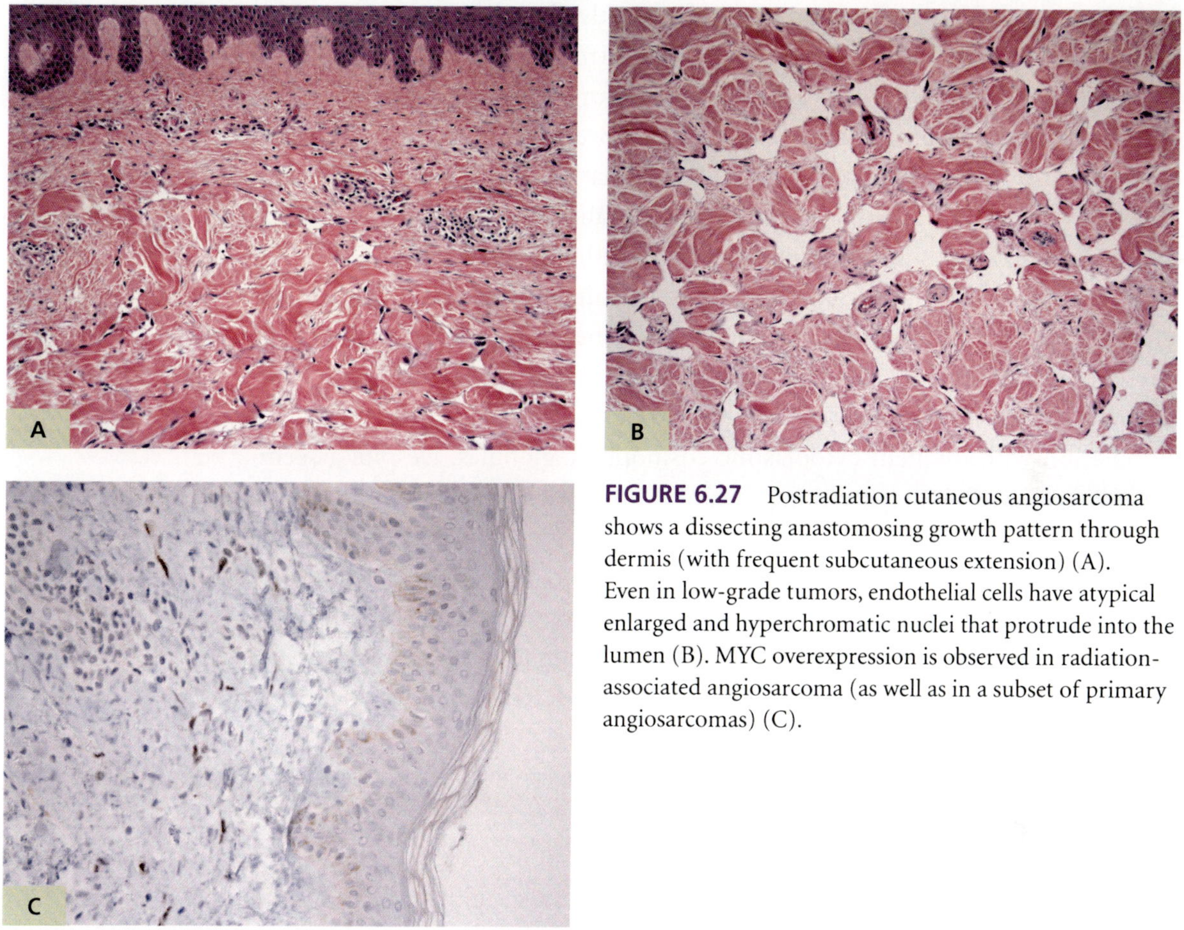

FIGURE 6.27 Postradiation cutaneous angiosarcoma shows a dissecting anastomosing growth pattern through dermis (with frequent subcutaneous extension) (A). Even in low-grade tumors, endothelial cells have atypical enlarged and hyperchromatic nuclei that protrude into the lumen (B). MYC overexpression is observed in radiation-associated angiosarcoma (as well as in a subset of primary angiosarcomas) (C).

KAPOSI SARCOMA

KS at all three stages (patch, plaque, and nodular) may show morphologic features worrisome for angiosarcoma. Despite frequently presenting as multifocal lesions and having some tendency for local recurrence (especially in the setting of AIDS), KS typically follows an indolent course, and is thus discussed here as a mimic of angiosarcoma. AIDS-associated KS is the most aggressive form, with frequent visceral involvement and poor response to treatment; however, the clinical context of HIV infection is informative. For the classic indolent, endemic African, and iatrogenic types of KS, despite being defined by three distinct clinical patient groups (respectively elderly Mediterranean, Eastern European, or Ashkenazi men; children and young adults of equatorial Africa without HIV infection; and solid-organ transplant patients undergoing immunosuppression), affected patients frequently show response to systemic chemotherapy and radiation. Patients with iatrogenic-type KS often show regression of lesions with decreased dosage of immunotherapy.

Both patch and plaque-stage KS can show overlapping features with low-grade angiosarcoma. Though confined to the dermis, the proliferating vessels can show dissecting growth through collagen, and the proliferating vascular spaces are lined by a single layer of atypical endothelial cells (**Figure 6.28**). The proliferating vessels may dissect around pre-existing normal vessels and adnexa creating the "promontory sign," which can also be seen in angiosarcoma. The presence of a lymphoplasmacytic infiltrate and hemosiderin deposition is characteristic of KS. In the plaque stage, KS shows a more prominent spindle cell population with frequent cytoplasmic eosinophilic globules. Despite a seemingly dissecting growth pattern, significant endothelial atypia and multilayering are absent (and if present, should prompt the consideration of angiosarcoma). Furthermore, despite the growth pattern of dissection through dermal collagen, the proliferating vessels in patch and plaque-stage KS are typically oriented parallel to the overlying epidermis, which is distinct from the irregular shapes and orientation of dissecting vascular channels of angiosarcoma.

The fascicular growth pattern and slit-like vasoformative spaces of nodular KS can be worrisome for high grade angiosarcoma, especially because mitotic activity can be high. In cutaneous sites, nodular Kaposi sarcoma tends to form an exophytic, well-circumscribed nodule, often with an overlying epidermal collarette. The spindle cells of nodular KS show at most mild cytologic atypia,

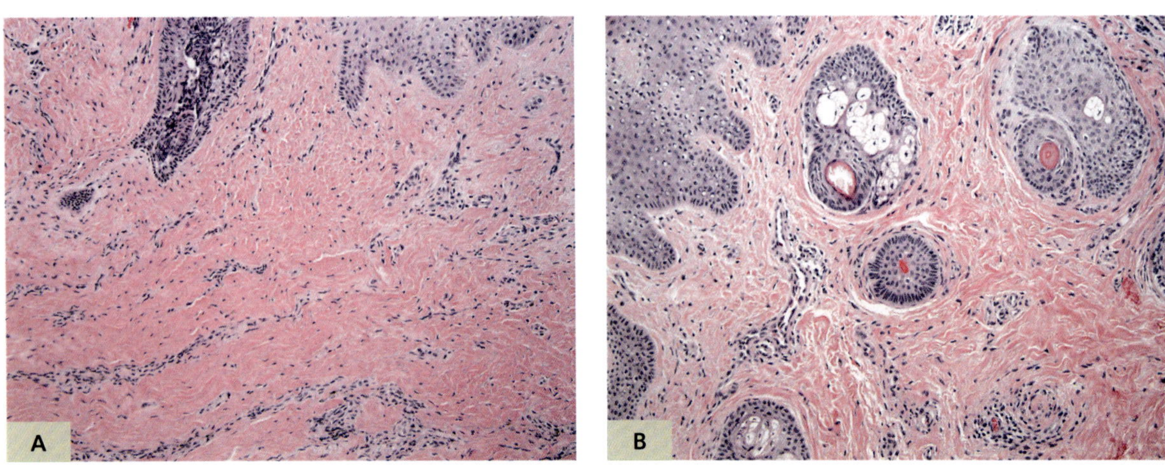

FIGURE 6.28 In patch-stage Kaposi sarcoma, the proliferating vessels can show dissecting growth through collagen (A). Vessels may dissect around pre-existing normal vessels and skin adnexa and are lined by a single layer of atypical endothelial cells (B).

and comprise a uniform population with at least focal eosinophilic hyaline globules present both in the cytoplasm and extracellularly (**Figure 6.29**). Lymphoplasmacytic aggregates can also be present in nodular KS. Nodular KS can be distinguished from angiosarcoma by its characteristic nodular appearance and circumscription and absence of significant cytologic atypia and atypical mitotic figures. HHV-8 immunohistochemistry can be employed to distinguish between these possibilities, as nuclear HHV-8 staining is expected in all clinical variants of KS but is absent in angiosarcoma.

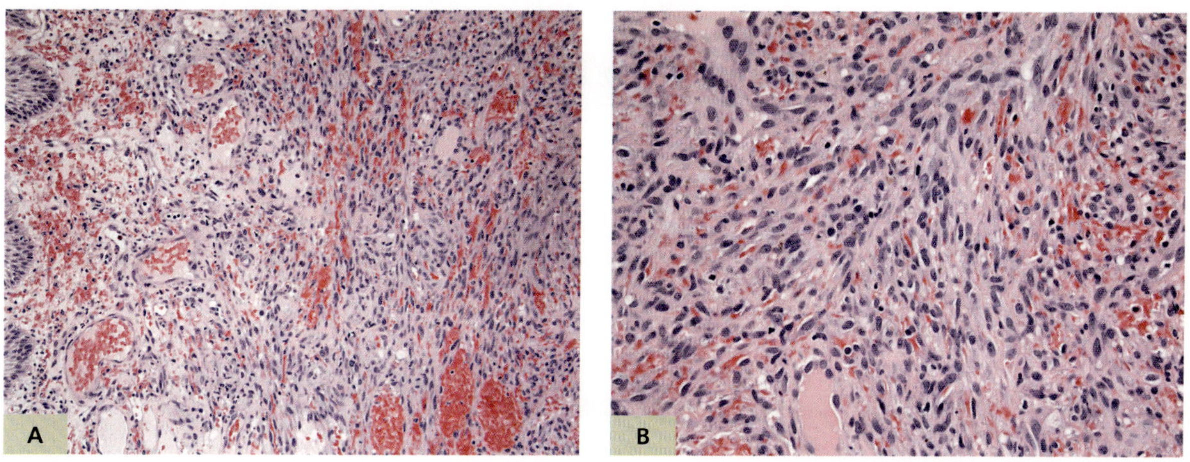

FIGURE 6.29 In nodular Kaposi sarcoma, a uniform population of mildly atypical spindle cells show fascicular and solid growth and numerous slit-like vasoformative spaces (A). Tumor cells may show focal eosinophilic hyaline globules both in the cytoplasm and extracellularly (B).

7

Mimics of Neuroectodermal Neoplasms

- TRAUMATIC NEUROMA
- SOLITARY CIRCUMSCRIBED NEUROMA
- DEGENERATIVE ATYPIA IN SCHWANNOMA (AND OTHER BENIGN NERVE SHEATH TUMORS)
- CELLULAR SCHWANNOMA
- EPITHELIOID SCHWANNOMA
- DIFFUSE NEUROFIBROMA
- PLEXIFORM NEUROFIBROMA
- HYBRID NERVE SHEATH TUMORS

Tumors of neuroectodermal differentiation include central and peripheral nerve sheath tumors and melanocytic neoplasms. Most neuroectodermal tumors in soft tissue differentiate toward Schwann cells; the two most common tumors are neurofibroma (**Figure 7.1**) and schwannoma (**Figure 7.2**). Immunohistochemistry can be useful in identifying differentiation in nerve sheath tumors: S-100 protein is positive in both neurofibroma and schwannoma, while epithelial membrane antigen (EMA) and claudin-1 are positive in perineurial cells (which are mesenchymal in origin). While schwannomas are diffusely S-100 positive, the extent of S-100 staining in neurofibroma is less, typically 30% to 70% of tumor cells. Neurofilament protein (NFP) highlights axons that are prevalent in neurofibroma, in comparison to schwannomas in which axons are absent or scarce (286).

Special considerations for benign peripheral nerve sheath tumors include clinical correlation and exclusion of transformation to malignant peripheral nerve sheath tumor (MPNST). In patients with type 1 neurofibromatosis, neurofibromas are more commonly multiple and more deeply seated than

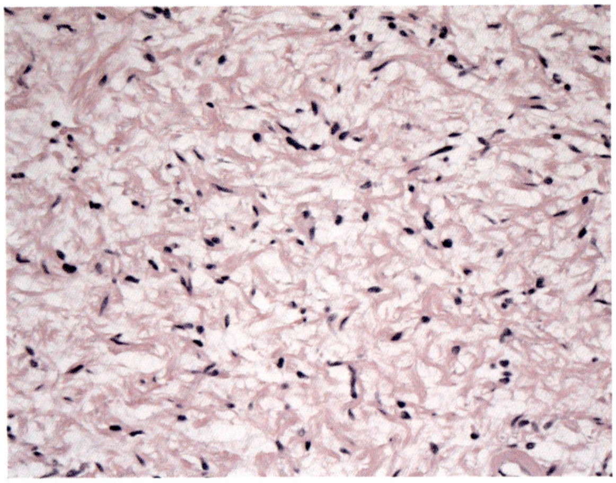

FIGURE 7.1 Neurofibroma. Tumor cells have ovoid and spindled, often comma-shaped nuclei, with abundant interspersed collagen fibers.

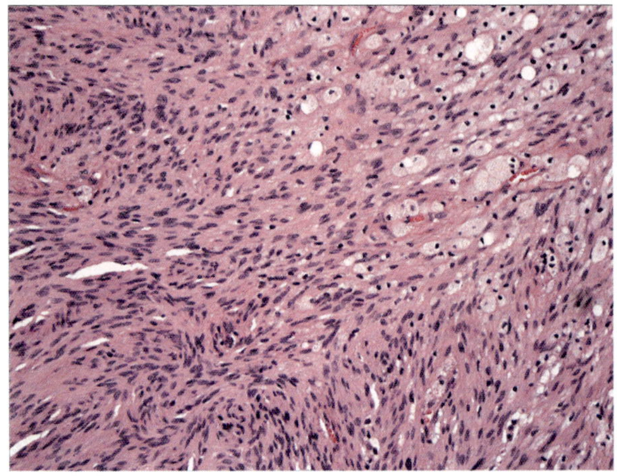

FIGURE 7.2 Schwannoma characteristically shows varying hypercellular and hypocellular patterns of spindle cells with ovoid nuclei and palely eosinophilic, fibrillary cytoplasm. Clusters of lipid-laden histiocytes are common.

sporadic neurofibromas. Plexiform neurofibromas occur almost exclusively in patients with type 1 neurofibromatosis (see section "*Plexiform Neurofibroma*"). Malignant transformation is exceedingly rare in schwannoma, while neurofibroma shows an overall small risk for transformation to MPNST. Most cases of malignant transformation in neurofibroma manifest as conventional MPNST; however, malignant neoplasms that arise in association with schwannoma include epithelioid schwannoma and epithelioid angiosarcoma. MPNST can be challenging to diagnose, given its typical limited expression of (or entire lack of staining for) the neuroectodermal markers S-100 and SOX10.

TRAUMATIC NEUROMA

Reactive lesions such as traumatic neuroma are rarely confused with malignant neoplasms, but may occasionally show morphologic overlap with benign nerve sheath tumors. Traumatic neuromas typically develop in response to injury, most commonly amputation or laceration on the extremities. Lesions show disorderly organization of normal nerve sheath components embedded in a collagenous stroma, with a variable admixture of nerve fibers, Schwann cells, and perineurial cells (**Figure 7.3**). In the absence of clinical history, traumatic

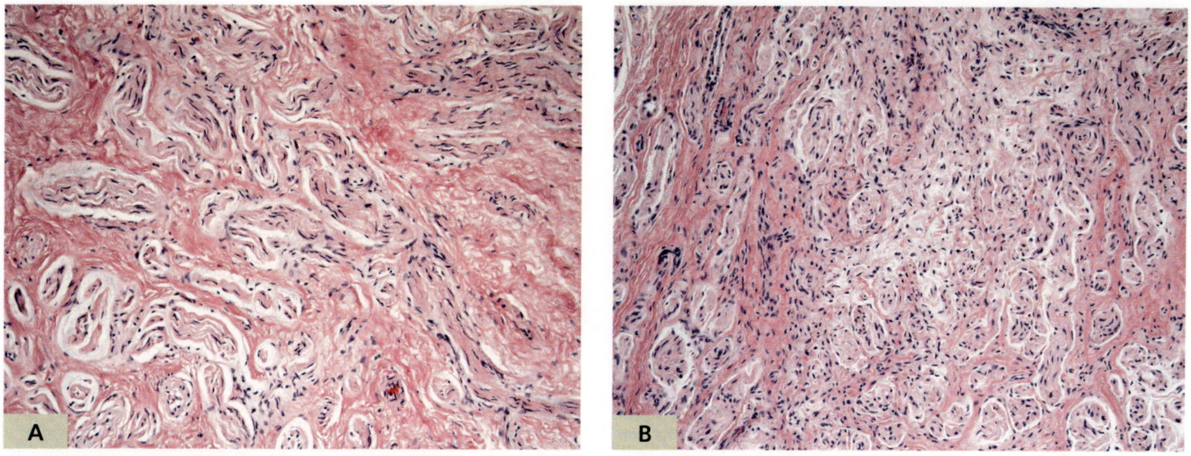

FIGURE 7.3 Traumatic neuroma is comprised of a disorderly organization of normal nerve sheath components embedded in a collagenous stroma, with a variable admixture of nerve fibers, Schwann cells, and perineurial cells (A). Stromal hyalinization and myxoid change are common (B).

neuromas may be mistaken for a benign nerve sheath neoplasm, such as a plexiform neurofibroma or schwannoma depending on the histologic appearances and most prominent components.

SOLITARY CIRCUMSCRIBED NEUROMA

Solitary circumscribed neuromas (also known as palisaded encapsulated neuromas) are small dermal lesions that are most common on the face, though they may rarely occur in mucosal sites. Lesions have a partial perineurial capsule, are often associated with a nerve, and contain a population of pale Schwann cells growing in fascicles within a collagenous stroma (**Figure 7.4**). The fascicular growth of Schwann cells raises the possibility of cellular schwannoma; however, within a solitary circumscribed neuroma there is a prominent axonal component that is NFP positive. Solitary circumscribed neuromas often show clefting between fascicles, and lack the hyalinized thick-walled vessels and alternating Antoni A and Antoni B areas that are characteristic of schwannoma.

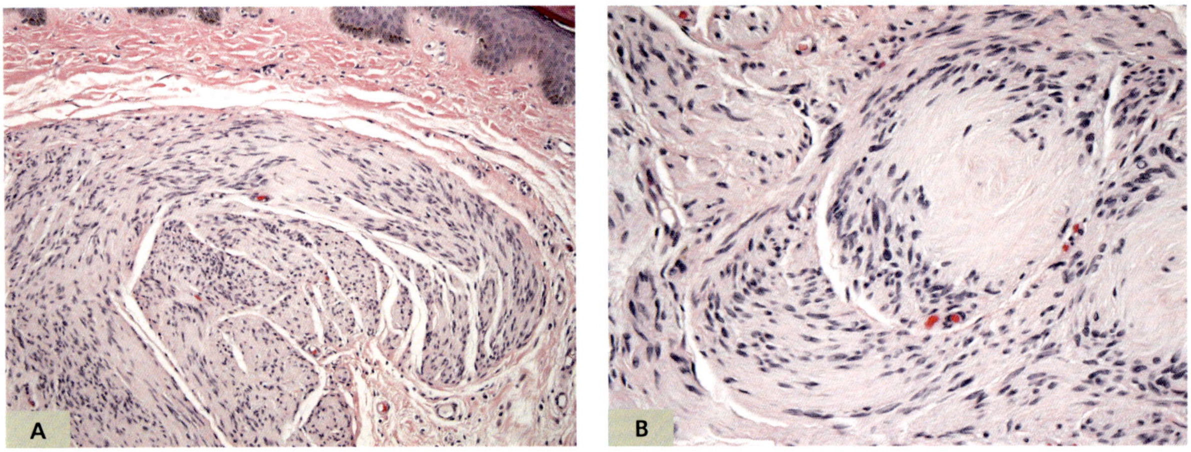

FIGURE 7.4 Solitary circumscribed neuromas are well-circumscribed (with a partial perineurial capsule) and contain a population of pale Schwann cells growing in fascicles within a collagenous stroma (A). Lesional Schwann cells have palely eosinophilic fibrillary cytoplasm, and clefting is common between fascicles (B).

DEGENERATIVE ATYPIA IN SCHWANNOMA (AND OTHER BENIGN NERVE SHEATH TUMORS)

Schwannoma can undergo degenerative changes resulting in scattered pleomorphic and atypical Schwann cells, cystic degeneration, necrosis, and calcification; such tumors are often referred to as "ancient schwannoma." Furthermore, schwannomas can show mitotic activity, which may be especially worrisome in combination with degenerative atypia; however, high mitotic counts and atypical forms are exceptional. The atypical degenerative cells are hyperchromatic, but lack prominent nucleoli; nuclear pseudoinclusions and "smudgy" chromatin are characteristic features (**Figure 7.5**). Degenerative nuclear atypia should be distinguished from "malignant epithelioid change" in schwannoma, in which there are large epithelioid cells with vesicular nuclei and prominent nucleoli (**Figure 7.6**). "Malignant epithelioid change" in a schwannoma typically follows a benign course when resected, but may be a precursor to malignant transformation of a schwannoma to epithelioid MPNST or epithelioid angiosarcoma (287).

Degenerative atypia can be seen in other benign peripheral nerve sheath tumors. In a neurofibroma with degenerative nuclear atypia, its typical immunohistochemical pattern of less extensive S-100 staining may raise the possibility of MPNST. In such cases, careful attention should be paid for features of malignant change in neurofibroma: increased cellularity, diffuse atypia, and mitotic activity (**Figure 7.7**). Soft tissue perineurioma can also show degenerative atypia

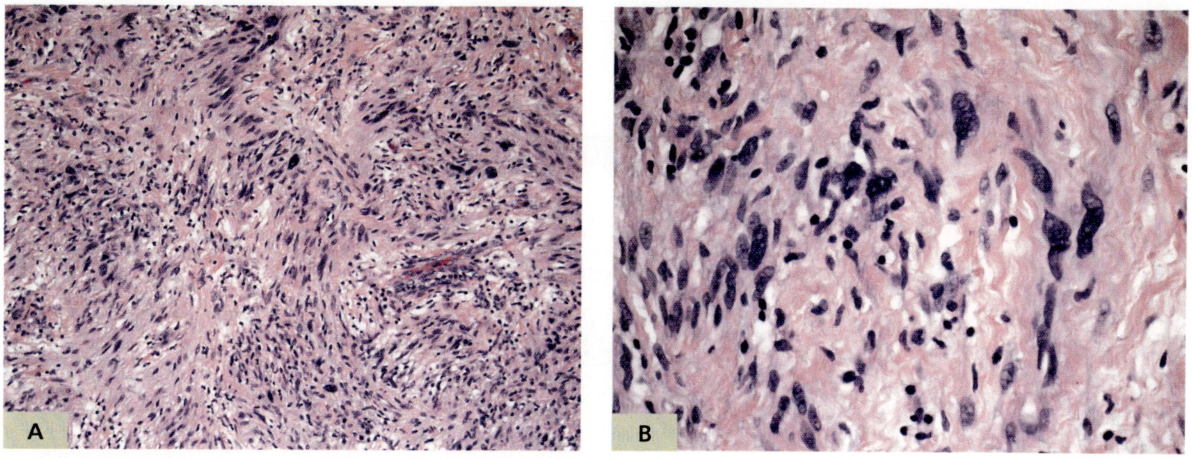

FIGURE 7.5 Degenerative changes in a schwannoma ("ancient Schwannoma") results in scattered pleomorphic and atypical Schwann cells (A). The atypical degenerative cells are hyperchromatic with "smudgy" chromatin and frequent nuclear pseudoinclusions (B).

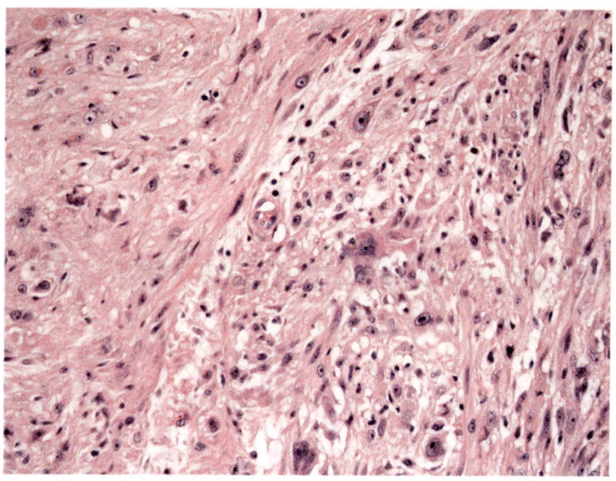

FIGURE 7.6 "Malignant epithelioid change" in a schwannoma. Large epithelioid cells with vesicular nuclei and prominent nucleoli are scattered throughout the tumor.

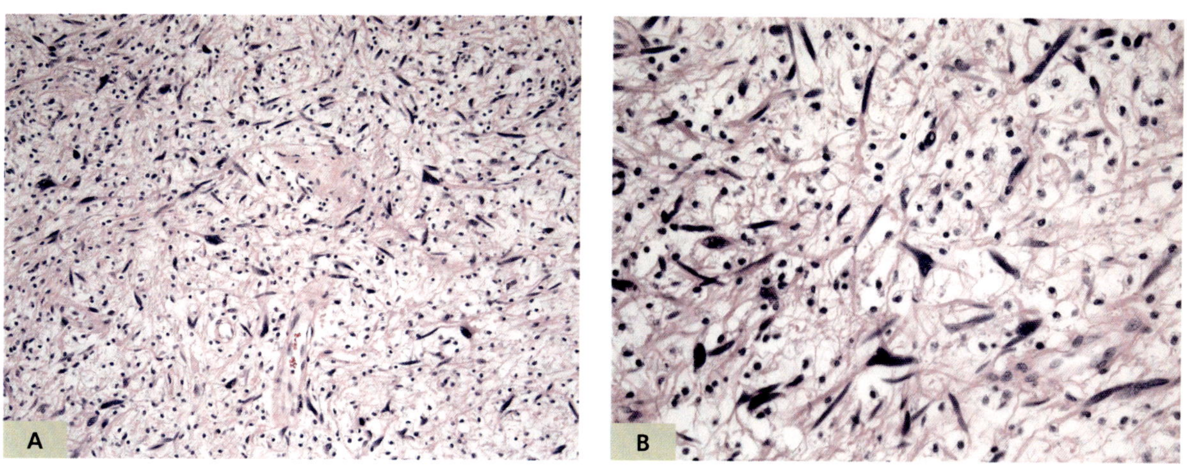

FIGURE 7.7 Malignant transformation in neurofibroma shows increased cellularity, diffuse atypia, and mitotic activity (A). Cytologic atypia is diffuse, and nuclei are hyperchromatic, enlarged, and atypical (B).

(249), but can be distinguished from MPNST by its typical storiform growth pattern and positivity for EMA and claudin-1.

CELLULAR SCHWANNOMA

Cellular schwannoma, which was discussed in Chapter 5 as a mimic of leiomyosarcoma, most commonly occurs in retroperitoneal or mediastinal locations. Tumors can be large and are typically encapsulated and associated with a nerve, although lesions in upper aerodigestive and gastrointestinal sites are frequently unencapsulated but well-circumscribed. A plexiform growth pattern can be observed in infants. Cellular schwannomas are hypercellular with a fascicular growth pattern of Schwann cells; Antoni B areas are scarce if present (**Figure 7.8**). Increased mitotic activity (but no atypical mitotic figures) is common. The increased mitotic rate and occasional degenerative atypia of cellular schwannoma may raise the possibility of MPNST. Features that favor cellular schwannoma over MPNST are circumscription or encapsulation, a lymphocytic infiltrate at the periphery, clusters of foamy histiocytes, thick-walled hyalinized blood vessels, and strong diffuse S-100 staining. MPNST characteristically shows varying hypercellular and hypocellular areas, with perivascular accentuation of cellularity (**Figure 7.9**). MPNST almost never shows uniform S-100 expression (only focal staining is observed in less than 50% of cases).

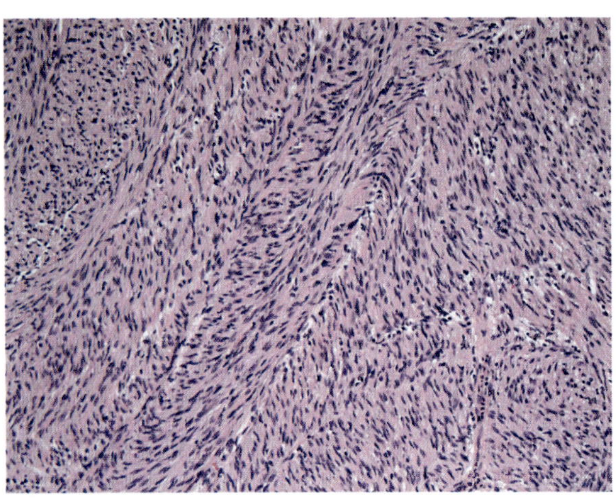

FIGURE 7.8 Cellular schwannomas are hypercellular with a fascicular growth pattern of Schwann cells, with absent or only rare Antoni B areas.

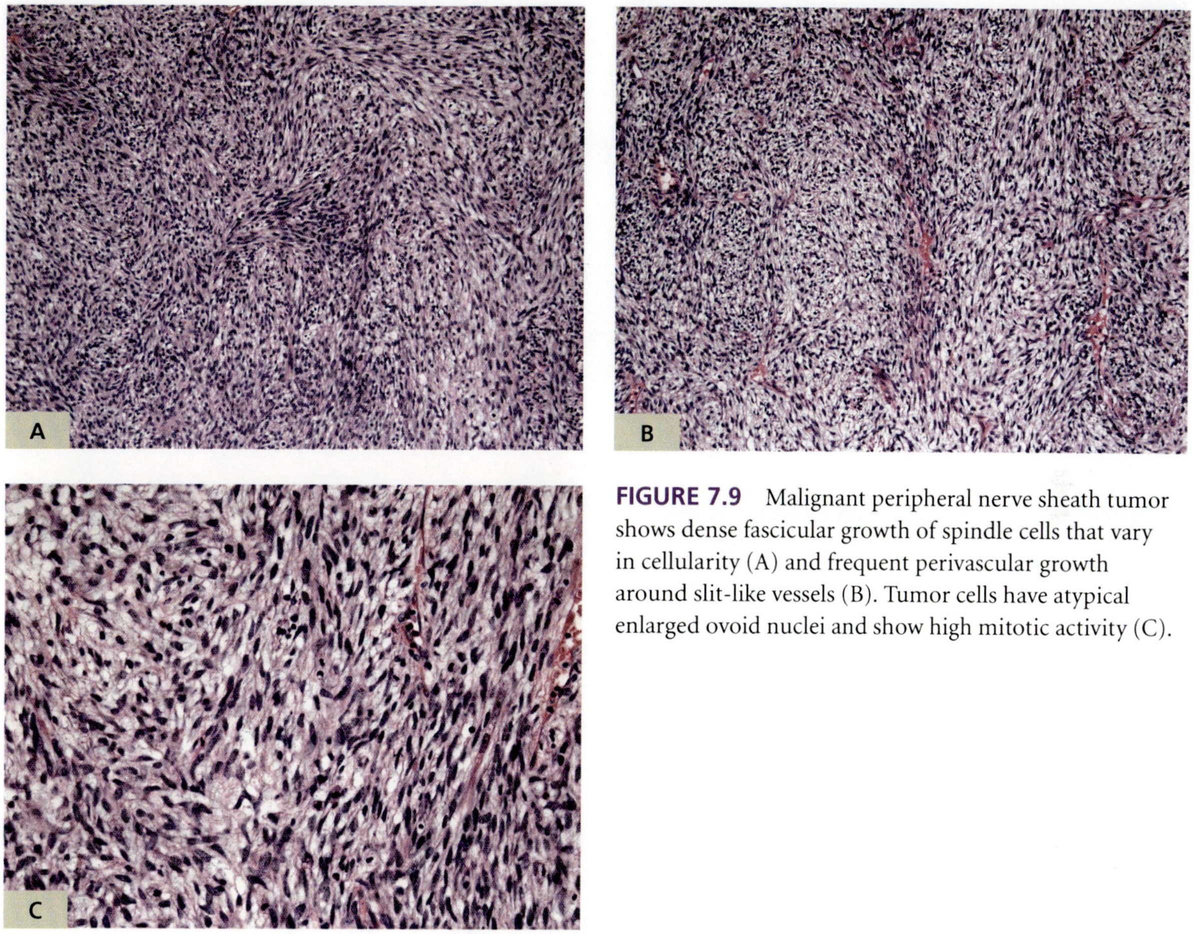

FIGURE 7.9 Malignant peripheral nerve sheath tumor shows dense fascicular growth of spindle cells that vary in cellularity (A) and frequent perivascular growth around slit-like vessels (B). Tumor cells have atypical enlarged ovoid nuclei and show high mitotic activity (C).

EPITHELIOID SCHWANNOMA

The epithelioid variant of schwannoma is rare, and has a distinctive histopathologic appearance of epithelioid tumor cells with variable amounts of amphophilic-to-eosinophilic cytoplasm, arranged in a multilobular growth pattern and a frequently fibrous or myxoid stroma (**Figure 7.10A, B**). Tumors are well-circumscribed and often have a perineurial capsule (**Figure 7.10C**), and mostly occur as dermal or subcutaneous lesions in the limbs (288–291). Areas of conventional schwannoma may be focally present. Epithelioid schwannoma may be particularly difficult to distinguish from low-grade epithelioid MPNST. Immunohistochemistry cannot reliably distinguish the two: both epithelioid

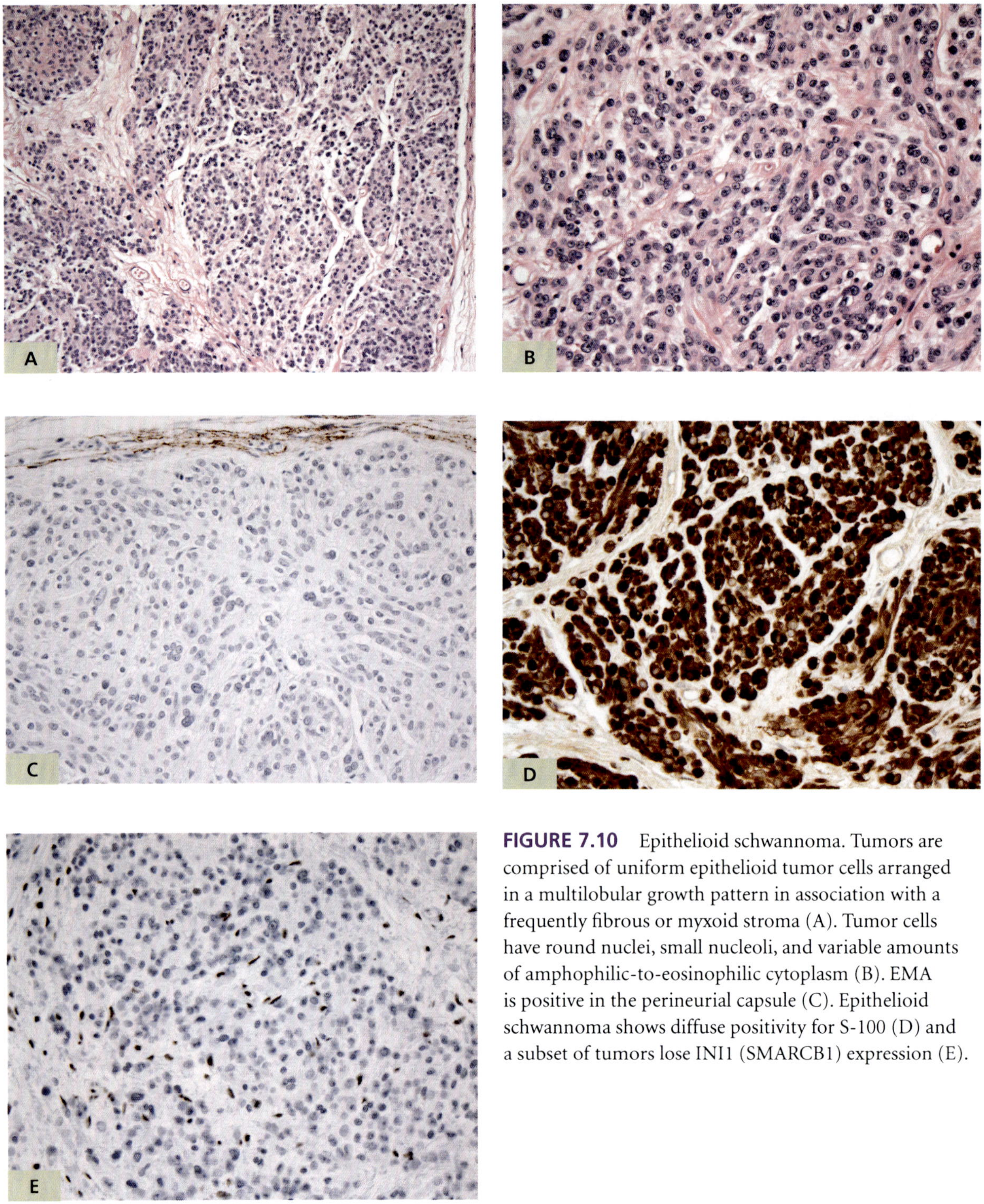

FIGURE 7.10 Epithelioid schwannoma. Tumors are comprised of uniform epithelioid tumor cells arranged in a multilobular growth pattern in association with a frequently fibrous or myxoid stroma (A). Tumor cells have round nuclei, small nucleoli, and variable amounts of amphophilic-to-eosinophilic cytoplasm (B). EMA is positive in the perineurial capsule (C). Epithelioid schwannoma shows diffuse positivity for S-100 (D) and a subset of tumors lose INI1 (SMARCB1) expression (E).

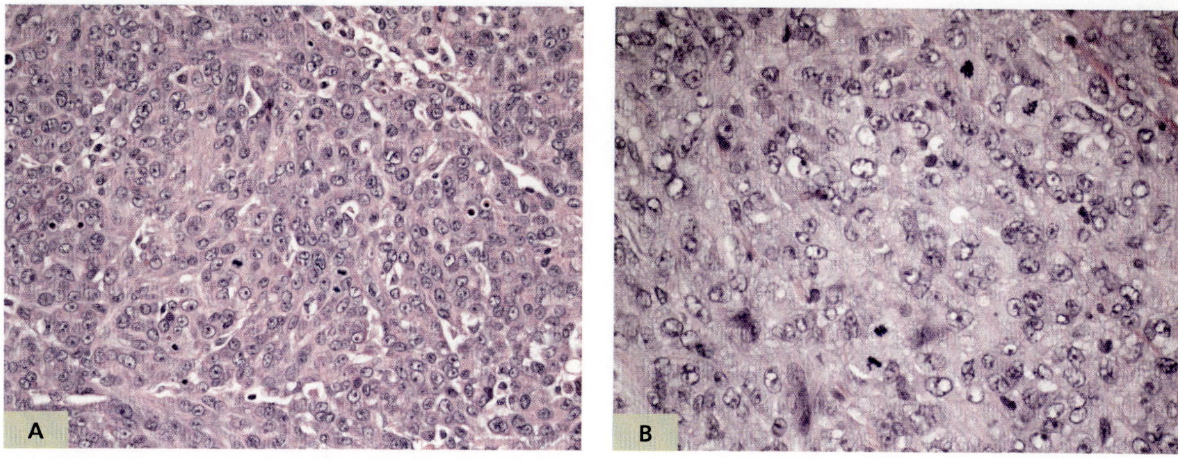

FIGURE 7.11 Epithelioid MPNST is characterized by diffuse atypia, pleomorphism, and frequent mitotic activity (A), and tumor cells have enlarged vesicular nuclei with prominent nucleoli and irregular nuclear membranes (B).

schwannoma and epithelioid MPNST are diffusely positive for S-100, and a subset of both tumor types lose INI1 (SMARCB1) expression (secondary to deletions on chromosome 22q) (**Figure 7.10D, E**). The distinction is based on morphologic features. Epithelioid schwannoma may show degenerative nuclear atypia, but the presence of diffuse atypia, pleomorphism, vesicular nuclei, prominent nucleoli, or atypical mitotic figures should prompt the diagnosis of epithelioid MPNST (**Figure 7.11**). Distinction between epithelioid variants of schwannoma and MPNST is important given the propensity of the latter for recurrence and metastasis (292).

DIFFUSE NEUROFIBROMA

Owing to its infiltrative growth pattern, diffuse neurofibroma may be worrisome for MPNST. Diffuse neurofibroma has a nearly negligible risk of malignant transformation, even for tumors occurring in patients with type 1 neurofibromatosis. Lesions are most common on the trunk, grossly appear plaque-like, and histologically show diffuse growth through the dermis and subcutis. Meissnerian corpuscles are a key feature of diffuse neurofibroma (**Figure 7.12**), and hypertrophic and edematous nerves are commonly dispersed through the tumor. Cytologic atypia, mitoses, and necrosis are absent. Careful microscopic examination will identify most cases of diffuse neurofibroma.

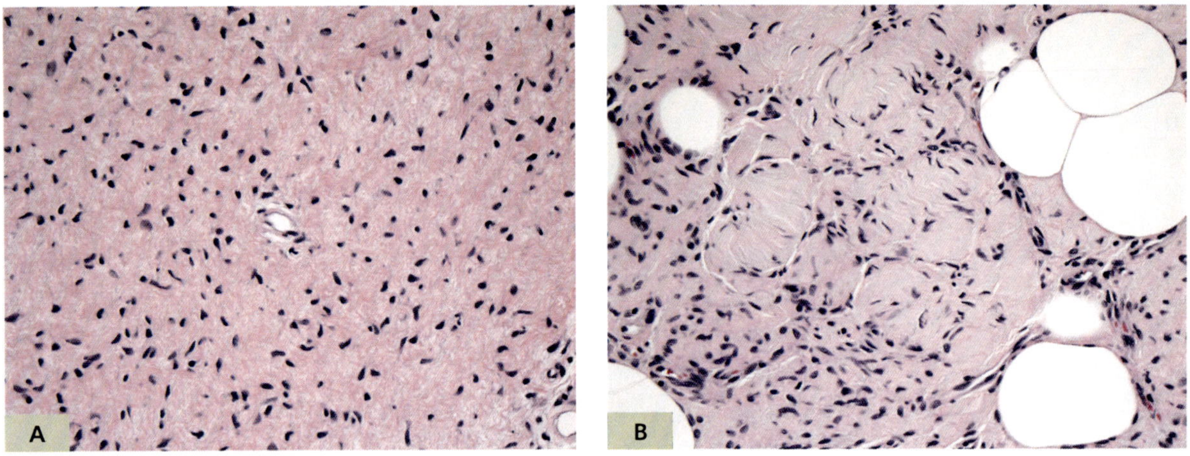

FIGURE 7.12 Diffuse-type neurofibroma is comprised of an infiltrative growth of conventional neurofibroma (A) and foci of Meissnerian corpuscles (B).

PLEXIFORM NEUROFIBROMA

Plexiform neurofibroma is essentially pathognomonic for type 1 neurofibromatosis. These lesions most commonly occur on the head and neck and clinically may be associated with thickened folded skin with variable hyperpigmentation. Some plexiform neurofibromas are present as a component of a hybrid tumor with diffuse neurofibroma. Plexiform neurofibroma is comprised of a neurofibromatous tumor component involving large bundles of expanded and edematous nerves (**Figure 7.13**). Myxoid change is frequent. Because plexiform neurofibroma has a risk for malignant transformation, careful histologic examination is required to exclude transformation to low-grade MPNST. Features of malignant transformation in the context of plexiform neurofibroma are any level of mitotic activity, increased cellularity, and cytologic atypia.

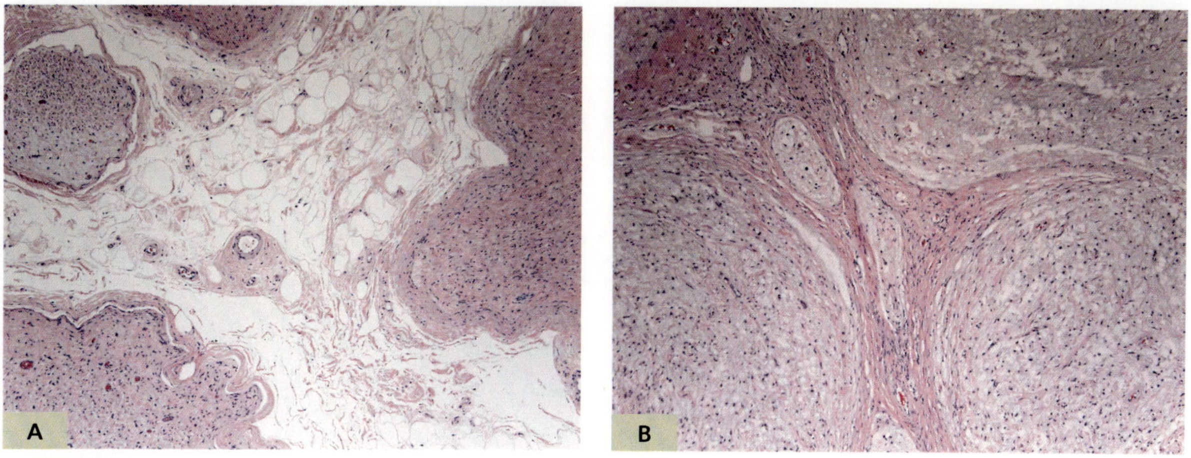

FIGURE 7.13 Plexiform neurofibroma is essentially pathognomonic for type 1 neurofibromatosis, and shows involvement of large bundles of nerves (A) that are expanded with edematous changes and prominent perineurium (B).

HYBRID NERVE SHEATH TUMORS

Hybrid nerve sheath tumors have been increasingly recognized, and occur at dermal or subcutaneous sites over a wide anatomic distribution. They show a benign clinical course similar to their component counterparts. Both hybrid schwannoma/perineurioma and schwannoma/neurofibroma can be challenging to recognize, and in some cases may be confused with MPNST. Hybrid schwannoma/perineurioma is most common, and typically occurs on the distal extremities in adults (293). Tumors are well-circumscribed and characterized by a storiform or fascicular architecture with alternating Schwann cells and perineurial cells (**Figure 7.14A**). Hybrid neurofibroma/schwannomas are more common in the setting of type 1 neurofibromatosis, and show a biphasic appearance in which schwannomatous nodules are interspersed within a

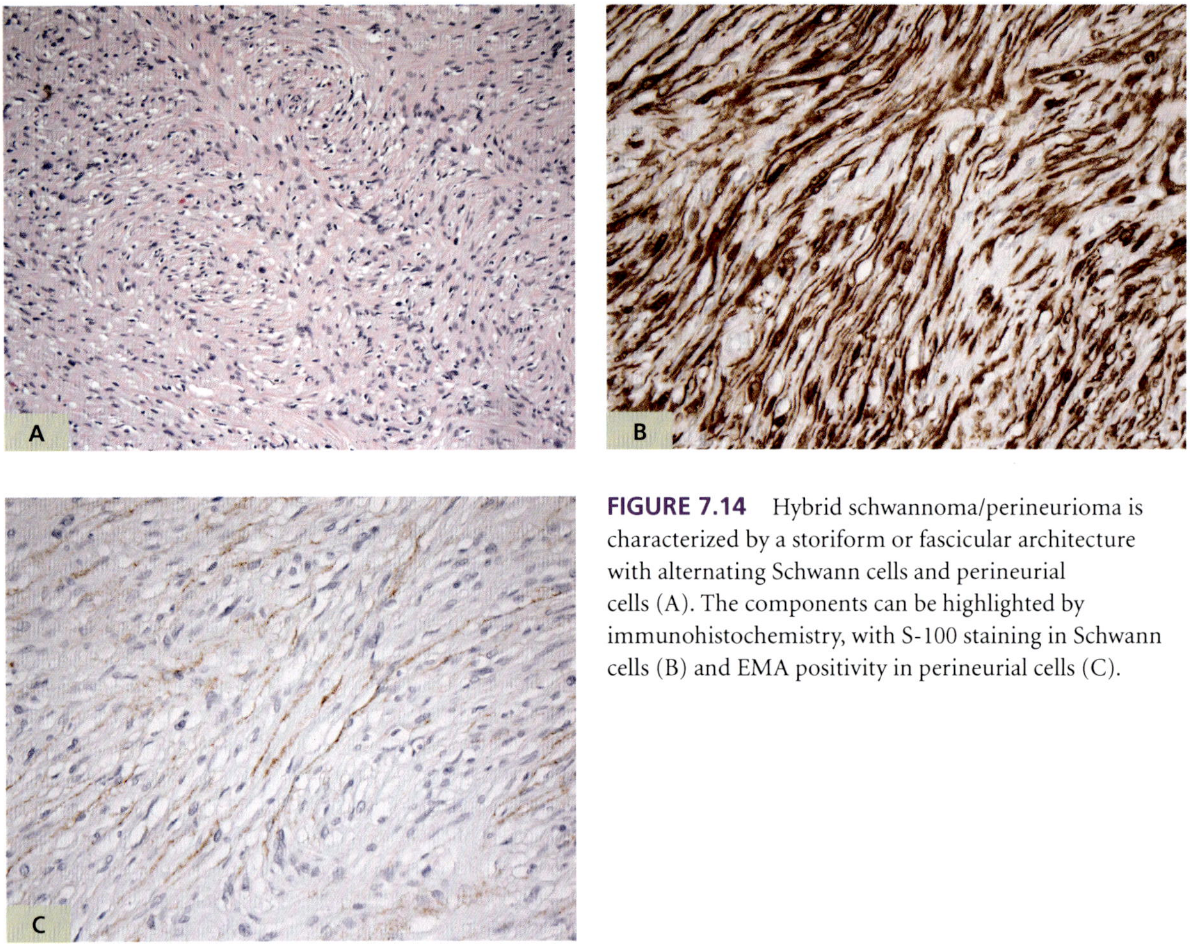

FIGURE 7.14 Hybrid schwannoma/perineurioma is characterized by a storiform or fascicular architecture with alternating Schwann cells and perineurial cells (A). The components can be highlighted by immunohistochemistry, with S-100 staining in Schwann cells (B) and EMA positivity in perineurial cells (C).

conventional or plexiform neurofibroma (294). The components in a hybrid nerve sheath tumor can be highlighted using immunohistochemistry: EMA and claudin-1 for perineurial cells and S-100 for Schwann cells (**Figure 7.14B, C**). The multifocal S-100 staining and fascicular pattern, which can occasionally appear hypercellular, may raise the possibility of MPNST. Significant cytological atypia, atypical mitotic figures, and necrosis are absent in hybrid nerve sheath tumors.

8

Mimics of Neoplasms of Uncertain Differentiation and Gastrointestinal Stromal Tumors

"Tumors of uncertain differentiation" as classified by the World Health Organization (WHO) are comprised of a diverse group of neoplasms, including myxomas, myoepithelial neoplasms of soft tissue, synovial sarcoma, epithelioid sarcoma, alveolar soft-part sarcoma, desmoplastic round-cell tumor, and perivascular epithelioid cell tumors (PEComa). Many tumors in this group have characteristic morphologic and immunophenotypic features and recurrent translocations. For instance, synovial sarcoma shows expression of TLE1, EMA and pan-keratin, and is characterized by the translocation t(X;18) (p11;q11) resulting in *SS18-SSX1* or *SS18-SSX2* fusion (295). In contrast, "unclassified/undifferentiated sarcomas" in the WHO classification scheme have no recognizable lines of differentiation (and are diagnoses of exclusion). Most of these tumors are high grade and are associated with a poor prognosis; tumors are currently subclassified according to predominant morphologic patterns: round cell, spindle cell, pleomorphic, or epithelioid.

Gastrointestinal stromal tumors (GIST) are the most common mesenchymal tumors in the gastrointestinal tract; most GISTs have spindle cell morphology, though epithelioid morphology and those with mixed spindle cell and epithelioid morphology are observed in up to a third of cases. Most GISTs are positive for KIT and DOG1, the latter being a highly sensitive and specific marker that is positive in up to a third of KIT-negative GISTs (296). GISTs are reported according to the National Comprehensive Cancer Network (NCCN) risk stratification scheme (297) based on anatomic site, tumor size, and mitotic count, features that have been shown in several large retrospective series to be highly predictive of malignant behavior (298,299). The majority of GISTs harbor mutations in *KIT*; tumors with mutations in exon 9 or 11 are the most responsive to the tyrosine kinase inhibitor imatinib; a smaller proportion of tumors have mutations in *PDGFRA*. Many "wild-type" GISTs that lack *KIT* and *PDGFRA* mutations are now classified as having succinate dehydrogenase (SDH) "deficiency" secondary to inactivation of *SDHA*, *B*, *C*, or *D* genes. SDH-deficient GISTs have predominantly epithelioid morphology, multinodular growth pattern within the gastric wall, and frequent nodal metastases; their behavior is not predicable by conventional NCCN risk stratification. SDH-deficiency can be identified by immunohistochemistry: loss of SDHB staining occurs in tumors with a mutation in any one of the *SDH* genes (or *SDHC* promoter hypermethylation), whereas loss of both SDHB and SDHA expression is seen only in the context of an *SDHA* mutation (300). Carney-Stratakis syndrome refers to patients with *SDH* germline mutations that develop GIST and paragangliomas.

MIMICS OF NEOPLASMS OF UNCERTAIN DIFFERENTIATION

ATYPICAL FIBROXANTHOMA

Atypical fibroxanthoma (AFX) is a dermal tumor of uncertain differentiation that arises in sun-damaged skin of elderly patients. Tumors present as rapidly growing, nodular or polypoid masses. When strictly defined, AFX is a benign lesion with essentially no risk for recurrence or metastasis with complete excision. Microscopically, AFX is completely confined to the dermis and has a smooth demarcation with normal dermis, and often appears to "push down" normal adnexal structures (**Figure 8.1A**). These exophytic tumors are often ulcerated and are partially surrounded by an epidermal collarette (**Figure 8.1B**). Solar elastosis is typically present adjacent to and compressed underneath tumors. AFX is comprised of sheets and fascicles of pleomorphic cells, which are variably epithelioid and spindled with occasional multinucleated forms (**Figure 8.1C**). The tumor cells are hyperchromatic and show significant nuclear pleomorphism, with single or multiple macronucleoli. A lymphocytic infiltrate and lipidized cells are often present within tumors. Mitotic activity is frequently high and atypical mitotic figures may be found. Despite the cytologic features and mitotic activity, AFX does

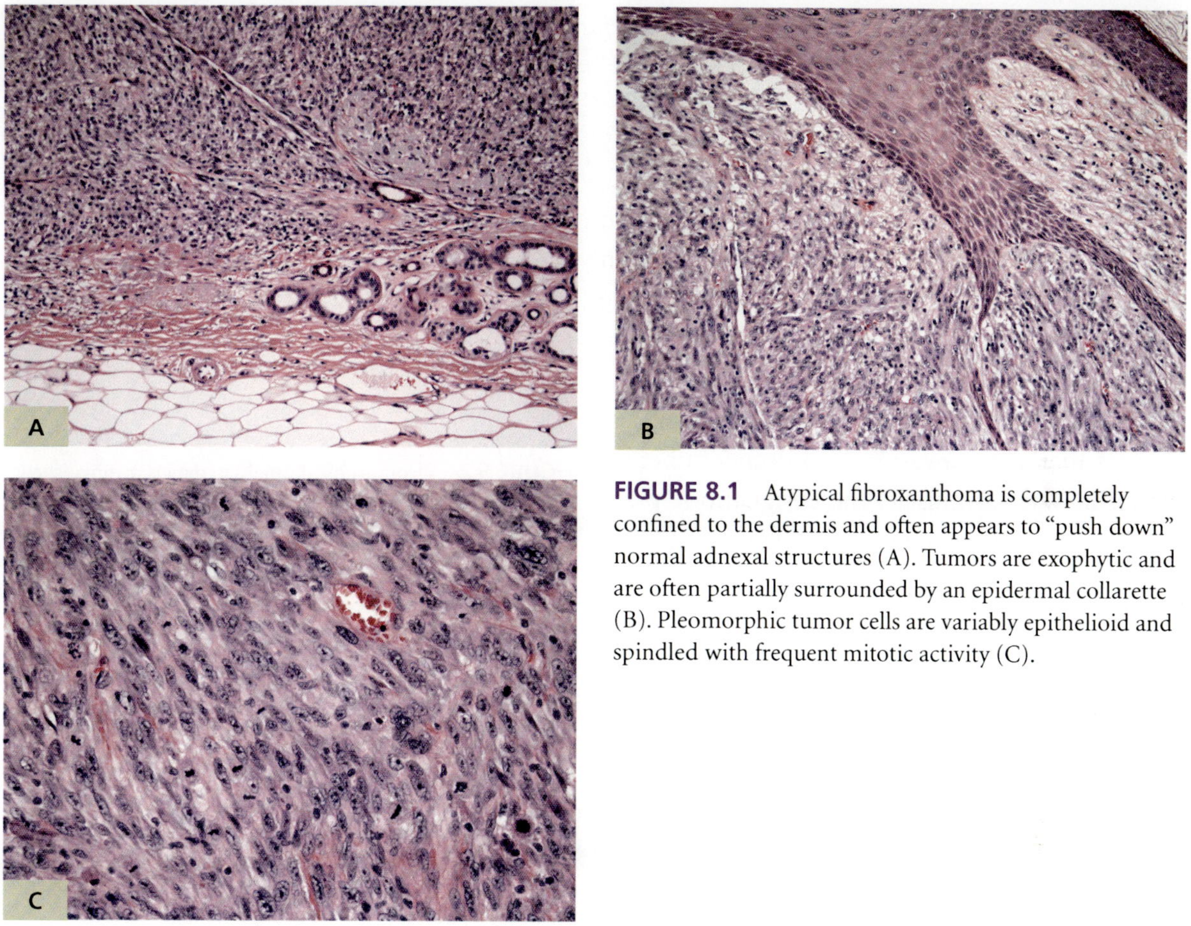

FIGURE 8.1 Atypical fibroxanthoma is completely confined to the dermis and often appears to "push down" normal adnexal structures (A). Tumors are exophytic and are often partially surrounded by an epidermal collarette (B). Pleomorphic tumor cells are variably epithelioid and spindled with frequent mitotic activity (C).

not show lymphovascular invasion, perineural invasion, or necrosis, and does not show invasion into subcutis, skeletal muscle, or fascia.

Based on its heterogeneous morphologies and high-grade cytologic features, the differential diagnosis of AFX may be broad and a comprehensive immunohistochemical panel is often necessary. Spindle cell squamous cell carcinoma and malignant melanoma should be excluded when encountering any pleomorphic dermal lesion in an elderly patient in sun damaged skin. Negativity for cytokeratins (including broad spectrum and high-molecular weight) and p63 will exclude squamous cell carcinoma, and melanoma markers S-100, SOX10, MART-1/Melan-A, HMB45, and MiTF should be negative. Careful examination of the epidermis to identify either high-grade squamous dysplasia or an in situ melanocytic component can help suggest an alternate diagnosis. Cutaneous angiosarcoma or atypical intradermal smooth muscle neoplasm (also known as cutaneous leiomyosarcoma), may also be considered. AFX will be negative for the endothelial markers CD31, CD34, and

ERG (although limited cytoplasmic staining for CD31 may occasionally be observed), and negative for myogenic markers desmin and caldesmon (although Smooth Muscle Actin [SMA] may sometimes show focal nonspecific staining).

For pleomorphic dermal tumors in which all specific lines of differentiation have been excluded, the diagnosis of AFX should only be applied when the tumor is completely confined to the dermis and there is no necrosis and lymphovascular or perineural invasion. For identical tumors that show invasion into deeper subcutis, fascia, or skeletal muscle, the designation "pleomorphic dermal sarcoma" should be applied (301) (**Figure 8.2**). Pleomorphic dermal sarcomas have a small but definite risk for recurrence (up to 30%) and metastasis (up to 15%).

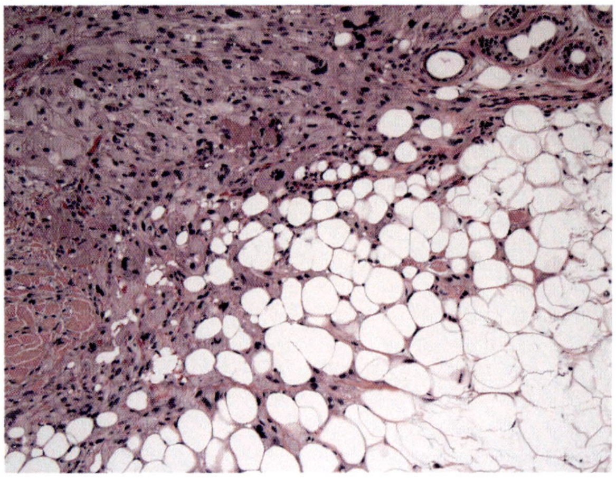

FIGURE 8.2 Pleomorphic dermal sarcoma is distinguished from atypical fibroxanthoma by invasion into deeper subcutis, fascia, or skeletal muscle.

ANGIOMYOFIBROBLASTOMA

Angiomyofibroblastoma is a fibroblastic/myofibroblastic tumor that occurs in the vulvovaginal region of reproductive-aged women (though has rarely been reported in men). Tumors show benign behavior and surgical excision is curative. Lesions are typically small (less than 5.0 cm) and well-circumscribed. Histologically, ovoid, plump, and stellate tumor cells are embedded in a myxoid stroma, with concentric growth around thin-walled capillaries (**Figure 8.3**). Lesions must be distinguished from deep (aggressive) angiomyxoma, a locally infiltrative, nonmetastasizing neoplasm that occurs in the pelvic and perineal sites most commonly in women. Deep angiomyxoma can be large infiltrative tumors that are disfiguring, with high morbidity associated with surgical resection. Recurrence secondary to incomplete resection occurs in up to a third of patients. Deep angiomyxoma is relatively paucicellular, with spindled tumor cells embedded in a myxoid stroma (**Figure 8.4A**). The vessels in deep angiomyxoma are round with thick-walled, hyalinized walls, occasionally associated with concentric myoid bundles and collagenous stroma. The myofibroblasts in both angiomyofibroblastoma and aggressive angiomyxoma are positive for desmin but negative for SMA; however, deep angiomyxoma often shows rearrangement of *HMGA2*, which can be confirmed by cytogenetic or immunohistochemical studies (**Figure 8.4B**) (302,303).

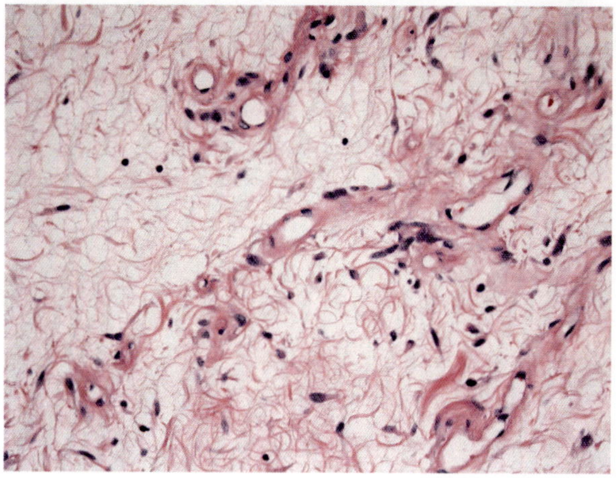

FIGURE 8.3 Angiomyofibroblastoma is comprised of ovoid, plump, and stellate tumor cells embedded in a myxoid stroma, with concentric growth around thin-walled capillaries.

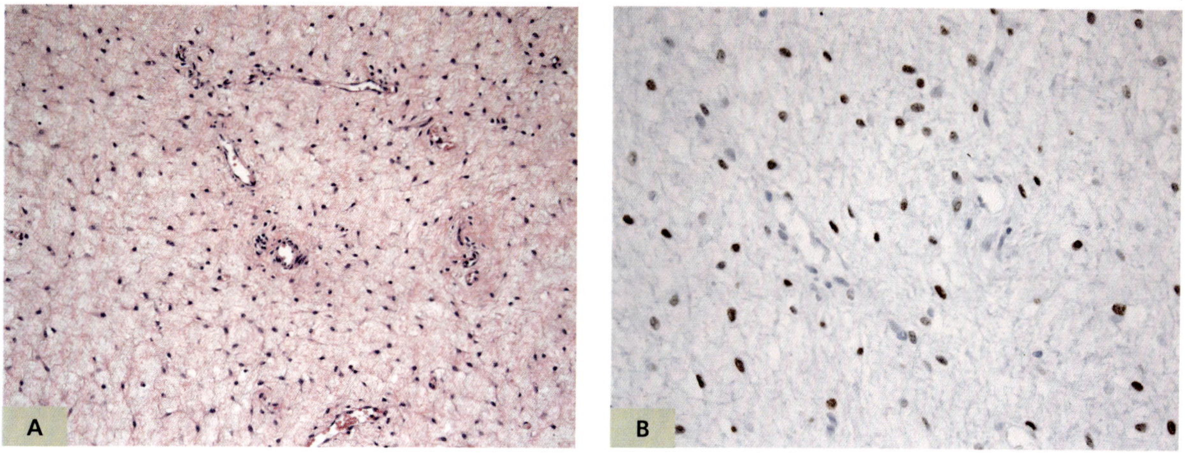

FIGURE 8.4 Deep ("aggressive") angiomyxoma is highly infiltrative and appears as a paucicellular proliferation of spindle cells embedded in a myxoid stroma that has round thick-walled vessels (A). HMGA2 is positive (B).

GRANULOMA ANNULARE

Granuloma annulare is a self-limited disorder that presents as groups of raised annular lesions most frequently on the hands and feet. Many patients have an associated systemic disease, including autoimmune diseases and hepatitis C. Rare cases may be disseminated, associated with diabetes mellitus, or in subcutaneous locations. Microscopically, the granulomatous lesions show a necrobiotic appearance: epithelioid to spindle shaped histiocytes arranged in a palisaded distribution around areas of altered dermal collagen appearing variably ropy and amorphous

(**Figure 8.5**). The granulomas are overall round in shape and are often associated with dermal mucin. Lymphocytic inflammatory infiltrate is common, but giant cells are rare.

There are overlapping features between granuloma annulare and other necrobiotic granulomatous dermatitides, namely necrobiosis lipoidica and rheumatoid nodule. The increased dermal mucin in granuloma annulare is a useful distinguishing feature from these other processes. Necrobiosis lipoidica is usually centered deeper in the dermis and the granulomas are often "laminated" with alternating areas of normal and abnormal collagen; lipid deposits are common and plasma cells can be more prominent. Rheumatoid nodules are larger and more deeply situated in deep dermis or subcutis over the extensor aspects of joints; nodules tend to be larger with frequent fibrin deposition within nodules (**Figure 8.6**). Correlation with clinical data and serologic studies is typically helpful.

Granuloma annulare must be distinguished from epithelioid sarcoma, some examples of which have a pseudogranulomatous growth pattern. Epithelioid sarcoma is most common in the distal extremities in younger patients (teens and young adults), and presents as solitary or multiple firm nodules. Microscopically, epithelioid sarcoma is comprised of nodules of spindled and epithelioid cells arranged around central areas of necrosis (**Figure 8.7A, B**). Lymphocytes are often present. The tumor cells have abundant pale-to-eosinophilic cytoplasm and large nuclei with vesicular chromatin and small nucleoli, and tend to show low mitotic activity. The cytologic atypia is mild, but greater than the bland-appearing

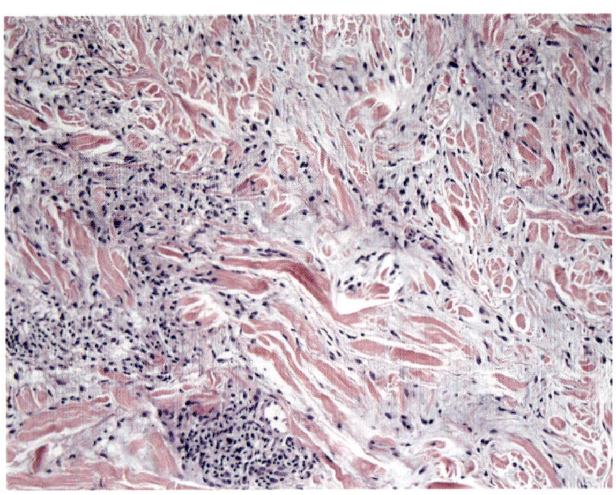

FIGURE 8.5 Granuloma annulare is a necrobiotic lesion characterized by epithelioid to spindled histiocytes palisaded around altered dermal collagen and dermal mucin. A lymphocytic inflammatory infiltrate is common.

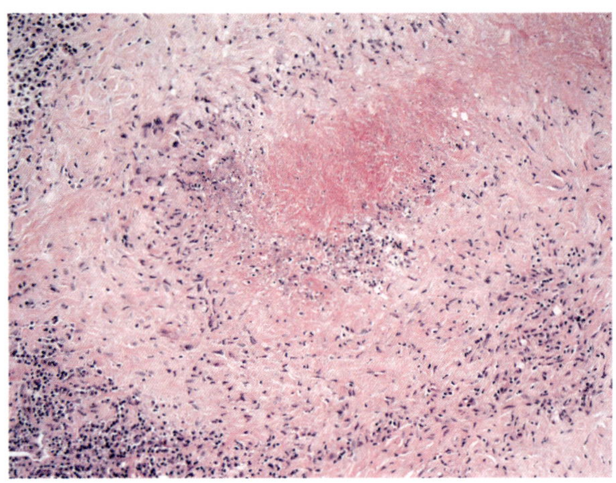

FIGURE 8.6 Rheumatoid nodules show palisaded spindled and epithelioid histiocytes around granular necrotic and fibrinoid debris. Multinucleated giant cells are common.

histiocytes of granuloma annulare. The nodules in epithelioid sarcoma often fuse to form large serpiginous areas, and when deep-seated may infiltrate along fascial planes, in contrast to the round and more superficially situated granulomas in granuloma annulare. Dystrophic calcifications and metaplastic osteoid formation may occasionally be seen in epithelioid sarcoma. Immunohistochemistry for histiocytic markers (CD68, CD163) will be positive in granuloma annulare, and epithelioid sarcoma shows a distinctive profile of positivity for EMA, cytokeratin (**Figure 8.7C**), and CD34 (the latter in approximately half of cases), and loss of nuclear expression of SMARCB1/INI1 (**Figure 8.7D**) (304). Epithelioid sarcoma shows a propensity for recurrence and metastasis, including to lymph nodes.

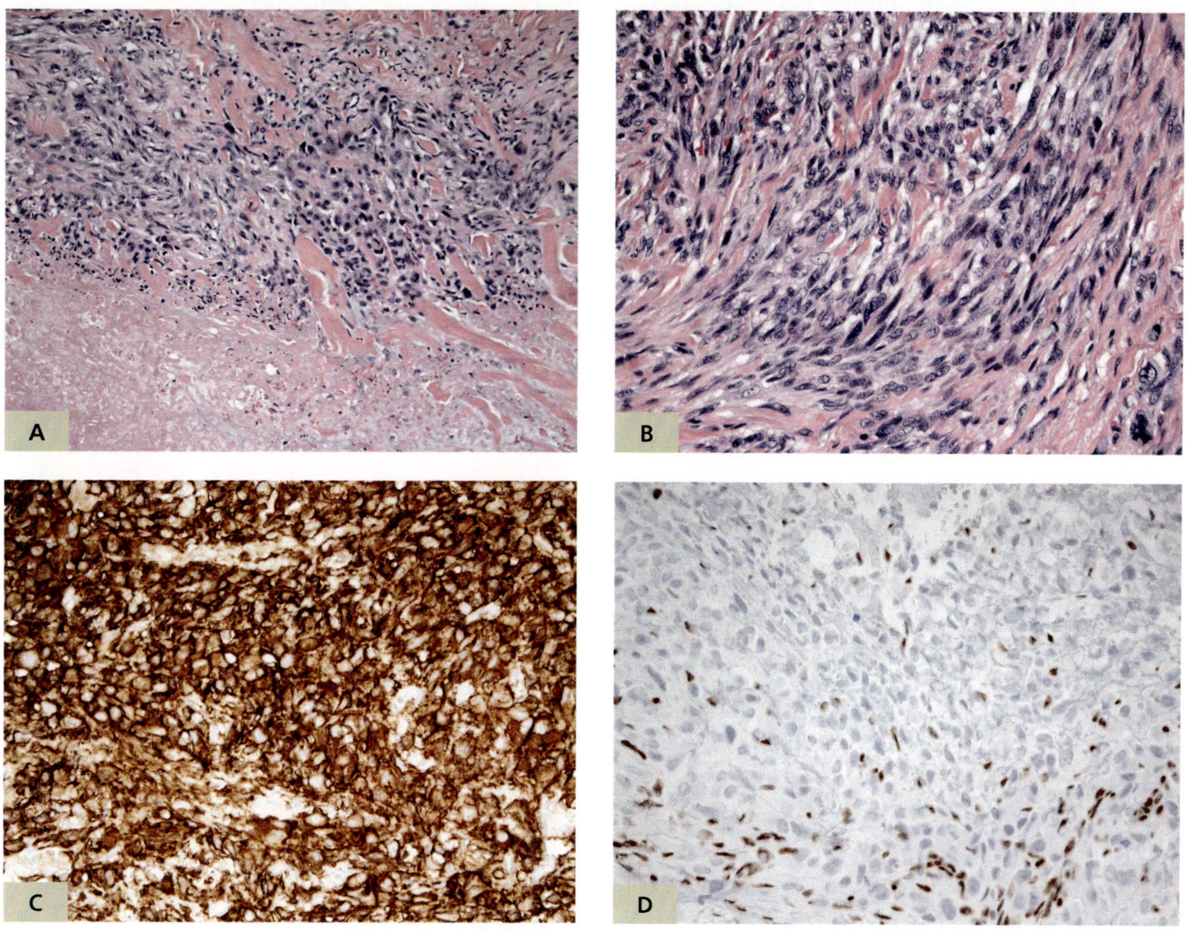

FIGURE 8.7 Epithelioid sarcoma can show a pseudogranulomatous growth pattern with nodules of spindled and epithelioid cells arranged around central areas of necrosis (A). Tumor cells have abundant palely eosinophilic cytoplasm and large nuclei with vesicular chromatin and small nucleoli (B). Epithelioid sarcoma is positive for keratin (C) and CD34, and shows loss of nuclear expression of SMARCB1/INI1 (D).

ANEURYSMAL, CELLULAR, AND DEEP VARIANTS OF FIBROUS HISTIOCYTOMA

Several variants of fibrous histiocytoma (also known as dermatofibroma) may mimic angiomatoid fibrous histiocytoma (AFH). Fibrous histiocytomas present as firm round dermal papules or nodules of the trunk and extremities, and are comprised of spindled cells growing in a haphazard, vaguely storiform or fascicular pattern with collagen entrapment at the periphery of the lesion and overlying epidermal hyperplasia. The spindled cells are variably plump and elongated with ovoid vesicular nuclei and indistinct cytoplasm; foamy histiocytes and giant cells may be present. The aneurysmal variant shows central blood-filled spaces (**Figure 8.8**), while the cellular variant is much more cellular with fascicular growth (**Figure 8.9**). The deep variant is usually subcutaneous, and rarely in visceral or intramuscular sites. The presence of necrosis in up to one-fifth of cases of cellular fibrous histiocytoma may raise concern for malignancy; however, metastasis is exceptional (305) and recurrence is seen in up to 20% of cases only after incomplete excision.

Aneurysmal fibrous histiocytoma, and less commonly the cellular and deep variants, may show overlapping morphologic features with AFH, which is a tumor of uncertain histogenesis. AFH most commonly arises in the extremities or trunk in superficial soft tissue of children and young adults. Tumors are well-circumscribed, multinodular masses surrounded by a thick fibrous pseudocapsule and a dense lymphoplasmacytic infiltrate, often with germinal center

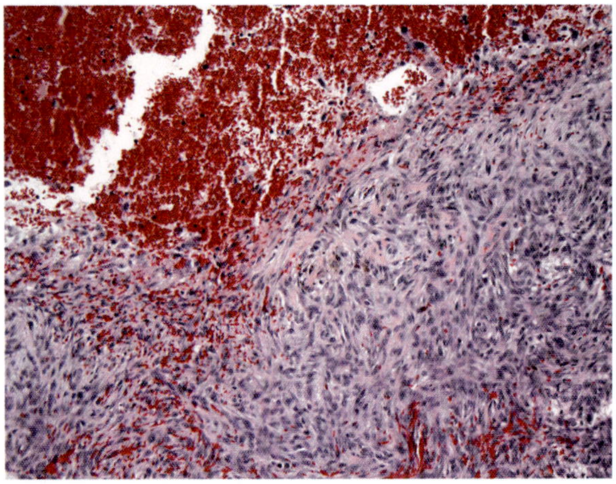

FIGURE 8.8 The aneurysmal variant of fibrous histiocytoma is comprised of spindle cells arranged in a variably storiform and fascicular growth pattern with central blood-filled spaces.

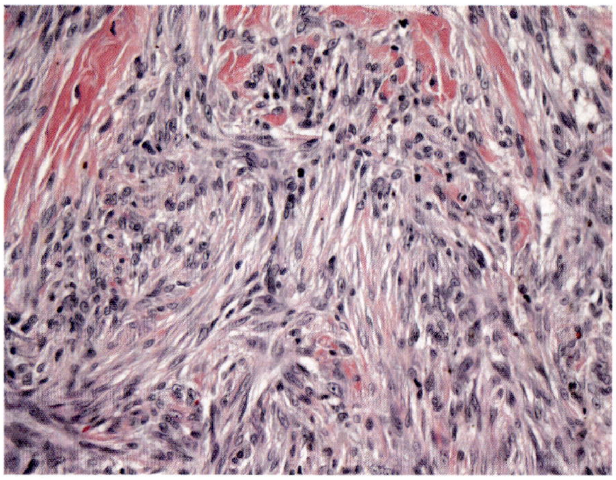

FIGURE 8.9 Cellular benign fibrous histiocytoma shows a more cellular fascicular growth pattern and frequent peripheral collagen entrapment.

formation (that may resemble a lymph node from low power) (**Figure 8.10A**). Masses are most commonly cystic with blood-filled spaces, and hemosiderin deposition within the tumor and pseudocapsule is seen. The tumor cells are variably spindled, ovoid, and round, with palely eosinophilic cytoplasm and uniform vesicular nuclei having small to indistinct nucleoli (**Figure 8.10B**). Tumor cells are arranged in sheets but can show vaguely storiform growth. Mitotic activity may be present, but only rare cases show significant nuclear pleomorphism and hyperchromatic nuclei. Occasional variants are "solid" and lack the central cystic hemorrhagic areas, which may be confused with cellular or deep fibrous histiocytoma. Aneurysmal fibrous histiocytoma typically shows

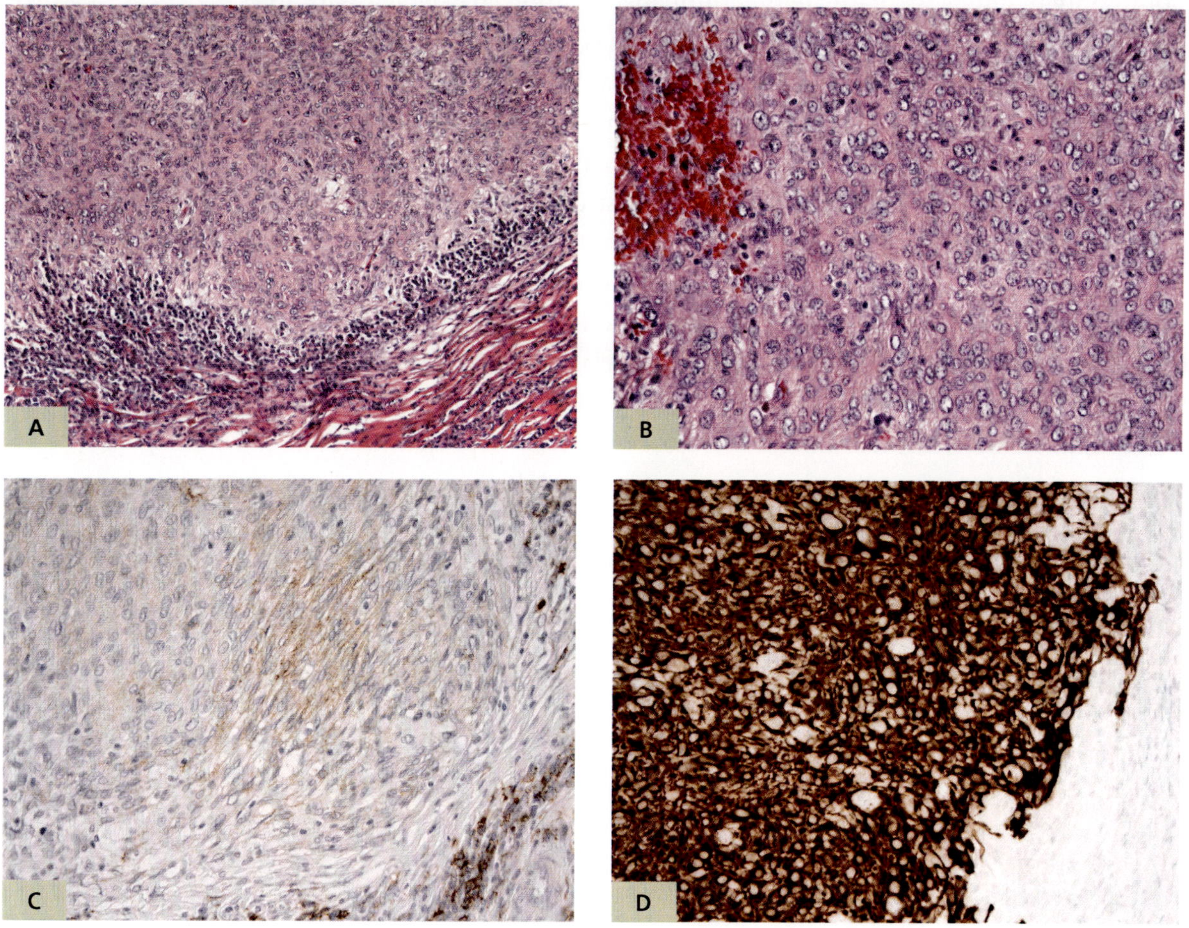

FIGURE 8.10 Angiomatoid fibrous histiocytomas are multinodular with a thick fibrous pseudocapsule and a dense lymphoplasmacytic infiltrate (A). Tumor cells are variably spindled, ovoid, and round, with palely eosinophilic cytoplasm and uniform vesicular nuclei having small to indistinct nucleoli, and surround central cystic hemorrhagic areas (B). Tumor cells are often positive for EMA (C) and desmin (D).

a more polymorphous appearance than AFH, with frequent foamy histiocytes and giant cells, and lacks a prominent pseudocapsule and dense peripheral lymphocytic infiltrate. AFH shows a somewhat unusual immunophenotype with frequent staining for EMA and desmin (**Figure 8.10C, D**); AFH is negative for SMA, which can be positive in fibrous histiocytoma. The diagnosis of AFH can also be confirmed by demonstration of *EWSR1* gene rearrangement, most commonly fused with *CREB1* (306).

SOFT TISSUE CHONDROMA

Soft tissue chondroma arises as small painless masses in acral locations, most commonly in adults with a male predominance. Tumors are benign with low rates of recurrence after resection. Chondromas are usually small, solitary masses comprised of multilobular growth of hyaline cartilage, with benign-appearing chondrocytes in single lacunae (**Figure 8.11A**). However, a range of appearances may be seen, including cases with ossification, fibrosis, and "grungy" calcifications (**Figure 8.11B**). Myxoid stromal change may be seen in which the chondrocytes adopt more spindled and stellate shapes. Osteoclast-like giant cells may be frequent. Soft tissue chondroma is associated with rearrangement of the *HMGA2* locus on chromosome 12q15 (307,308).

Cases of soft tissue chondroma having osteoclast-like giant cells and extensive grungy calcifications may resemble phosphaturic mesenchymal tumor. Phosphaturic mesenchymal tumors are most frequently reported in adults in

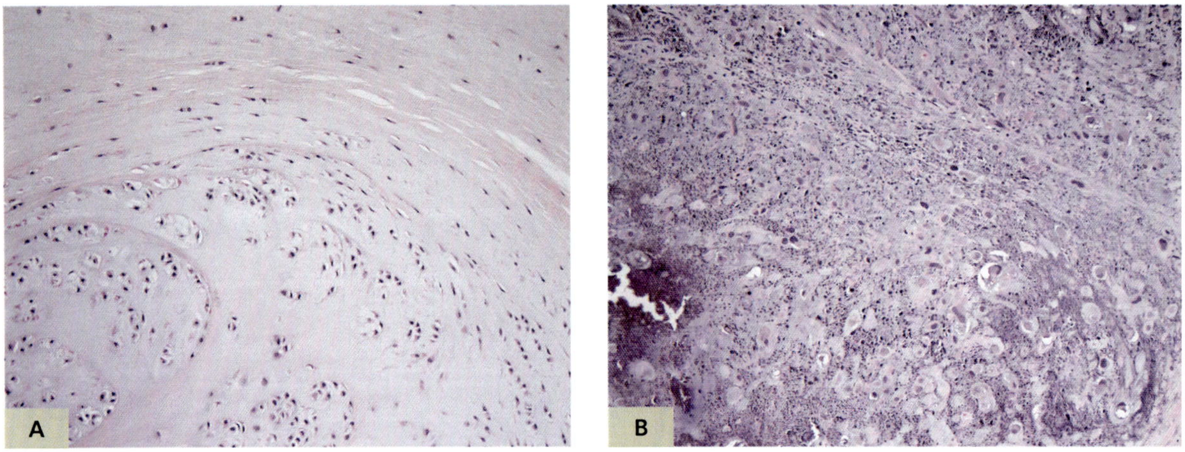

FIGURE 8.11 Soft tissue chondroma is comprised of multilobular growth of hyaline cartilage with benign-appearing chondrocytes in lacunae (A). Some examples may show extensive calcification (B).

any anatomic site, and are associated with tumor-induced osteomalacia secondary to the production of fibroblast growth factor 23 (FGF23) (309,310). The *FN1-FGFR1* fusion gene has recently been identified in phosphaturic mesenchymal tumor (311). Tumors are comprised of nodules of bland, predominantly spindled cells with an extensive capillary network (some appearing hemangiopericytoma-like), and a distinctive pattern of "grungy" calcification that appears gray-to-purple and fibrillary (**Figure 8.12**). Osteoclast-like giant cells, chondro-osseous metaplasia, and histiocytes are often present. Soft tissue chondroma lacks a prominent spindle cell component.

CELLULAR NEUROTHEKEOMA

Cellular neurothekeoma occurs most frequently on the head and neck and upper extremities of young adults, with a female predominance. This benign cutaneous tumor of uncertain histogenesis appears as nests and lobules of spindled and epithelioid cells that are separated by dense hyalinized collagen (**Figure 8.13**). The tumor cells have palely eosinophilic cytoplasm with ovoid nuclei and occasional small nucleoli; significant cytologic atypia and pleomorphism are usually absent, although when present do not seem to confer risk for malignant behavior (312). Within the nests, tumor cells have ill-defined cytoplasmic borders and appear somewhat syncytial. Osteoclast-like giant cells may be present. Lesions may show a somewhat infiltrative appearance with

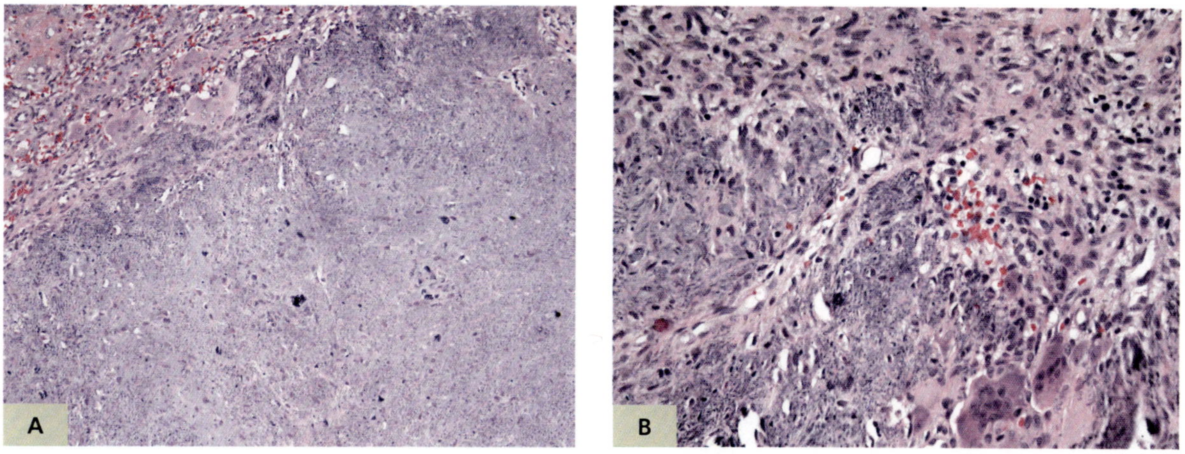

FIGURE 8.12 Phosphaturic mesenchymal tumor is composed of spindle cells with an extensive capillary network and an extensive basophilic calcified matrix (A). Tumors have a distinctive pattern of "grungy" calcification that appears gray-to-purple and fibrillary, and osteoclast-like giant cells and histiocytes are common (B).

extension into subcutaneous tissue. Cellular neurothekoma is positive for the nonspecific markers NKI-C3, NSE, and SMA.

The differential diagnosis may include cutaneous PEComa and cutaneous clear cell sarcoma of soft tissue. Cutaneous PEComa is rare, is usually associated with benign behavior (313), and shows a similar nested growth pattern of epithelioid cells with variably granular eosinophilic or clear cytoplasm (**Figure 8.14**). Distinction from cellular neurothekeoma is usually straightforward by immunohistochemical stains: while both entities may be positive for SMA, cutaneous PEComa is consistently positive for HMB-45.

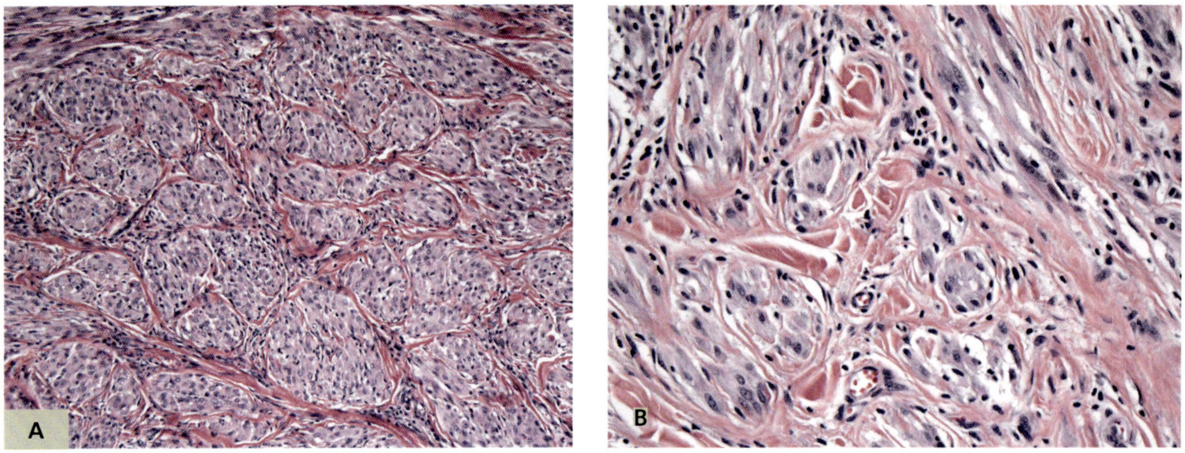

FIGURE 8.13 Cellular neurothekeoma appears as nests and lobules of spindled and epithelioid cells that are separated by dense hyalinized collagen bands (A). Tumor cells have palely eosinophilic and syncytial cytoplasm with ovoid nuclei and occasional small nucleoli (B).

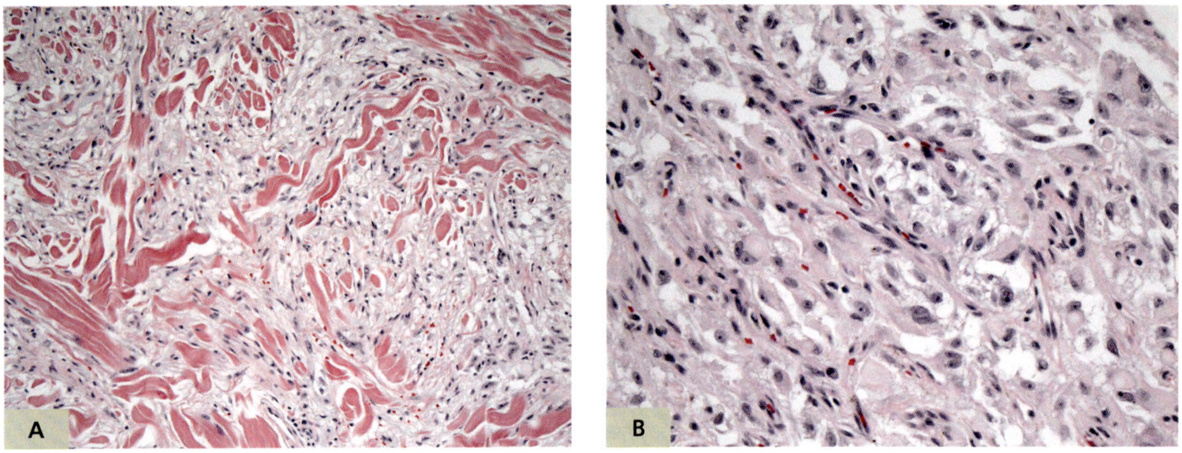

FIGURE 8.14 Cutaneous PEComa shows a nested growth pattern (A) of epithelioid cells with variably granular eosinophilic or clear cytoplasm and large-round nuclei with prominent nucleoli (B).

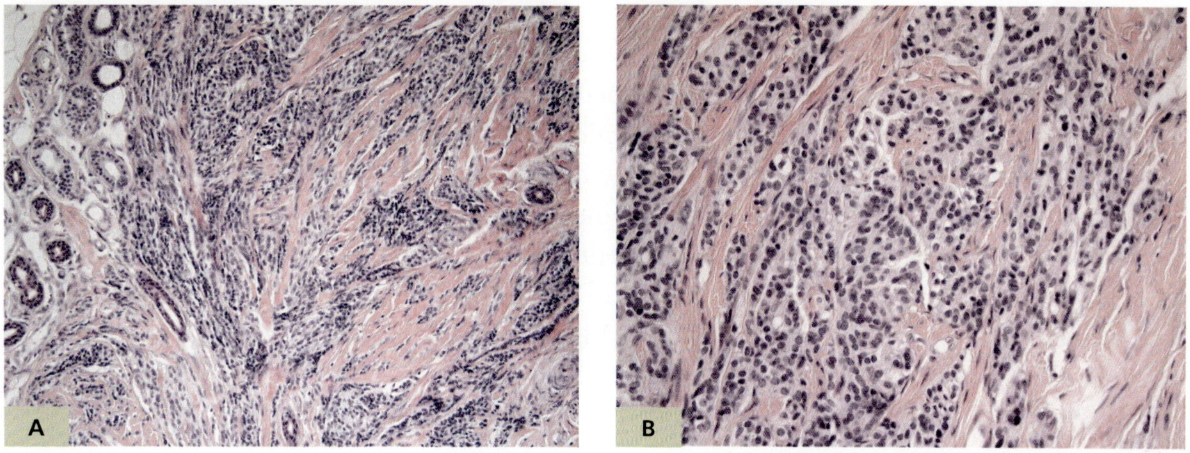

FIGURE 8.15 Clear cell sarcoma in dermal locations show an infiltrative nested growth of polygonal, epithelioid, or spindle cells separated by fibrous septa (A), with palely eosinophilic-to-amphophilic tumor cells having vesicular nuclei and macronucleoli (B).

Clear cell sarcoma arising in cutaneous locations has also been described (314), and is associated with a risk of recurrence and metastasis (including to lymph nodes). Clear cell sarcoma is most frequent in the extremities of young adults, and is associated with the translocation t(12;22) (q13;q12) resulting in *EWSR1-ATF1* gene fusion (315,316). While clear cell sarcoma also shows a distinct nested growth of polygonal, epithelioid, or spindle cells separated by fibrous septa, the tumor cells have more vesicular nuclei and macronucleoli (**Figure 8.15**). The cytoplasm is uniformly palely eosinophilic or amphophilic. Wreath-like giant cells are common in clear cell sarcoma, in contrast to the osteoclast-like giant cells in a subset of cellular neurothekeomas. In addition to molecular studies to confirm *EWSR1* gene rearrangement, immunohistochemistry is also helpful, which will show S-100 and HMB-45 reactivity in clear cell sarcoma.

MYOEPITHELIOMA OF SOFT TISSUE

Myoepithelioma of soft tissue can occur in a wide range of anatomic sites but is most frequent in the limbs and trunk. Tumors are typically well-circumscribed masses. Prognosis is excellent, with recurrence seen in up to 20% of cases (especially after incomplete resection) and rare metastases (317). Tumors show trabecular, nested, and reticular growth patterns within a variably myxoid and hyalinized stroma (**Figure 8.16A, B**). Tumor cells show spindle and epithelioid morphology with uniform nuclei, indistinct nucleoli, and eosinophilic-to-clear cytoplasm. Nuclear atypia, necrosis, and significant mitotic activity are absent in most cases. "Hyaline cells," or plasmacytoid cells with dense eosinophilic cytoplasmic inclusions, may be seen. Myoepithelioma may also have tumor cells with abundant cytoplasmic clearing, predominantly spindle cell morphology, areas of solid growth, and adipocytic, chondro-osseous, and squamous metaplasia. Similar to their salivary gland counterparts, myoepithelioma of soft tissue often shows intratumoral heterogeneity and variable staining for cytokeratin, EMA, S-100, GFAP, and p63 (**Figure 8.16C, D**). *EWSR1* translocation (and rarely alternate *FUS* rearrangement) is common in myoepithelial neoplasms (including myoepithelioma) (318–324).

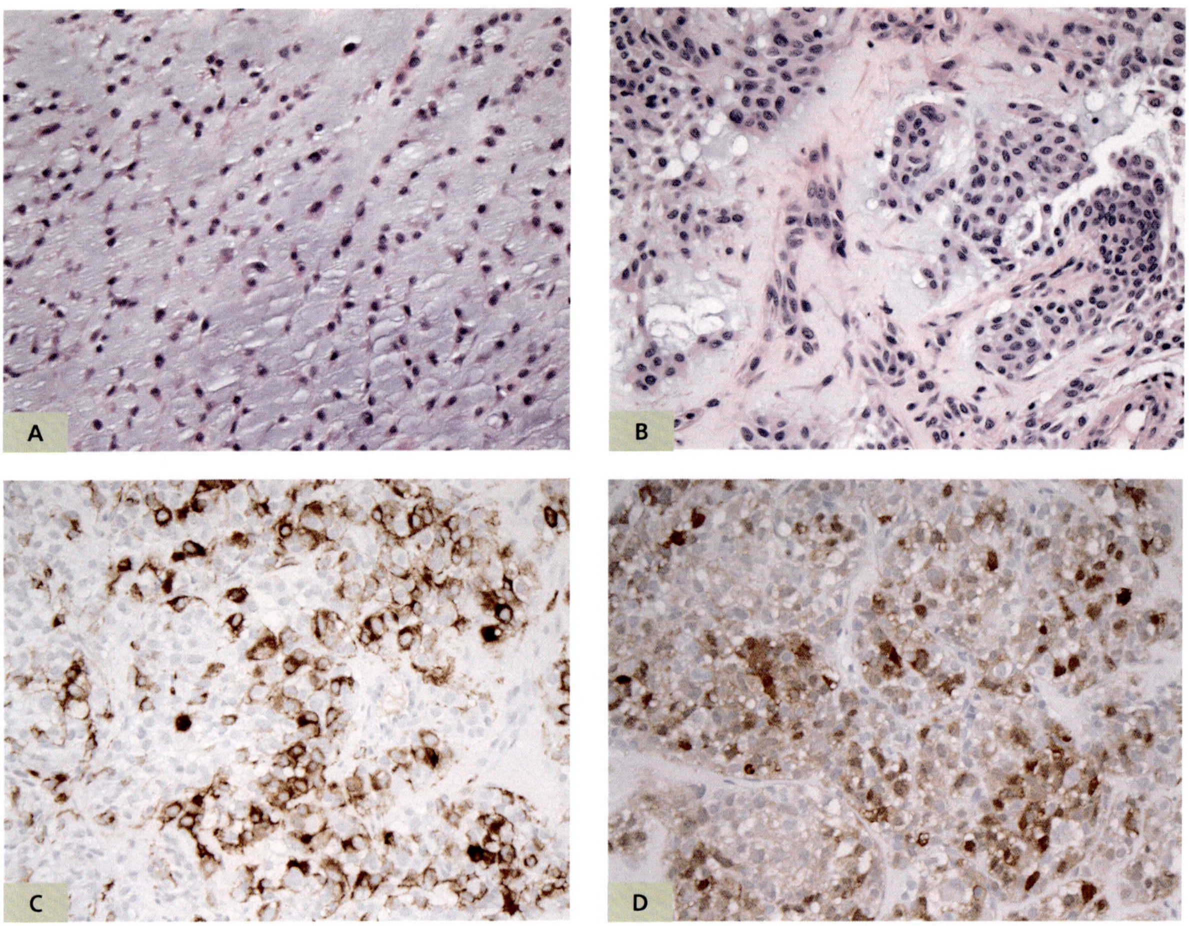

FIGURE 8.16 Myoepithelioma can show variable growth patterns of spindle and epithelioid cells with uniform nuclei, indistinct nucleoli, and eosinophilic-to-clear cytoplasm, including reticular (A) and nested (B) architecture, within a myxoid and hyalinized stroma. The immunophenotype may be variable, but keratin (C) and S-100 (D) positivity are frequent.

Distinction between myoepithelioma and myoepithelial carcinoma of soft tissue is based solely on the presence of cytologic atypia (317), in contrast to their salivary gland counterparts in which malignancy is based on invasive growth. Tumors classified as myoepithelial carcinoma have moderate-to-severe nuclear atypia, with vesicular nuclei and prominent nucleoli or coarse chromatin (**Figure 8.17**). Cytologic atypia has been shown to be a reliable predictor of aggressive behavior (317); myoepithelial carcinomas are associated with a recurrence rate of 40% and distant metastasis in 30% to 50% of affected patients (317,325).

Monomorphic cases of myoepithelioma may resemble ossifying fibromyxoid tumor (OFMT) on morphologic and immunohistochemical grounds. OFMT occurs in adults and arises most frequently as subcutaneous masses in the thigh and head and neck. OFMT is a well-circumscribed multilobular mass; the majority of cases have an incomplete peripheral shell of metaplastic bone (**Figure 8.18A**). Within the lobules, tumor cells are arranged in cords and trabeculae with a variable fibromyxoid stroma (**Figure 8.18B**). The tumor cells appear uniform with ovoid-to-round nuclei and palely eosinophilic cytoplasm. Mitotic activity and pleomorphism are rare (except in malignant variants). OFMT is positive for desmin and S-100, and variable expression of cytokeratin and Glial fibrillary acidic protein (GFAP) is seen. Most cases of myoepithelioma show some architectural and cytologic heterogeneity, and areas of cleared cells and nested and solid growth may aid in the distinction. Myoepithelioma is typically negative for desmin. Challenging cases may require cytogenetic studies for either *EWSR1* gene rearrangement in myoepithelioma, or *PHF1* rearrangement in OFMT (326,327). OFMT has a potential for recurrence, typically over a protracted clinical course of up to 20 years.

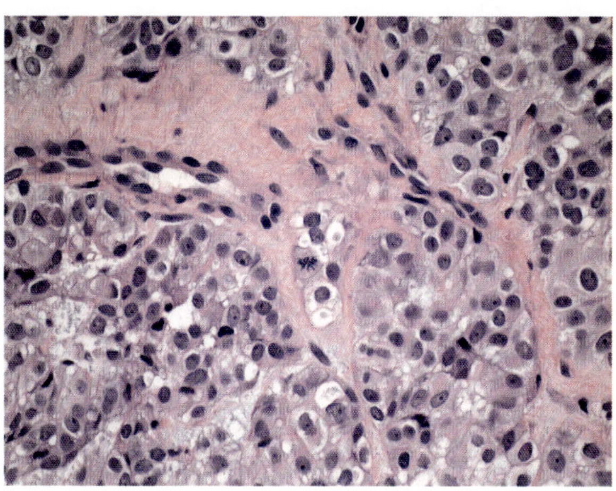

FIGURE 8.17 Cytologic atypia is the single criterion for malignancy in myoepithelial neoplasms, and tumors classified as myoepithelial carcinoma have moderate-to-severe nuclear atypia, with vesicular nuclei and prominent nucleoli or coarse chromatin. Mitotic activity is present.

Extraskeletal myxoid chondrosarcoma (EMC) arises predominantly in adults as deep-seated masses in the proximal limb, and has a significant risk of recurrence and metastasis (up to 50%). EMC shares morphologic and immunohistochemical features with myoepithelioma, and is also associated with *EWSR1* translocation. EMC is a multinodular tumor with a uniform tumor cell population arranged in cords and strands embedded in a myxoid stroma (**Figure 8.19**). Tumor cells have round nuclei with small nucleoli and

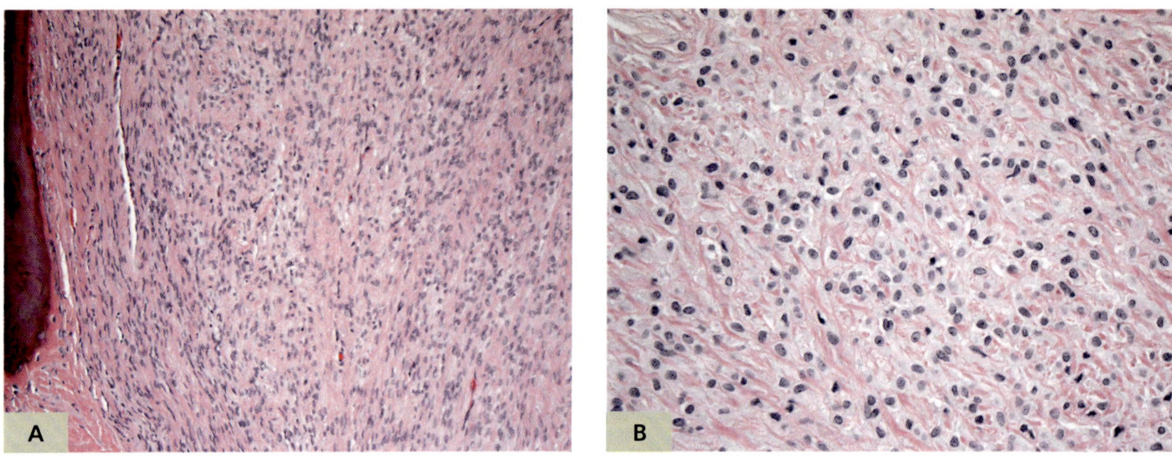

FIGURE 8.18 Ossifying fibromyxoid tumor (OFMT) is lobulated and often has an incomplete peripheral shell of metaplastic bone (A). Within the lobules, uniform tumor cells with ovoid-to-round nuclei and palely eosinophilic cytoplasm are arranged in cords and trabeculae with a variable fibromyxoid stroma (B).

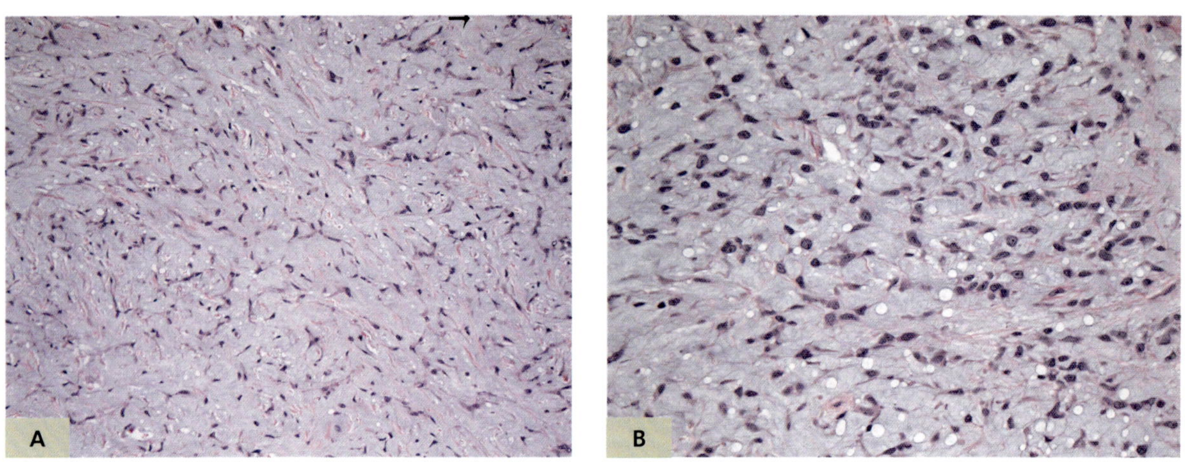

FIGURE 8.19 Extraskeletal myxoid chondrosarcoma (EMC) is composed of a uniform tumor cell population arranged in cords and strands embedded in a myxoid stroma (A). Tumor cells have round nuclei with small nucleoli and eosinophilic cytoplasm that extends into delicate processes creating its distinctive reticular growth pattern (B).

eosinophilic cytoplasm that extends into delicate processes to "reach out" to adjacent cells, creating its distinctive reticular growth pattern. The nodules appear overall hypocellular, but show slightly more hypercellularity at the periphery of nodules. S-100 positivity is seen in a small subset of EMC, and Epithelial Membrane Antigen (EMA) staining may also occasionally be seen; negativity for cytokeratin, GFAP, and p63 will help distinguish most cases from myoepithelioma. Both myoepithelioma and EMC are characterized by *EWSR1* gene fusions. While the fusion partners are varied in myoepithelioma (including *POU5F1*, *PBX1*, *ZNF444*, *ATF1*, and *PBX3* (319,320,328)), EMC is characterized by the translocation t(9;22) (q22;q11) resulting in *NR4A3-EWSR1* (or rearrangements of *NR4A3* with other fusion partners) (329,330); Fluorescence in situ hybridization (FISH) testing for *NR4A3* rearrangement can be performed to confirm the diagnosis of EMC.

SCHWANNOMA

Cellular schwannoma (discussed in Chapters 5 and 7; see Figures 5.7 and 7.8) in somatic soft tissue sites may occasionally mimic synovial sarcoma. Synovial sarcoma most frequently arises in the deep tissues of the limbs in young adults (though nearly all anatomic sites have been described). Survival at five years is approximately 40%, and recurrences and distant metastases are common. Monophasic synovial sarcoma shows fascicular growth of spindle cells with uniform tapering nuclei and poorly defined cytoplasm; within the fascicles the nuclei tend to overlap (**Figure 8.20A, B**). Biphasic synovial sarcoma shows epithelial differentiation most frequently as glandular structures lined by cuboidal or columnar epithelium, and may be only focally present. The stroma is variably collagenous, often appearing wiry in between tumor cells, and large dystrophic calcifications are common. In contrast to the thick-walled hyaline vessels seen in schwannoma, synovial sarcoma is characterized by frequent thin-walled, dilated hemangiopericytoma-like vessels. Synovial sarcoma typically shows multifocal positivity for EMA and cytokeratin, and diffuse nuclear staining for TLE1 (331) (**Figure 8.20C**). While schwannoma may occasionally show focal cytokeratin positivity (particularly retroperitoneal examples), staining for EMA and TLE1 will be negative in tumor cells and S-100 will be diffusely positive. The diagnosis of synovial sarcoma can be further supported by molecular studies to confirm *SS18* rearrangement.

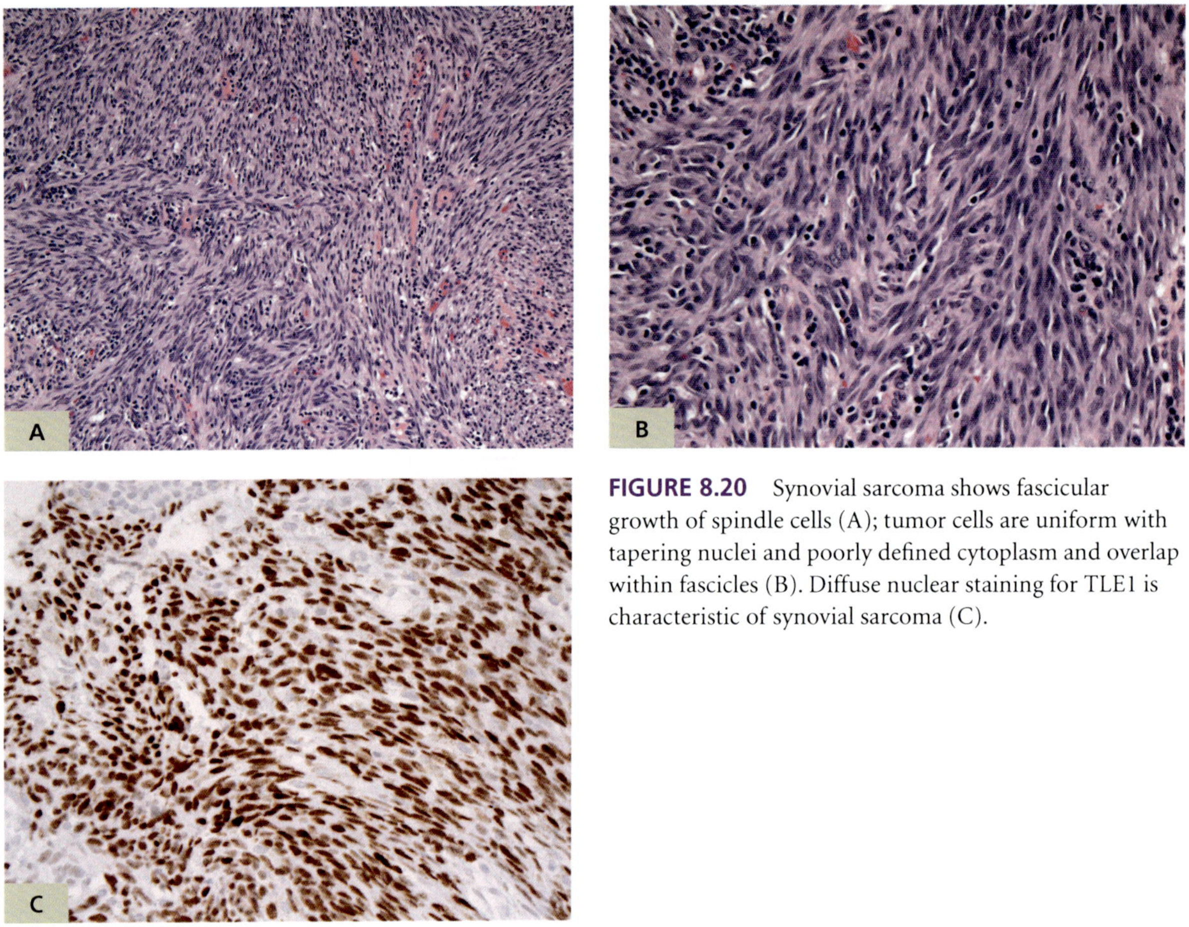

FIGURE 8.20 Synovial sarcoma shows fascicular growth of spindle cells (A); tumor cells are uniform with tapering nuclei and poorly defined cytoplasm and overlap within fascicles (B). Diffuse nuclear staining for TLE1 is characteristic of synovial sarcoma (C).

MIMICS OF GASTROINTESTINAL STROMAL TUMORS

SCHWANNOMA

Schwannomas in the gastrointestinal tract are typically well-circumscribed but unencapsulated, and can mimic GIST, especially in small-biopsy specimens. Gastrointestinal schwannomas usually arise in the stomach. These benign tumors are comprised of bland-appearing plump spindle cells arranged in fascicles; gastric schwannomas typically lack the classic alternating hypercellular (Antoni A) and hypocellular (Antonio B) areas of peripheral schwannomas. Tumor cells have mild nuclear variability, indistinct nucleoli, and palely eosinophilic cytoplasm (**Figure 8.21A**). A dense peripheral lymphoid infiltrate is often present, a helpful

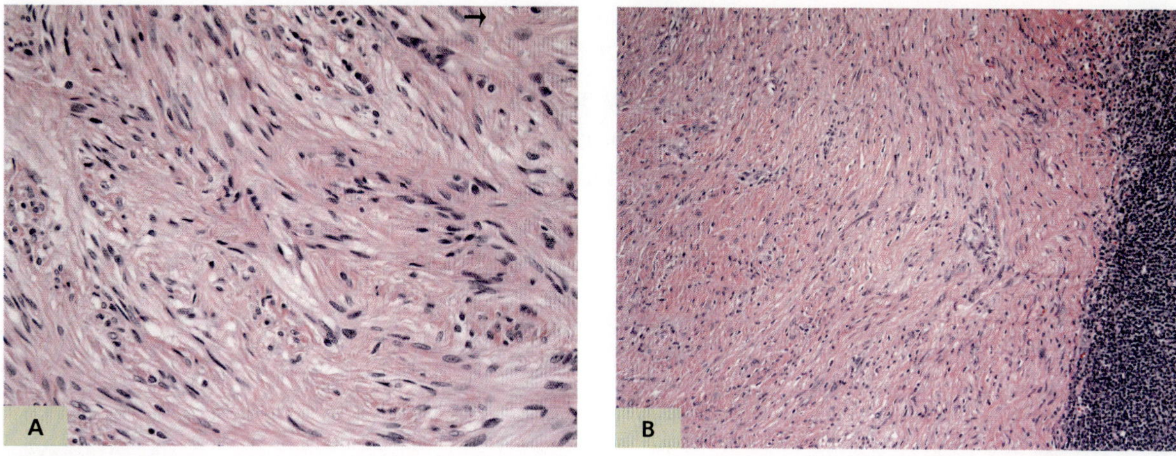

FIGURE 8.21 Gastric schwannomas are typically more cellular and lack the classic alternating hypercellular (Antoni A) and hypocellular (Antonio B) areas (A). While most tumors are unencapsulated, a dense peripheral lymphoid infiltrate is often present (B).

clue to the diagnosis of gastric schwannoma (**Figure 8.21B**). Most schwannomas lack mitotic activity, and diffuse severe cytologic atypia is not observed, although degenerative nuclear activity and occasional mitotic figures may be seen.

Gastric schwannomas may resemble spindle cell GIST, owing to shared features of uniform cytomorphology, general lack of significant atypia, and pale cytoplasm. GIST typically shows a more uniformly cellular growth pattern and lacks stromal collagen fibers often seen in schwannomas (**Figure 8.22A**). Other features favoring GIST include paranuclear vacuoles (most commonly in gastric tumors) (**Figure 8.22B**). This differential diagnosis can easily be resolved by immunohistochemistry: S-100 will be diffusely positive in schwannoma, whereas KIT and DOG1 are positive in GIST (**Figure 8.22C**).

LEIOMYOMA

Leiomyomas may also arise within the wall of the gastrointestinal tract (especially esophagus and proximal stomach) and show some morphologic overlap with spindle cell GIST. Leiomyomas are well-circumscribed and are comprised of intersecting fascicles of brightly eosinophilic spindle cells having blunt-ended (ie, cigar-shaped) nuclei (**Figure 8.23A, B**). Fascicles cut in cross-section may resemble the morphology of epithelioid GIST. Tumors are positive for SMA, desmin, and caldesmon, and negative for KIT and DOG1. The spindle cell tumors in GIST tend to be less brightly eosinophilic.

When encountering the differential diagnosis in an esophageal tumor, leiomyoma should be favored as spindle cell GIST in the esophagus is rare. The presence of numerous intratumoral KIT-positive mast cells and interstitial cells of Cajal within esophageal mural leiomyomas (which may be mistaken for KIT-positive tumor cells) is a diagnostic pitfall (**Figure 8.23C**) (332).

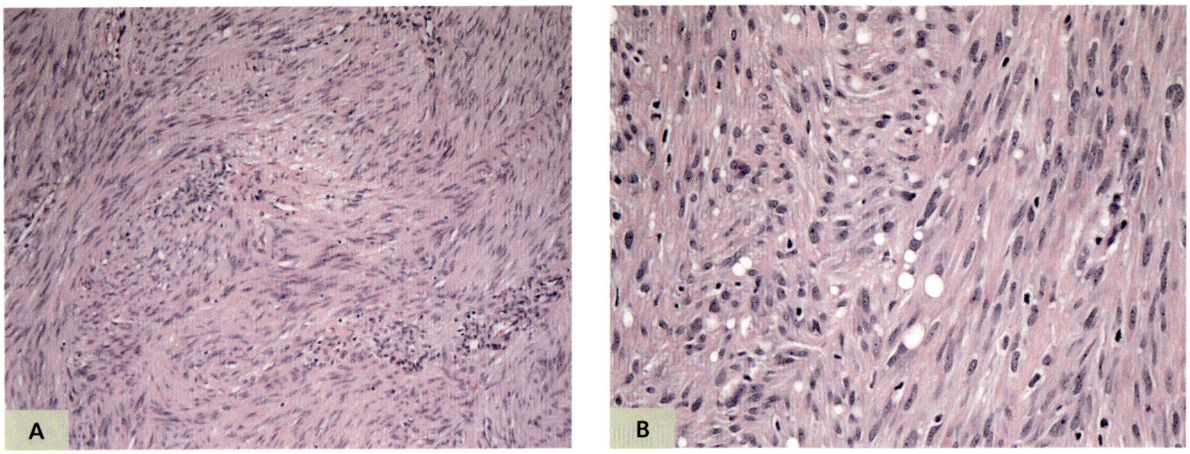

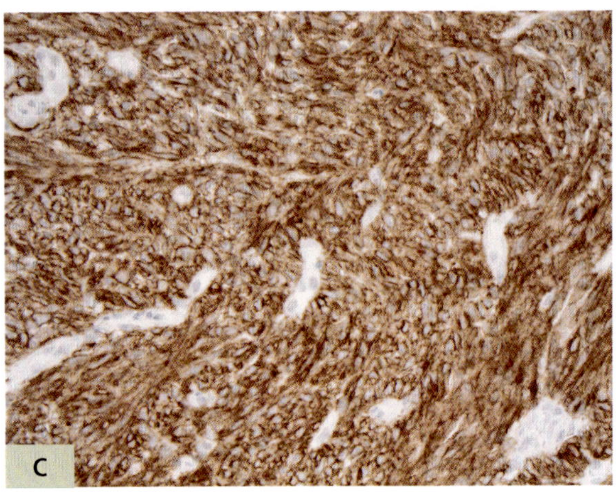

FIGURE 8.22 Spindle cell gastrointestinal stromal tumor (GIST) shows a uniform population of spindle cells with ovoid nuclei and palely eosinophilic syncytial cytoplasm (A). Paranuclear vacuoles are commonly seen in gastric tumors (B). DOG1 is diffusely positive in GIST (C).

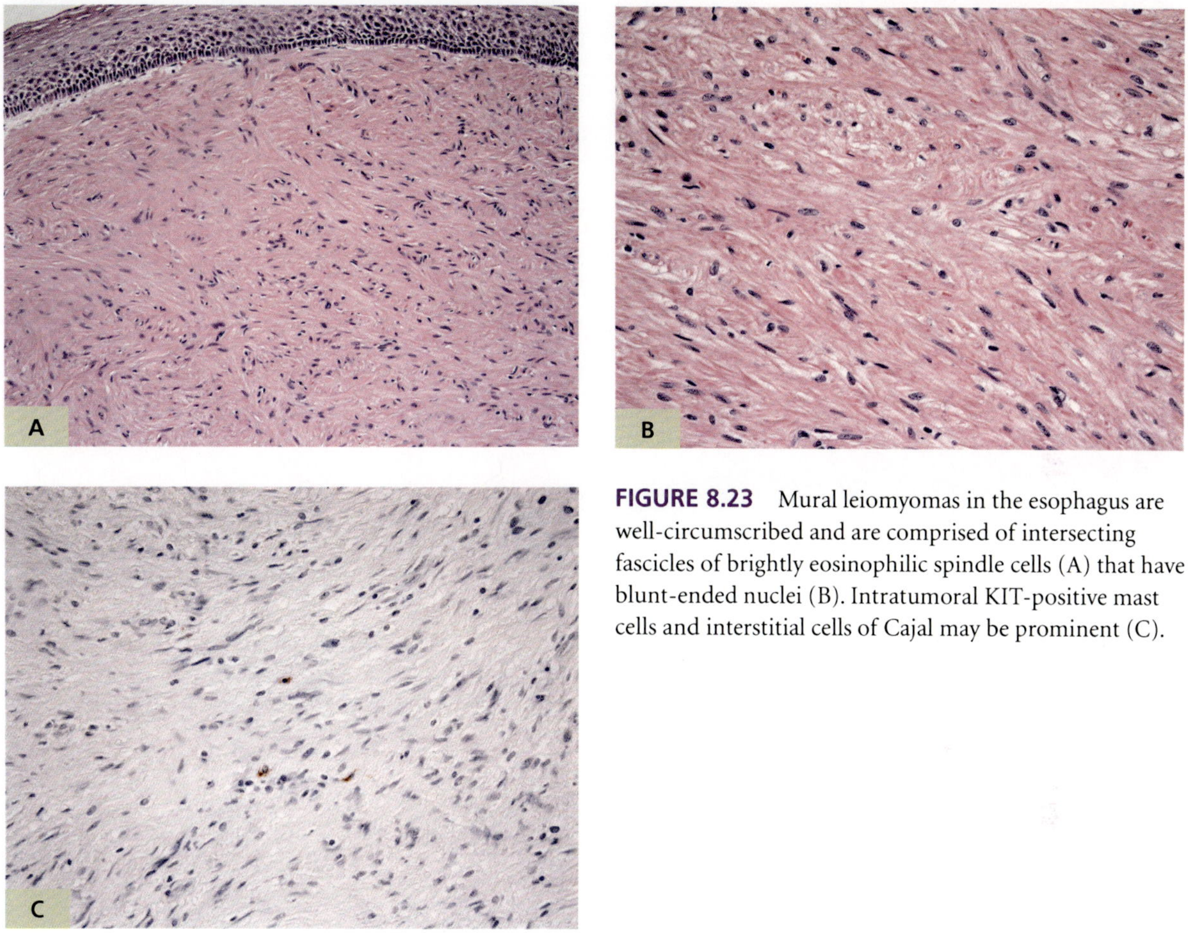

FIGURE 8.23 Mural leiomyomas in the esophagus are well-circumscribed and are comprised of intersecting fascicles of brightly eosinophilic spindle cells (A) that have blunt-ended nuclei (B). Intratumoral KIT-positive mast cells and interstitial cells of Cajal may be prominent (C).

9 Mimics of Osseous Neoplasms

- MYOSITIS OSSIFICANS
- GIANT CELL REPARATIVE GRANULOMA
- GIANT CELL TUMOR OF BONE
- ANEURYSMAL BONE CYST
- OSTEOID OSTEOMA AND OSTEOBLASTOMA
- SUBUNGAL EXOSTOSIS
- BIZARRE PAROSTEAL OSTEOCHONDROMATOUS PROLIFERATION
- OSTEOCHONDROMA
- FIBROUS DYSPLASIA
- DESMOPLASTIC FIBROMA

Evaluation of primary osseous neoplasms (and extra-osseous tumors with bone formation) requires careful correlation of histologic findings with clinical and radiographic data. Many primary bone tumors are strictly defined by clinicopathologic features and anatomic distribution; in the vast majority of cases, radiographic features correlate well with benignity or malignancy. Many benign tumors, typically characterized by slow growth, are well-circumscribed with a sclerotic periphery on radiographs; in contrast, malignant tumors show a permeative or destructive growth pattern, corresponding to infiltrative margins on histology. The clinical context informs the differential diagnosis. Conventional osteosarcoma is more common in males between the second and fourth decades, and is usually centered in the metaphysis. Secondary osteosarcoma can arise in the setting of Paget disease or after radiation therapy.

The diagnosis of osteosarcoma is based on the presence of osteoid matrix production by tumor cells, so-called "malignant" osteoid. The osteoid appears intimately associated with tumor cells (usually having high grade cytological features), and has a lace-like delicate quality (**Figure 9.1A, B**). Mineralization is variable, and osteoid may be present as trabeculae. Tumors having extensive

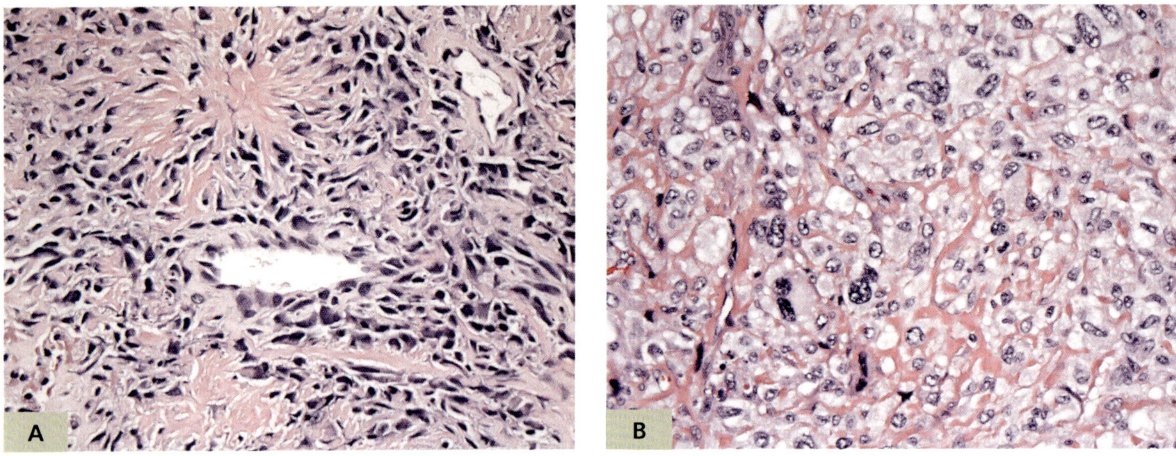

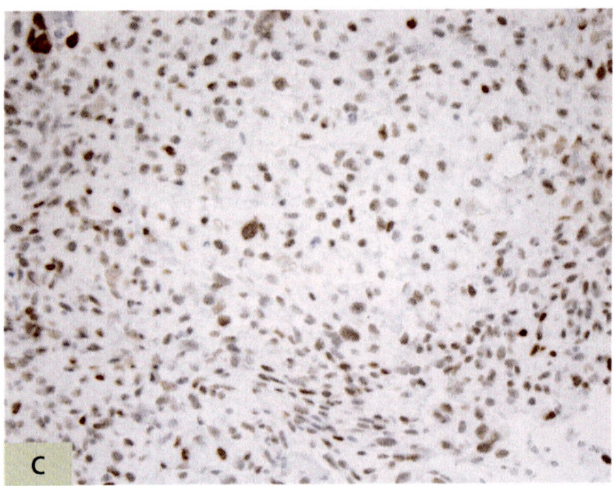

FIGURE 9.1 Osteosarcoma is characterized by osteoid matrix production by malignant tumor cells (A); the malignant osteoid is dense and surrounds tumor cells with a lace-like quality (B). Osteoblastic differentiation can be confirmed by SATB2 positivity (C).

stromal hyalinization resembling osteoid deposition can mimic osteosarcoma. Immunohistochemistry for SATB2 may be helpful in confirming osteoblastic differentiation in this context, though nuclear staining is seen in both benign and malignant bone-forming tumors (**Figure 9.1C**) (333). Osseous metaplasia is a common feature of both benign and malignant neoplasms, and several sarcoma types (eg, dedifferentiated liposarcoma, malignant peripheral nerve sheath tumor [MPNST]) can show heterologous chondro-osseous differentiation that mimics osteosarcoma or chondrosarcoma. Notably, there are several subtypes of osteosarcoma that are characterized by low-grade cytology, including parosteal osteosarcoma and low-grade central osteosarcoma.

MYOSITIS OSSIFICANS

Myositis ossificans is a benign tumor that arises most commonly in the deep-soft tissue of the extremities and truncal region of young adults. Tumors often develop over a short period of time (sometimes with a reported history of trauma) and can be associated with pain; approximately a third of cases spontaneously regress. A characteristic peripheral, eggshell-like rim of delicate calcification encircling an area of lucency often enables recognition via radiographic studies. On histologic examination, an overall appearance of zonation is evident at low power, where there is mature woven bone at the periphery with more immature bone centrally (**Figure 9.2A**). In the central areas of the lesion, the immature bone is associated with hemorrhagic changes, a cellular proliferation of spindled myofibroblasts, and osteoclast-like giant cells (**Figure 9.2A**). The spindle cell component resembles nodular fasciitis, growing in loose fascicles, and similarly can exhibit mitotic activity (although atypical mitoses are absent). Osteoblasts rimming the edges of bony trabeculae are a common feature (**Figure 9.2C**).

The central areas of myofibroblastic proliferation and immature bone may lead to concern for extraskeletal osteosarcoma, which may be difficult to distinguish in small biopsy samples. In contrast to conventional osteosarcoma of bone, extraskeletal osteosarcoma tends to affect an older patient population, including

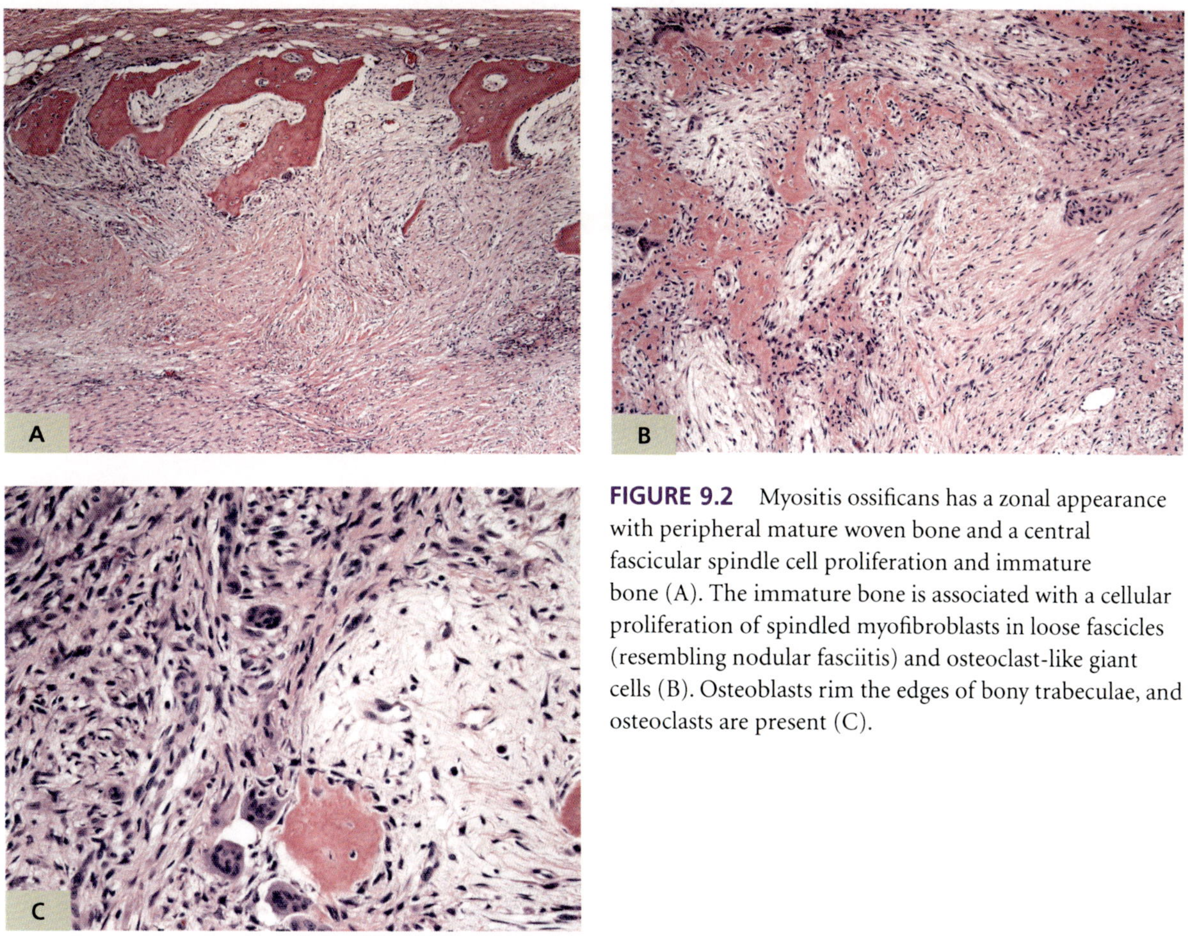

FIGURE 9.2 Myositis ossificans has a zonal appearance with peripheral mature woven bone and a central fascicular spindle cell proliferation and immature bone (A). The immature bone is associated with a cellular proliferation of spindled myofibroblasts in loose fascicles (resembling nodular fasciitis) and osteoclast-like giant cells (B). Osteoblasts rim the edges of bony trabeculae, and osteoclasts are present (C).

those with prior local radiation therapy. Correlation with radiographic studies can exclude the possibility of soft tissue extension of a primary osseous osteosarcoma. Cytologic atypia is absent in myositis ossificans; the characteristic pattern of zonation is a particularly helpful diagnostic feature for myositis ossificans.

GIANT CELL REPARATIVE GRANULOMA

Giant cell reparative granulomas are benign proliferations that arise predominantly in the head and neck in either intraosseous mandibular or maxillary sites (termed central giant cell reparative granuloma) or adjacent sinonasal or oral soft tissues (termed peripheral giant cell reparative granuloma). Tumors are most common in women below the age of 30 years. Central, intraosseous tumors radiographically appear as lytic lesions. Tumors are comprised of aggregates and sheets of osteoclast-like giant cells, fibrous stroma and areas of hemorrhage (**Figure 9.3**). Bland fibroblast-type cells comprise the stromal component; giant cells tend to cluster around the areas of hemorrhage. Although mitoses may be frequent, atypical mitotic forms and cytologic atypia are lacking. Curettage is the treatment of choice; central tumors are more likely to recur (up to 15%) than peripheral giant cell reparative granulomas, which rarely recur.

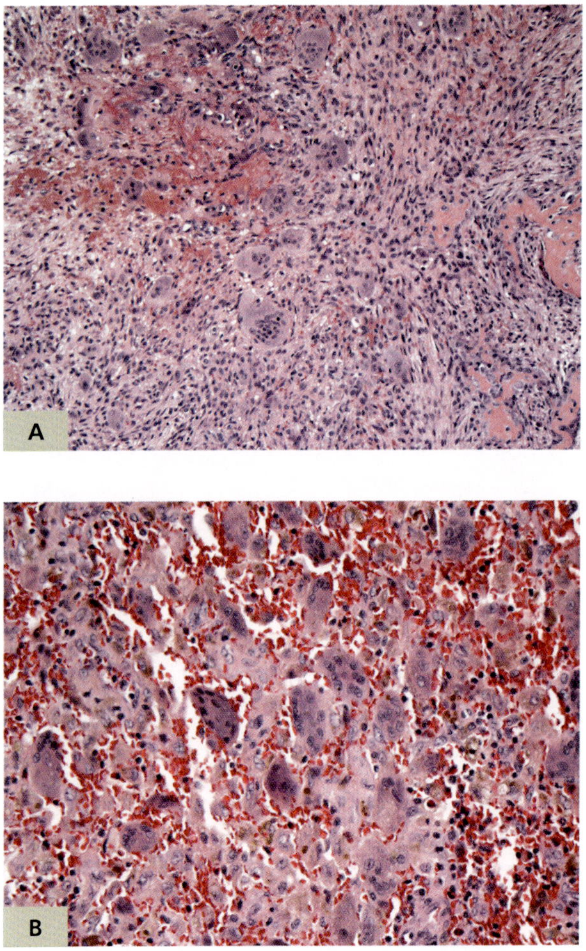

FIGURE 9.3 Giant cell reparative granuloma may be intraosseous (A) and is comprised of numerous osteoclast-like giant cells, bland fibroblasts, and areas of hemorrhage (B).

Brown tumor of hyperparathyroidism is nearly morphologically identical to giant cell reparative granuloma; the diagnosis of brown tumor must be confirmed by either clinical symptoms or laboratory features of hyperparathyroidism (increased calcium, phosphate, alkaline phosphatase, and parathyroid hormone). In addition to appearing as a lytic mass on imaging studies (often in the vertebral bodies), there is usually radiographic evidence of diffuse osteopenia in the phalanges and skull. A distinctive feature of brown tumor is the presence of active bone resorption, with osteoclasts arranged around bony trabeculae in adjacent normal bone. Careful clinical and radiographic correlation is required for accurate diagnosis.

Giant cell reparative granuloma may also mimic aneurysmal bone cyst (ABC), giant cell tumor of bone, or osteosarcoma. Zonation of giant cells around areas of hemorrhage favors giant cell reparative granuloma, and the absence of cytologic atypia and "malignant" osteoid excludes osteosarcoma. Notably, approximately half of gnathic osteosarcomas are chondroblastic in type (334). Anatomic location is helpful: giant cell tumor of bone arises in the epiphysis of skeletally mature young adults, and ABC is most frequent in the metaphysis of long bones in young adults. Confirmation of the defining *USP6* gene rearrangement is diagnostic of ABC.

GIANT CELL TUMOR OF BONE

Giant cell tumor of bone is a locally aggressive neoplasm of uncertain histogenesis that occurs in young adults (more often in women) with mature skeletons (ie, closed epiphyseal growth plates) during the third and fourth decades. Most tumors arise in the epiphysis of long bones, although sacral tumors are not infrequent. The typical radiographic appearance is a purely lytic, poorly defined lesion extending to the end of the bone. Grossly, most giant cell tumors are dark brown-red fleshy masses with occasional cystic areas. Tumors are comprised of a mononuclear cell population of round-to-ovoid cells, with osteoclast-type giant cells interspersed uniformly among the mononuclear cells (**Figure 9.4**).

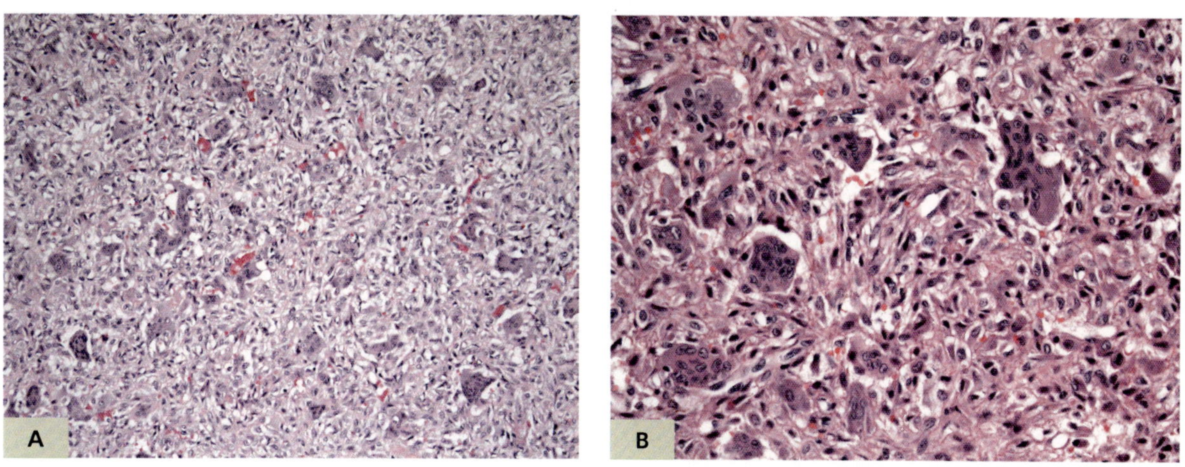

FIGURE 9.4 Giant cell tumor of bone typically arises in the epiphysis of skeletally mature long bones. Tumors are comprised of a mononuclear ovoid-to-round cell population and interspersed osteoclast-type giant cells (A). The mononuclear cells may show fascicular growth, and giant cells may have numerous nuclei that resemble those in the mononuclear cell component (B).

Aggregates of foamy macrophages are common. The mononuclear cells may occasionally appear spindled with storiform growth; however, cytologic atypia and pleomorphism are absent. At the interface with soft tissue, there is sometimes formation of an ossified peripheral shell. Foci of lymphovascular invasion may be seen (but do not confer aggressive behavior). Giant cell tumors of bone have a significant risk of local recurrence. Metastases of histologically benign giant cell tumors occasionally occur.

Histologically, giant cell tumors may resemble ABC, a benign neoplasm with a small risk of recurrence (see section *"Aneurysmal Bone Cyst"*); correlation with radiographic studies may be helpful. Some cases of giant cell tumor show bone formation, which may be worrisome for osteosarcoma. However, the bony trabeculae in giant cell tumor appear reactive (often rimmed by osteoblasts) and lace-like osteoid is absent; overt features of malignancy (nuclear atypia, atypical mitotic figures, necrosis) are absent. Correlation with clinical and radiographic data is helpful, as most osteosarcomas arise in the metaphysis.

ANEURYSMAL BONE CYST

ABC may occur as primary tumors in bone or less often in soft tissue. Tumors usually arise during the first two decades in life, and are slightly more common in females. ABC most commonly arises in the metaphysis of long bones and in the dorsal aspect of vertebrae. Tumors appear nearly purely lytic, asymmetric lesions on radiographs, and may be variably well-circumscribed or infiltrative. Fluid–fluid levels are characteristic, and are best appreciated on MRI. Tumors are cavitary with thin septa separating pools of blood or serum. The pools are of varying sizes, and the septa lack an epithelial or endothelial lining. Within the septa are spindle cells, osteoclast-like giant cells, and capillaries (**Figure 9.5**). Reactive woven bone is also present within the septa, rimmed by osteoblasts. Although the spindle cells are often mitotically active, atypical forms and cytologic atypia are lacking. The solid variant of ABC has areas of more solid growth of spindle cells (**Figure 9.6**). Most cases of primary ABC are characterized by translocations involving chromosome 17p13, which encodes the *USP6* gene; the most common fusion partner is *CDH11* encoded on 16q22 (335). Secondary ABC, which may be observed in many tumor types, including fibrous dysplasia, giant cell tumor of bone, and chondroblastoma, lacks *USP6* gene rearrangements. ABCs are benign, but may recur if incompletely excised.

Telangiectatic osteosarcoma is a rare subtype of osteosarcoma that has many overlapping radiographic and morphologic features with ABC. Tumors appear lytic and are usually centered on the metaphysis of long bones. They similarly appear to be cavitary hemorrhagic lesions, and the tumor cell population may be obscured by hemorrhage and superimposed reactive changes. However, recognition of the cytologically malignant tumor cells within the fibrous septa is diagnostic of telangiectatic osteosarcoma (**Figure 9.7**).

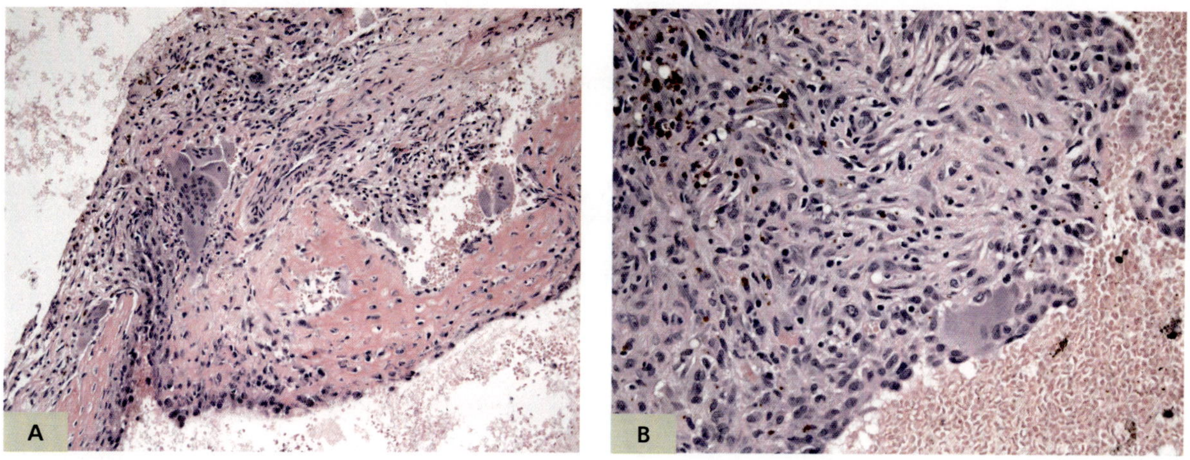

FIGURE 9.5 Aneurysmal bone cysts are cavitary with numerous pools of blood and serum separated by thin septa, within which are spindle cells, reactive bone, osteoclast-like giant cells, and capillaries (A). The spindle cell component may appear fascicular (B).

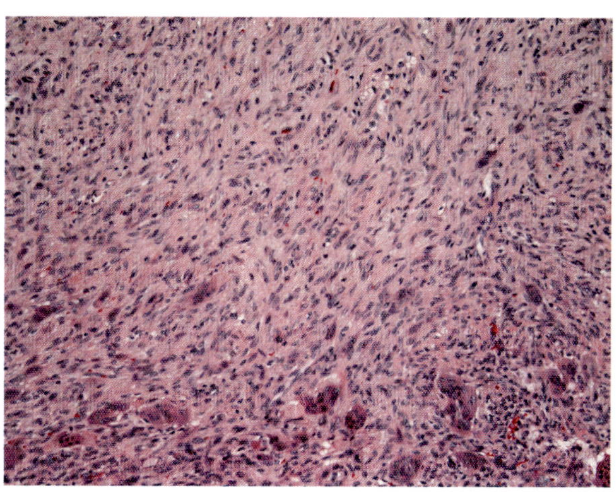

FIGURE 9.6 The solid variant of aneurysmal bone cyst has a predominance of solid growth of spindle cells.

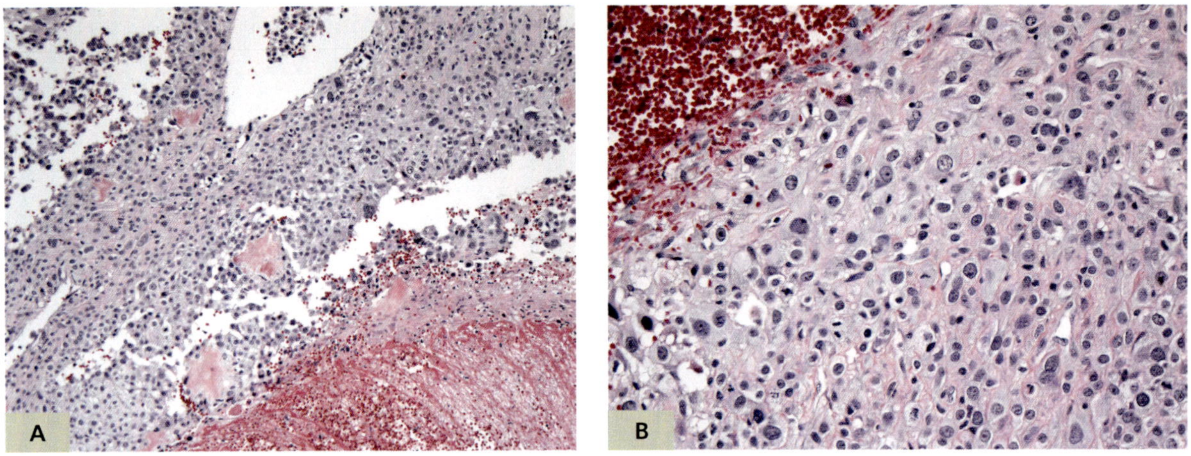

FIGURE 9.7 Telangiectatic osteosarcomas are cavitary hemorrhagic lesions (A). Cytologically malignant cells are present within the fibrous septa (B).

OSTEOID OSTEOMA AND OSTEOBLASTOMA

Osteoblastoma is a benign tumor that is more common in men and occurs most frequently in the spine. Osteoid osteomas are histologically identical lesions, and are defined as lesions smaller than 2 cm; most occur in the metaphysis or diaphysis of long bones and tend to be cortical based. Most osteoid osteomas are painful and are treated by either ablative therapy or resection, whereas osteoblastomas are resected. Recurrence is rare after complete resection. While radiographs of osteoid osteoma and osteoblastoma tend to show extensive sclerosis and a characteristically radiolucent nidus, it should be noted that a subset of osteoblastomas may show aggressive radiographic features.

Tumors are well circumscribed. Histologically, tumors are composed of anastomosing trabeculae of mature bone rimmed by a single layer of osteoblasts (**Figure 9.8**). Within the intertrabecular spaces is a fibrovascular stroma with bland appearing spindle cells. The central nidus is formed by the anastomosing unmineralized woven bone; toward the periphery the osteoid is mineralized and merges into normal host bone. The zonation of the bony trabeculae is especially distinctive for osteoblastoma.

The distinction between osteoblastoma and osteosarcoma may be challenging, especially in core needle biopsy samples. Osteosarcoma is characterized by a malignant tumor cell population, and the presence of solid growth of malignant cells with production of lace-like osteoid and permeation into pre-existing normal bone are diagnostic of osteosarcoma. Osteoblastoma does not show permeation into adjacent bone, but rather the bony trabeculae merge seamlessly at the periphery.

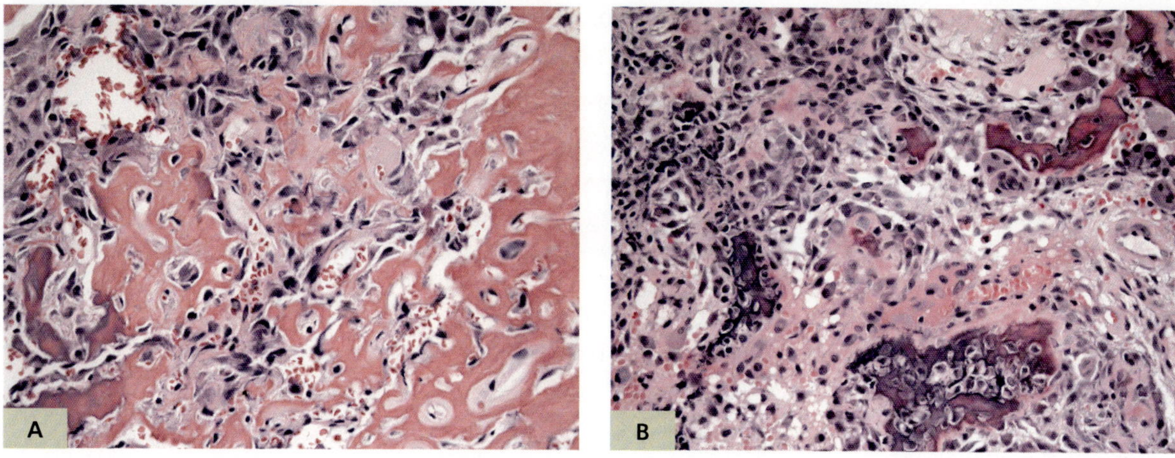

FIGURE 9.8 Osteoblastoma is comprised of anastomosing trabeculae of mature bone rimmed by a single layer of osteoblasts (A). Osteoblasts are numerous within a fibrovascular stroma (B).

SUBUNGAL EXOSTOSIS

Subungual exostosis is a benign proliferation that arises in the distal phalanx of the great toe of young adults, often associated with swelling, pain, and ulceration of the overlying skin. It is characterized by the translocation t(X;6)(q24-q26;q15-21)(336,337). Lesions appear as outgrowths of trabecular bone, but in contrast to osteochondroma, subungual exostosis lacks continuity with the underlying medullary cavity. Tumors show a transition from a bland spindle cell population to hyaline cartilage to trabecular bone (**Figure 9.9**). The spindle cells fill the intertrabecular spaces, and lack cytologic atypia. The proliferation of

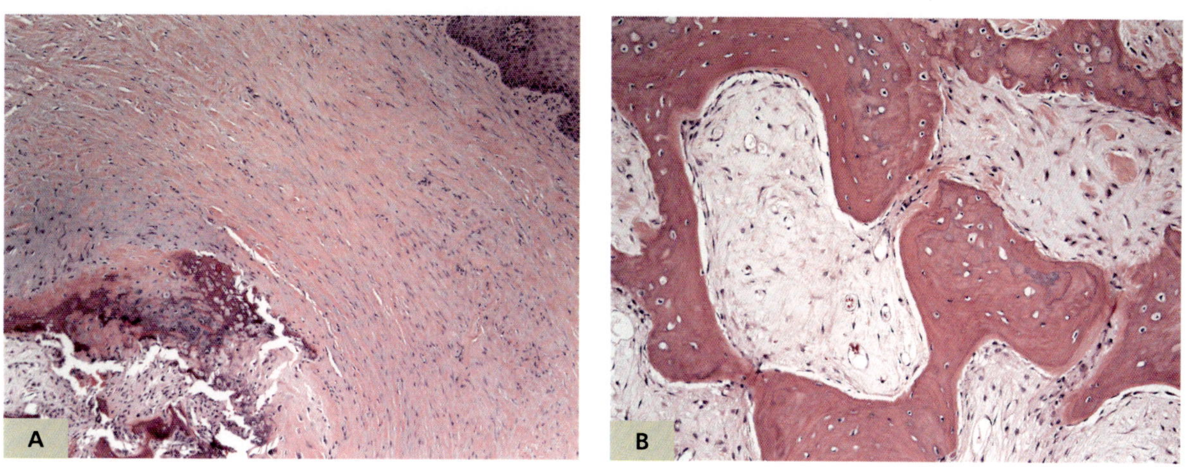

FIGURE 9.9 Subungual exostosis usually arises in the distal phalanx of the great toe, and shows a transition from a bland spindle cell population to hyaline cartilage to trabecular bone (A). A bland spindle cell proliferation fills the intertrabecular spaces (B); tumors are separate from the underlying medullary cavity.

spindle cells and bony trabeculae may mimic osteosarcoma; however, the distinct clinicopathologic features and absence of atypia (as well as the rarity of osteosarcoma on the distal digits) allow for straightforward distinction in most cases.

BIZARRE PAROSTEAL OSTEOCHONDROMATOUS PROLIFERATION

Bizarre parosteal osteochondromatous proliferation (BPOP) is a benign osteochondromatous neoplasm characterized by the translocation t(1;17)(q32;q21) (338). BPOP arises most commonly in the upper and lower digits, but can also occur in long bones in young adults. Tumors are attached by a bony stalk with a lobulated cartilaginous cap, but do not show continuity with the underlying cortical surface. BPOP is comprised of a haphazard and disorganized arrangement of a bland spindle cell population, hypercellular cartilaginous islands, and bony trabeculae (**Figure 9.10**). The chondrocytes are somewhat enlarged and show a distinctive blue-tinted mineralization (ie, "blue bone"). Recurrences are common.

The cortical-based location and admixture of hypercellular and enlarged chondrocytes admixed with osteoid and spindle cells of BPOP can mimic periosteal osteosarcoma. Periosteal osteosarcoma is a rare variant of osteosarcoma that arises on the surface of the bone, and occurs predominantly in diaphyseal location. In contrast to the characteristic involvement of the digits of BPOP, periosteal osteosarcoma occurs most frequently in the distal femur and tibia. Periosteal osteosarcoma appears as an intermediate grade osteosarcoma, with an atypical cartilaginous component transitioning to osteoid

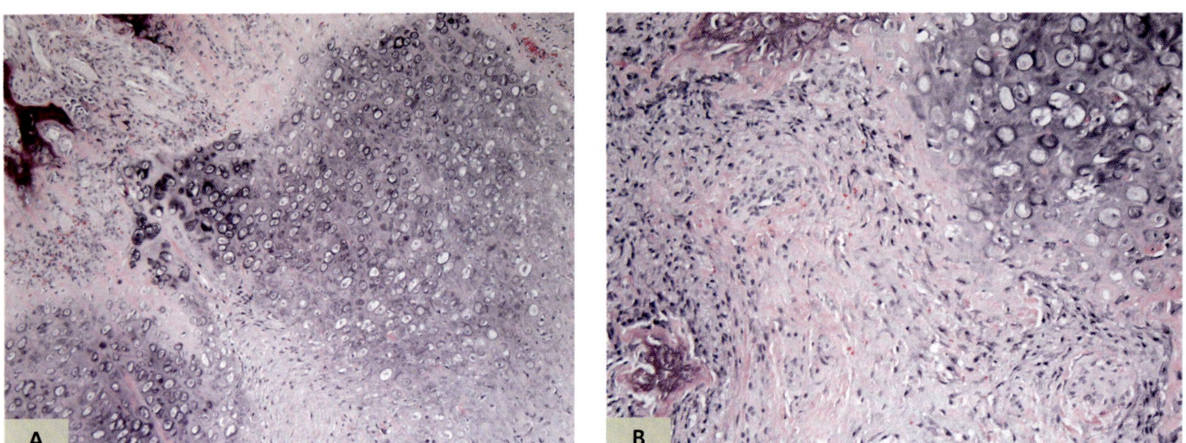

FIGURE 9.10 Bizarre parosteal osteochondromatous proliferation is comprised of a disorganized arrangement of a bland spindle cell population, hypercellular cartilaginous islands, and bony trabeculae (A). The enlarged chondrocytes show a distinctive blue-tinted mineralization pattern (B).

formation (**Figure 9.11**). In addition to the contrasting clinicopathologic features, BPOP can be distinguished by the absence of cytologic atypia and the dark-blue tinctorial quality of the cartilage.

OSTEOCHONDROMA

Osteochondroma, one of the most common benign primary bone tumors, most commonly arise in the metaphysis of long bones. Patients are typically young adults, and men are slightly more commonly affected than women. Sporadic osteochondromas have homozygous deletion of *EXT1* gene (339), and germline inactivating mutations or deletions of *EXT1*, *EXT2*, and *EXT3* genes characterize multiple osteochondromas, an autosomal dominant disease (340). Osteochondromas are chondroid neoplasms that appear as mushroom-like masses growing at an angle from the bone of origin. Radiographs demonstrate continuity between the tumor and underlying bone of both the cortical surface and the medullary cavity. Approximately 15% of patients have multiple lesions. Osteochondromas have a cartilaginous "cap" (less than 2.0 cm in maximum thickness) with benign-appearing chondrocytes often arranged in vertical columns as they undergo maturation toward the base and underlying marrow (**Figure 9.12A**). The maturing chondrocytes undergo endochondral ossification to form trabeculae, often appearing regular in size and spacing within the marrow (**Figure 9.12B**). Osteochondromas are benign, and are surgically resected when large and symptomatic.

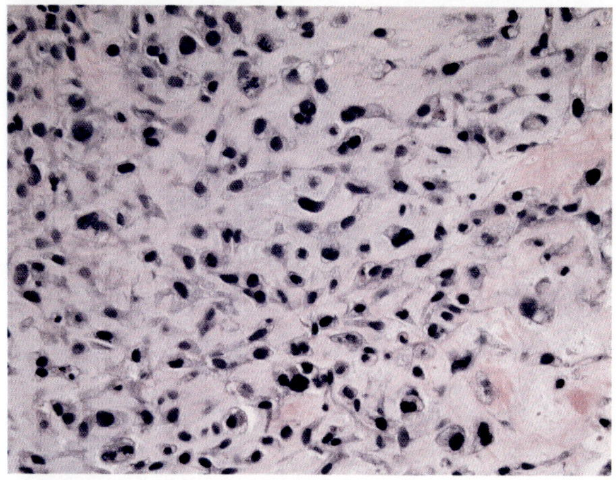

FIGURE 9.11 The rare variant periosteal osteosarcoma arises on the diaphyseal surface of the bone, most frequently in the distal femur and tibia. Periosteal osteosarcoma is composed of an atypical cartilaginous component transitioning to osteoid formation.

Osteochondromas may share morphologic features with benign entities such as BPOP and subungual exostosis, but are usually not a source of diagnostic confusion as osteochondromas are rare in the small bones of the hands and feet. Osteochondroma may mimic parosteal osteosarcoma. Parosteal osteosarcoma is a low-grade osteosarcoma that arises on the surface of long bones (predominantly on the posterior femur) of young adults, and women are affected slightly more than men. Tumors often show circumferential growth over the underlying bone, and appear as a heavily ossified mass attached to the cortex without invasion into the medullary

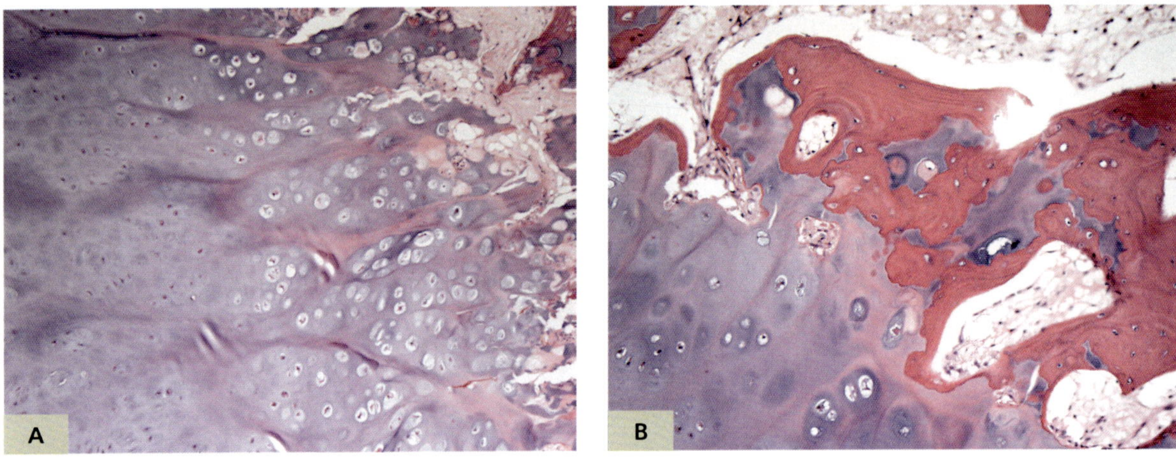

FIGURE 9.12 Osteochondroma has a cartilaginous "cap" with chondrocytes arranged in vertical columns that undergo maturation toward the base and underlying marrow (A). The maturing chondrocytes undergo endochondral ossification to form bony trabeculae (B).

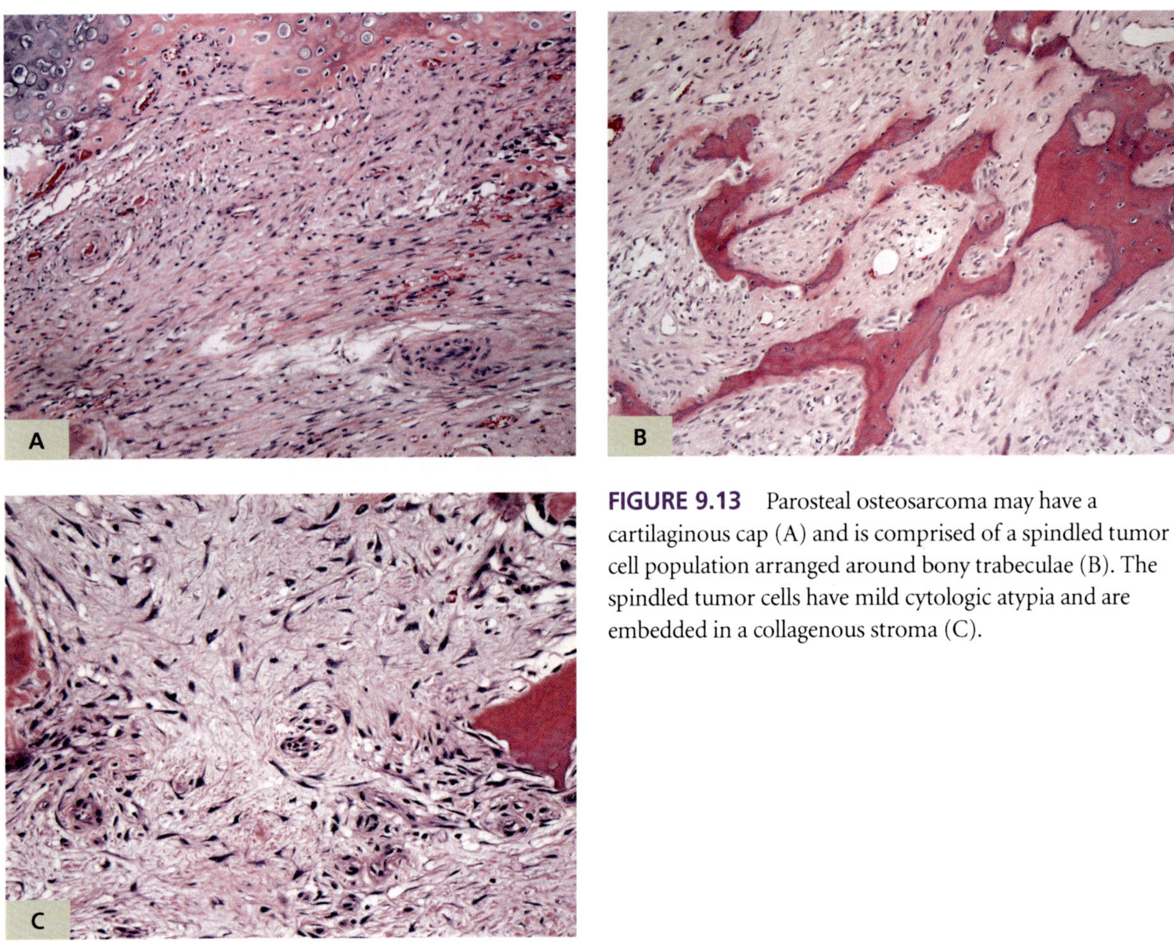

FIGURE 9.13 Parosteal osteosarcoma may have a cartilaginous cap (A) and is comprised of a spindled tumor cell population arranged around bony trabeculae (B). The spindled tumor cells have mild cytologic atypia and are embedded in a collagenous stroma (C).

space. Approximately 25% of tumors have a cartilaginous cap; however, underlying the cap is a spindle cell tumor population embedded in a collagenous stroma (**Figure 9.13**). The spindled tumor cells show relatively mild atypia and little mitotic activity but show infiltrative growth into adjacent soft tissue. Parosteal osteosarcoma is characterized by 12q13-15 amplification (which encodes *MDM2* and *CDK4*)(341). Immunohistochemistry for MDM2 and CDK4 is positive in the majority of parosteal osteosarcomas and is a helpful diagnostic tool (342).

FIBROUS DYSPLASIA

Fibrous dysplasia is a benign neoplasm that primarily affects patients during the first and second decades. Fibrous dysplasia may occur as monostotic or polyostotic disease, though presentation as solitary lesions is most common. Femur and craniofacial bones are the most commonly affected sites. Tumors are benign and prognosis is excellent when complete resection is achieved, although fibrous dysplasia may lead to secondary mass effects such as skeletal deformities. On radiology, tumors commonly appear as well-circumscribed lucent lesions with peripheral sclerosis and ground-glass matrix. Tumors are comprised of a patternless expansile growth of spindle cells and a network of irregular trabeculae of woven bone, centered within the medullary cavity. The trabeculae lack osteoblastic rimming, and show varying curvilinear and branching shapes (**Figure 9.14**). The spindle cell population appears fibroblastic and does not show cytologic atypia or significant mitotic activity. Fibrous dysplasia is associated with point mutations of the *GNAS* gene. Polyostotic disease is seen as part of the rare inherited diseases Mazabraud syndrome (with soft tissue myxomas) and McCune-Albright syndrome (with skin hyperpigmentation and endocrine abnormalities). Sarcomatous transformation is exceedingly rare.

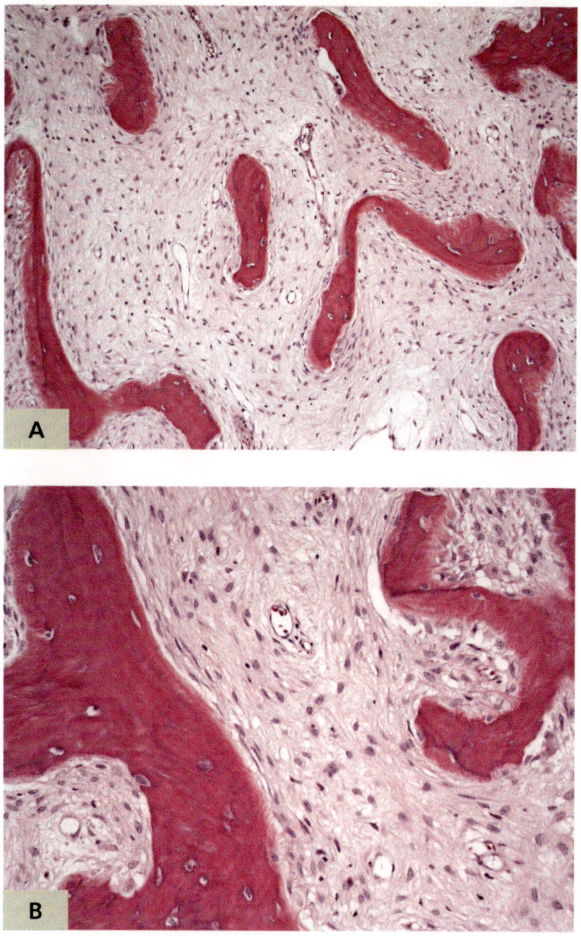

FIGURE 9.14 Fibrous dysplasia is comprised of a patternless expansile growth of bland spindle cells and a network of irregular trabeculae of woven bone (A). The bony trabeculae exhibit curvilinear and branching shapes and lack osteoblastic rimming (B).

Fibrous dysplasia has overlapping features with many benign neoplasms, including osteofibrous dysplasia and desmoplastic fibroma (see section "*Desmoplastic Fibroma*"). Osteofibrous dysplasia arises in the cortex of the proximal or mid-tibia in the same patient demographic as fibrous dysplasia, but the bony trabeculae are surrounded by osteoblasts and keratin-positive cells are found scattered in the fibrous areas (**Figure 9.15**).

It is important to distinguish fibrous dysplasia from low-grade central osteosarcoma, which occurs in the medullary cavity in the metaphysis of long bones (most commonly lower extremities). Radiographically, lesions appear lytic with partial adjacent sclerosis and varying features of permeation (indicative of slow but infiltrative growth). Tumors are comprised of a hypocellular fibroblastic spindle cell population with mild cytologic atypia and low mitotic activity (**Figure 9.16**). Atypical mitotic figures are rare, but when present, favor osteosarcoma. The spindle cells are arranged in loose fascicles and infiltrate pre-existing bone or adjacent soft tissue. Osteoid production is variable and frequently mimics the irregular curvilinear and branching shapes of fibrous dysplasia. The infiltrative growth is specific for low-grade central osteosarcoma; in

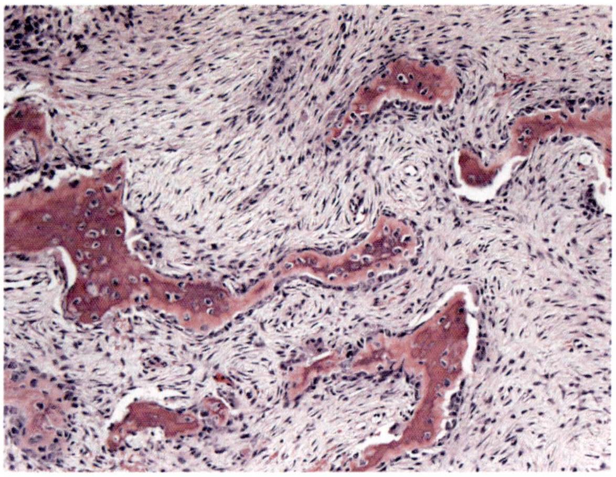

FIGURE 9.15 Osteofibrous dysplasia has bland spindle cells growing around bony trabeculae, which are surrounded by osteoblasts.

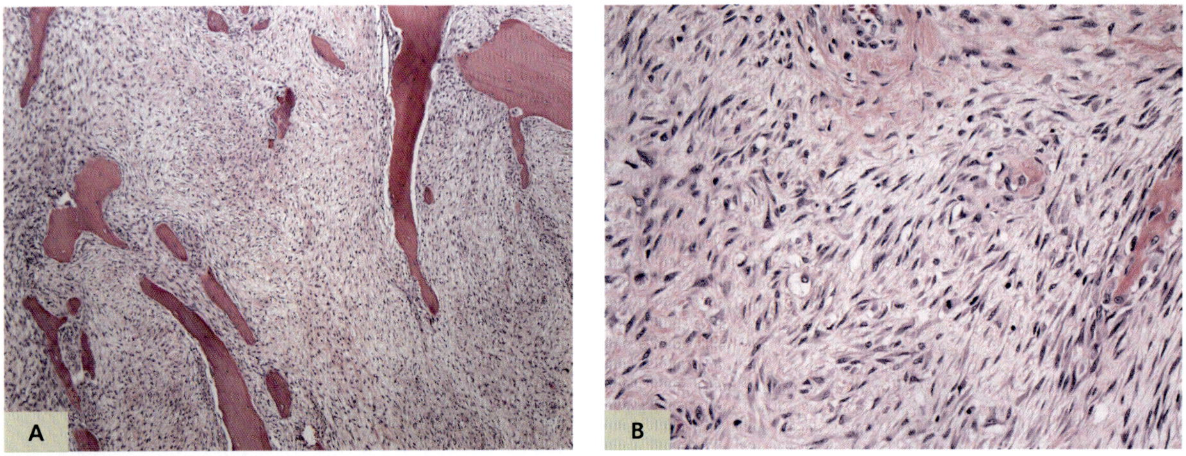

FIGURE 9.16 Low-grade central osteosarcomas are comprised of a hypocellular fibroblastic spindle cell population infiltrating between bony trabeculae (A), which is characterized by mild cytologic atypia and mitotic activity (B).

contrast, fibrous dysplasia is well-circumscribed. Similar to parosteal osteosarcoma, low-grade central osteosarcoma is associated with 12q13-15 amplification (343), and MDM2 and CDK4 are useful diagnostic markers (344). Although the prognosis of low-grade central osteosarcoma is excellent, with over 90% survival at five years, recurrence and progression (dedifferentiation) to high grade osteosarcoma is reported in 15% of patients.

DESMOPLASTIC FIBROMA

Desmoplastic fibroma is a rare lesion that has been reported in all skeletal locations, most commonly in the mandible, and appears morphologically similar to desmoid-type fibromatosis. The radiologic features may be misleading, appearing lytic and expansile (but nonmineralizing). The spindled tumor cells are arranged in long fascicles and whorls in a collagenous stroma; atypia is absent and mitoses are rare (**Figure 9.17**). Despite its likeness to desmoid-type fibromatosis, desmoplastic fibroma lacks *CTNNB1* mutations and immunohistochemistry for β-catenin is negative. Desmoplastic fibroma is a benign but locally aggressive neoplasm; recurrence is frequent.

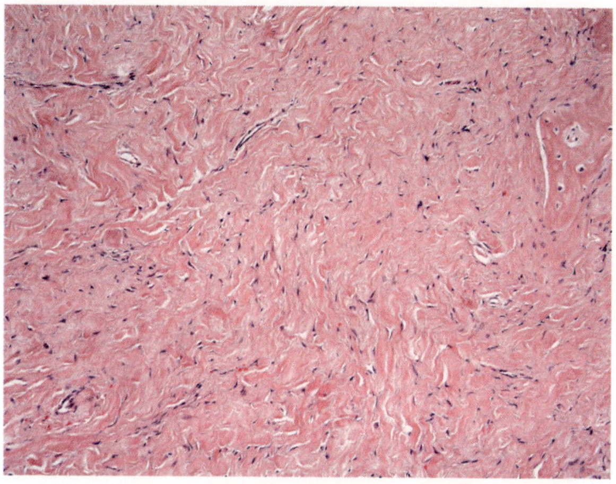

FIGURE 9.17 Desmoplastic fibroma appears morphologically similar to desmoid-type fibromatosis, with spindled tumor cells arranged in long fascicles and whorls in a collagenous stroma.

Desmoplastic fibroma may mimic the spindle cell component of low-grade central osteosarcoma; it may be difficult to distinguish the two in small biopsies. However, desmoplastic fibroma is not osteogenic, and it lacks cytologic atypia and infiltrative growth. MDM2 and CDK4 immunohistochemical stains will be positive in low-grade central osteosarcoma, but negative in desmoplastic fibroma.

10 Mimics of Cartilaginous Neoplasms

- OSTEOCHONDROMA
- CHONDROMA
- CHONDROMYXOID FIBROMA
- CHONDROBLASTOMA
- BIZARRE PAROSTEAL OSTEOCHONDROMATOUS PROLIFERATION
- SYNOVIAL CHONDROMATOSIS

Similar to osteogenic tumors of bone, the evaluation of cartilaginous neoplasms requires clinicopathologic and radiographic correlation. Patient demographics and tumor site can guide the differential diagnosis, and features such as destructive growth within bone or through the cortex, periosteal reaction, and the presence and distribution of cartilaginous matrix formation (appearing as mineralization) can be assessed on radiographs. Clinical data are informative. For instance, when considering the diagnosis of chondrosarcoma in an unusual location such as the digits, it is helpful to know whether the patient has multiple or prior enchondromas, which may be seen in certain syndromes associated with an increased risk for secondary chondrosarcoma, most frequently Ollier Disease (enchondromatosis) and Maffucci syndrome (enchondromatosis and soft tissue spindle cell hemangiomas).

The most important prognostic predictor for recurrence and metastasis of chondrosarcoma is the histologic grade, which is assigned on a three-tier system based on nuclear size, presence of hyperchromatic nuclei, cellularity, and mitotic count. The most recent World Health Organization (WHO) Classification in 2013 introduced the terminology "atypical cartilaginous tumor" (with analogy to "atypical lipomatous tumor") for grade I chondrosarcoma on the basis that these tumors have an excellent prognosis and show predominantly locally aggressive behavior but essentially no risk of metastasis, with five-year survival of 83% (345,346). Atypical cartilaginous tumor/grade I chondrosarcoma is characterized by moderately cellular tumors with a uniform population of slightly enlarged and occasionally binucleated chondrocytes; mitotic activity is absent (**Figure 10.1**). It can be extremely difficult to distinguish atypical cartilaginous tumor/grade I chondrosarcoma from enchondroma on histologic grounds alone. Thorough tissue sampling and histologic evaluation are also important, as foci of permeative growth into pre-existing bone or soft tissue (**Figure 10.2**) may be limited in extent, and some chondrosarcomas may show coexistence of various histologic grades. Grade II and grade III chondrosarcomas show progressively increased cellularity, nuclear atypia, and mitotic activity; myxoid stroma and hypercellular growth of spindled tumor cells at the edge of lobules are frequent (**Figure 10.3**). Grade II and grade III tumors show worse prognosis, with five-year survival rates of 83% and 43% and metastatic rates of 10% and 71%, respectively (345).

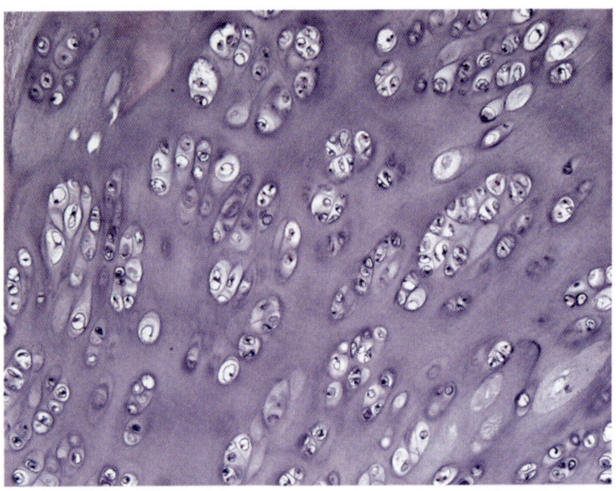

FIGURE 10.1 Atypical cartilaginous tumors/grade I chondrosarcomas are moderately cellular tumors with a relatively uniform population of slightly enlarged and occasionally binucleated chondrocytes that display mild cytologic atypia and show very low (if any) mitotic activity.

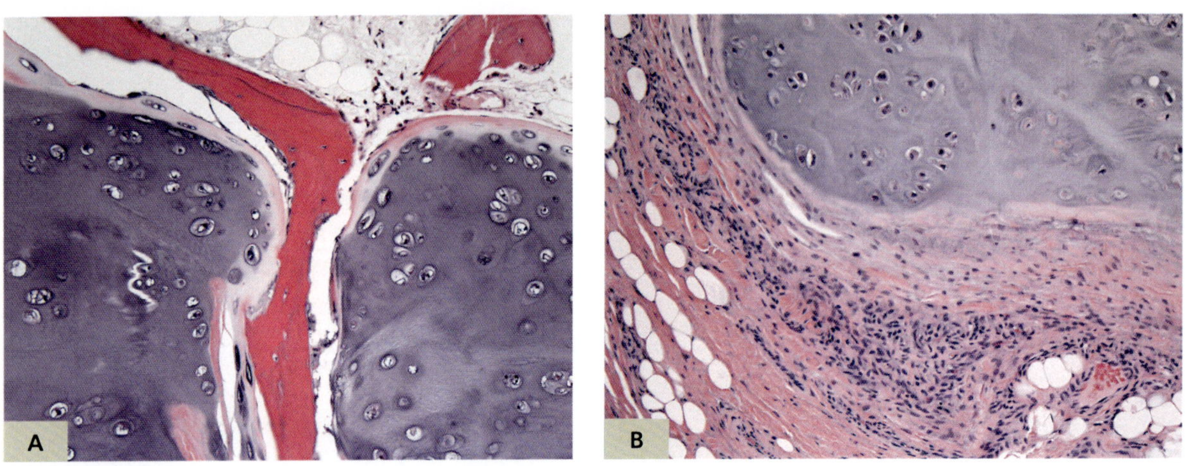

FIGURE 10.2 The diagnosis of atypical cartilaginous tumor/grade I chondrosarcoma requires foci of permeative growth into bone (A) or soft tissue (B).

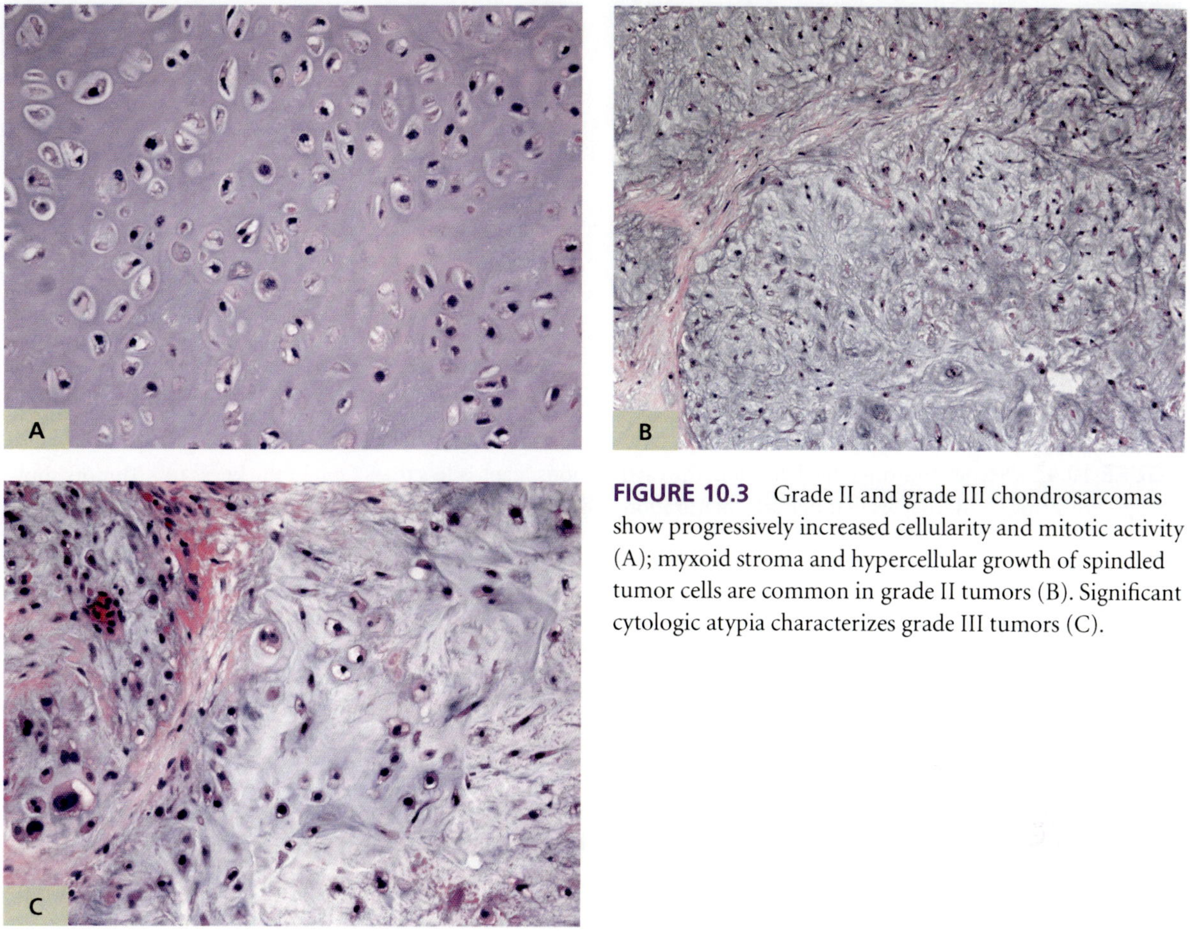

FIGURE 10.3 Grade II and grade III chondrosarcomas show progressively increased cellularity and mitotic activity (A); myxoid stroma and hypercellular growth of spindled tumor cells are common in grade II tumors (B). Significant cytologic atypia characterizes grade III tumors (C).

OSTEOCHONDROMA

Osteochondroma most commonly arises in the metaphysis of long bones in young adults (though they may also arise in the pelvis and scapula). Most cases present as a single lesion, although 15% of patients may have multiple lesions. Osteochondromas appear radiologically as bony pedunculated outgrowth from the bone, with continuity of the cortical surface and medullary space between the tumor and underlying bone. The cartilaginous "cap" is by definition less than 2 cm in thickness and is comprised of benign-appearing chondrocytes that undergo maturation and endochondral ossification to form trabeculae that merge into the marrow (**Figure 10.4**). Homozygous deletion of *EXT1* gene is present in sporadic osteochondromas (339). The autosomal dominant disease multiple osteochondromas (MO) results from germline inactivating mutations or deletions of *EXT1*, *EXT2*, and *EXT3* genes (340).

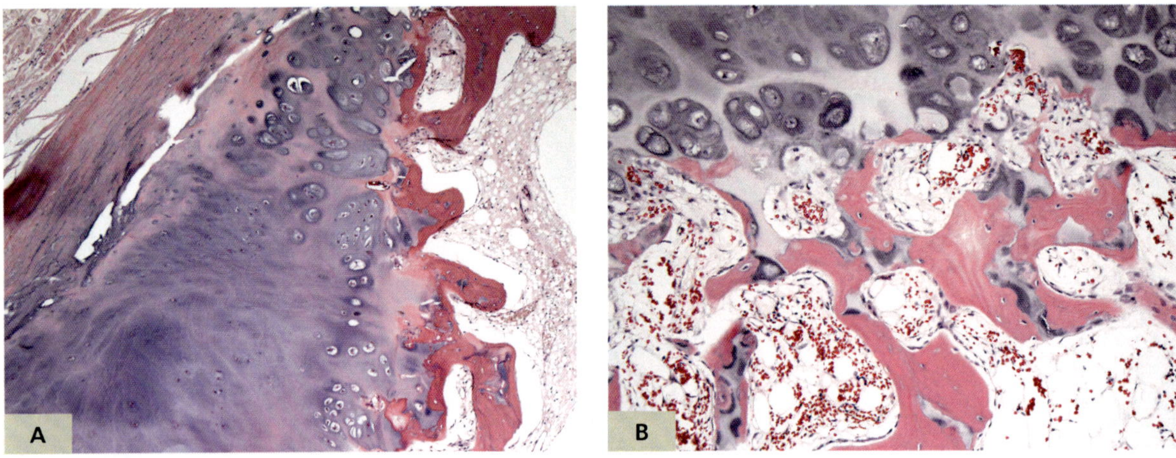

FIGURE 10.4 Osteochondroma. By definition, the cartilaginous "cap" is less than 2 cm in thickness (A). Tumors show benign-appearing chondrocytes that undergo maturation and endochondral ossification to form trabeculae that merge into the medullary cavity (B).

Osteochondromas are benign tumors, and are only surgically resected when tumors become large and symptomatic. However, a small percentage of tumors [1% of solitary tumors, 4%–5% of multifocal disease, and up to 5% of patients with MO (347–349)] undergo malignant transformation to secondary chondrosarcoma. Most cases of secondary chondrosarcoma are well-differentiated, and the distinction between osteochondroma and a low-grade chondrosarcoma may be difficult on histologic grounds and often requires thorough tissue sampling and correlation with radiographic features. The typically thin, smooth cartilaginous cap is usually 2 cm or less in maximum thickness; in the setting of malignant transformation the cap is increased in thickness and appears lobulated with irregular borders. Some cases may show myxoid change. The presence of permeation into bone or adjacent soft tissue is diagnostic of chondrosarcoma.

CHONDROMA

This group of benign tumors of hyaline cartilage may occur in the medullary cavity of the bone (enchondroma), on the surface of the bone (periosteal chondroma), or in soft tissue sites (soft tissue chondroma). Enchondromas and periosteal chondromas may occur in patients of all ages, and are most frequent in the short bones of the hand and in the upper and lower extremities; flat bones and craniofacial tumors are exceptional. Tumors are often in the metaphysis and are either centrally or eccentrically based; in short tubular bones, a pathologic fracture may result. Most tumors are less than 5 cm in size and on imaging are well-circumscribed, with variable mineralization patterns of small punctate calcifications that are trabecular, ring, and arc-like. Up to one-half of enchondromas and periosteal chondromas have heterozygous mutations in *IDH1* and *IDH2* genes (which are also present in central and periosteal chondrosarcomas) (350). Chondromas are benign lesions, with low rates of recurrence.

Chondromas show either a multinodular or lobular pattern, with hypocellular lobules of abundant cartilage matrix and intervening delicate fibrous septa. The chondrocytes are distributed in lacunae or embedded in the stroma, and are round with small nuclei and occasional nucleoli (**Figure 10.5**). Occasional cells are stellate or bipolar in shape or binucleated. Mitotic activity is absent. Periosteal chondromas are located underneath the periosteum and are sharply demarcated from the underlying cortex (**Figure 10.6**). Enchondromas and periosteal chondromas do not permeate into cortical or cancellous bone or into adjacent soft tissue. The distinction between enchondroma/periosteal chondroma and atypical cartilaginous tumor/grade I chondrosarcoma may be extremely difficult, and the diagnosis of malignancy requires the presence of permeation into bone or soft tissue (which may only be focally present). Notably, enchondromas in the small bones of the hands and feet and periosteal chondromas tend to be more hypercellular with occasional mild atypia and binucleation, and may suggest grade I–II chondrosarcoma (**Figure 10.7**). However, the diagnosis of chondroma is appropriate if the tumor is well-circumscribed and there is no

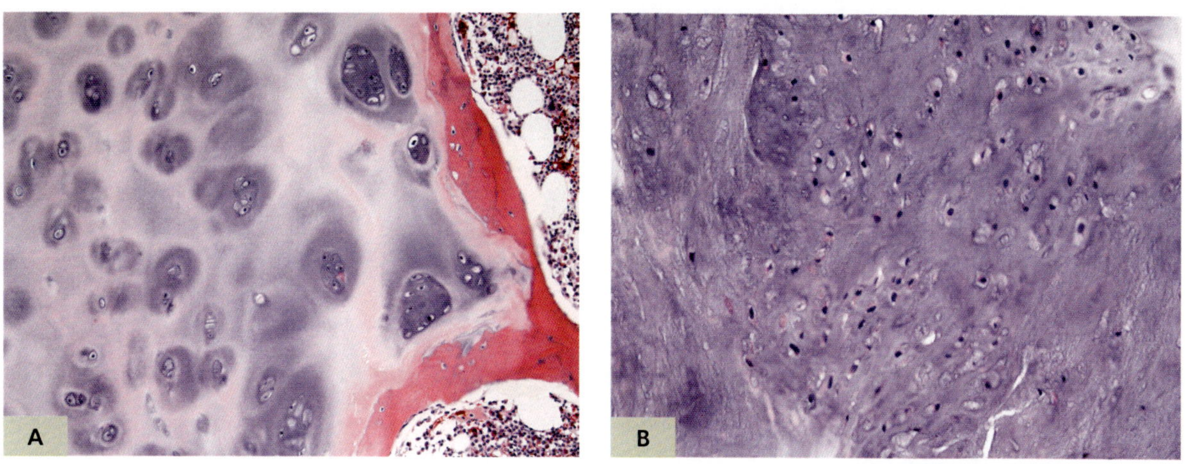

FIGURE 10.5 Enchondromas are well-circumscribed lobulated tumors with hypocellular lobules of benign chondrocytes (A) that are distributed in lacunae and are occasionally binucleated or show stellate or bipolar morphology (B).

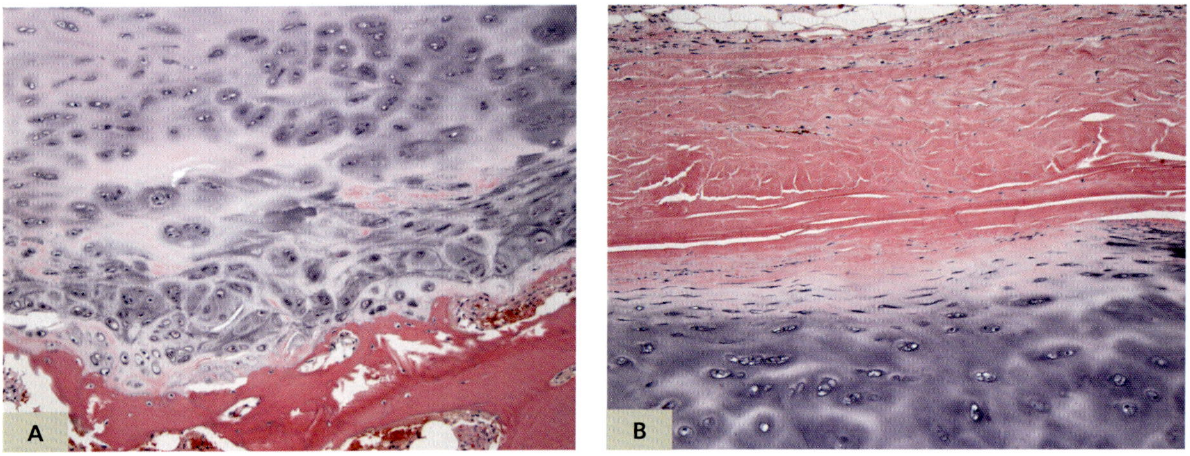

FIGURE 10.6 Periosteal chondromas are sharply demarcated from the underlying cortex (A) and lie underneath intact periosteum (B).

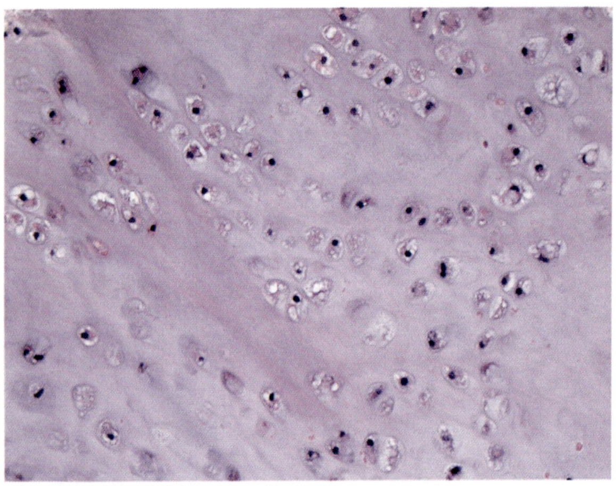

FIGURE 10.7 Enchondromas in the small bones of the hands and feet tend to be more hypercellular with occasional mild atypia and binucleation.

extension into soft tissue, although cortical thinning may be seen in tumors at these sites. For soft tissue chondroma, clinical and radiographic correlation will help exclude metastatic chondrosarcoma to soft tissue sites or extraosseous extension of chondrosarcoma. Of note, conventional chondrosarcoma does not arise primarily in soft tissue.

CHONDROMYXOID FIBROMA

Chondromyxoid fibroma is a rare benign cartilaginous tumor that most commonly occurs during the second and third decades. Tumors most frequently arise on the metaphysis of long bones of the lower extremities. Tumors appear on x-ray as well-circumscribed lytic defects with a sclerotic border. Microscopically, chondromyxoid fibroma shows a multilobular growth pattern; within the lobules the spindled-to-stellate tumor cells are embedded in a myxoid matrix and show higher cellularity at the periphery of the lobules (**Figure 10.8**). Tumor cells have indistinct to eosinophilic cytoplasm with occasional bipolar and multipolar extensions. The tumor cells appear uniform, although occasional cases may show enlarged, hyperchromatic nuclei. Mitotic activity is generally lacking. The stroma is myxoid; hyaline cartilage is absent. Frequent aberrations of chromosome 6 have been reported (351). Chondromyxoid fibroma shows an excellent prognosis, although 15% of cases may show local recurrence.

The differential diagnosis includes chondroblastoma (see "*Chondroblastoma*" section) or grade III chondrosarcoma. Chondroblastomas do not show a lobular growth pattern, and can be recognized by the mononuclear cell population with longitudinal grooves and distinct "chicken-wire" calcification pattern. The lobular growth pattern, myxoid stroma, and hypercellularity at the periphery of the lobules of chondromyxoid fibroma may mimic grade III chondrosarcoma. However, chondrosarcoma is more common in older patients and is more frequent in the diaphysis of long bones; radiographic images usually show aggressive features (such as destructive growth). The presence of diffuse cytologic atypia, increased mitotic activity, and atypical mitotic figures favors the diagnosis of grade III chondrosarcoma, which will lack the central hypocellular areas within lobules.

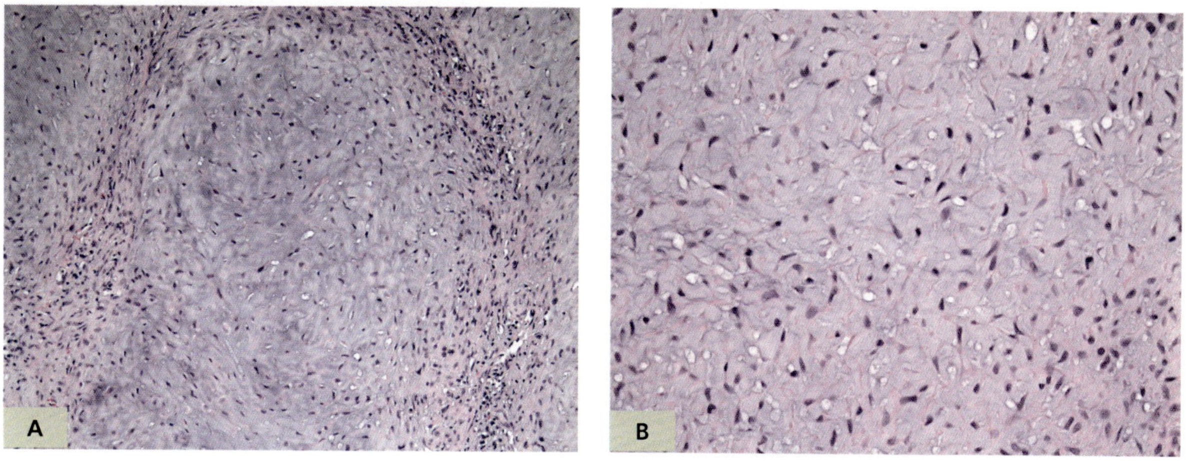

FIGURE 10.8 Chondromyxoid fibroma shows a multilobular growth pattern with spindled-to-stellate tumor cells embedded in a myxoid matrix and increased cellularity at the periphery of the lobules (A). Tumor cells are relatively uniform with indistinct to eosinophilic cytoplasm and occasional bipolar and multipolar extensions (B).

CHONDROBLASTOMA

Chondroblastoma is a rare benign neoplasm that typically arises in the epiphysis of long bones in prepubertal patients (ie, before epiphyseal growth plates have closed). Males are affected more frequently than females. Tumors most commonly have the radiographic appearance of a lytic, well-circumscribed, and often lobular lesion with a thin sclerotic rim. Microscopically, lesions are comprised of predominantly sheet-like growth of ovoid, round, and polygonal cells with ovoid nuclei surrounded by a moderate amount of basophilic cytoplasm (**Figure 10.9A**). The nuclei are bland and have indistinct-to-small nucleoli and longitudinal grooves (**Figure 10.9B**). The tumor cells are associated with a stromal matrix with a variably chondroid, osseous, and fibrous appearance.

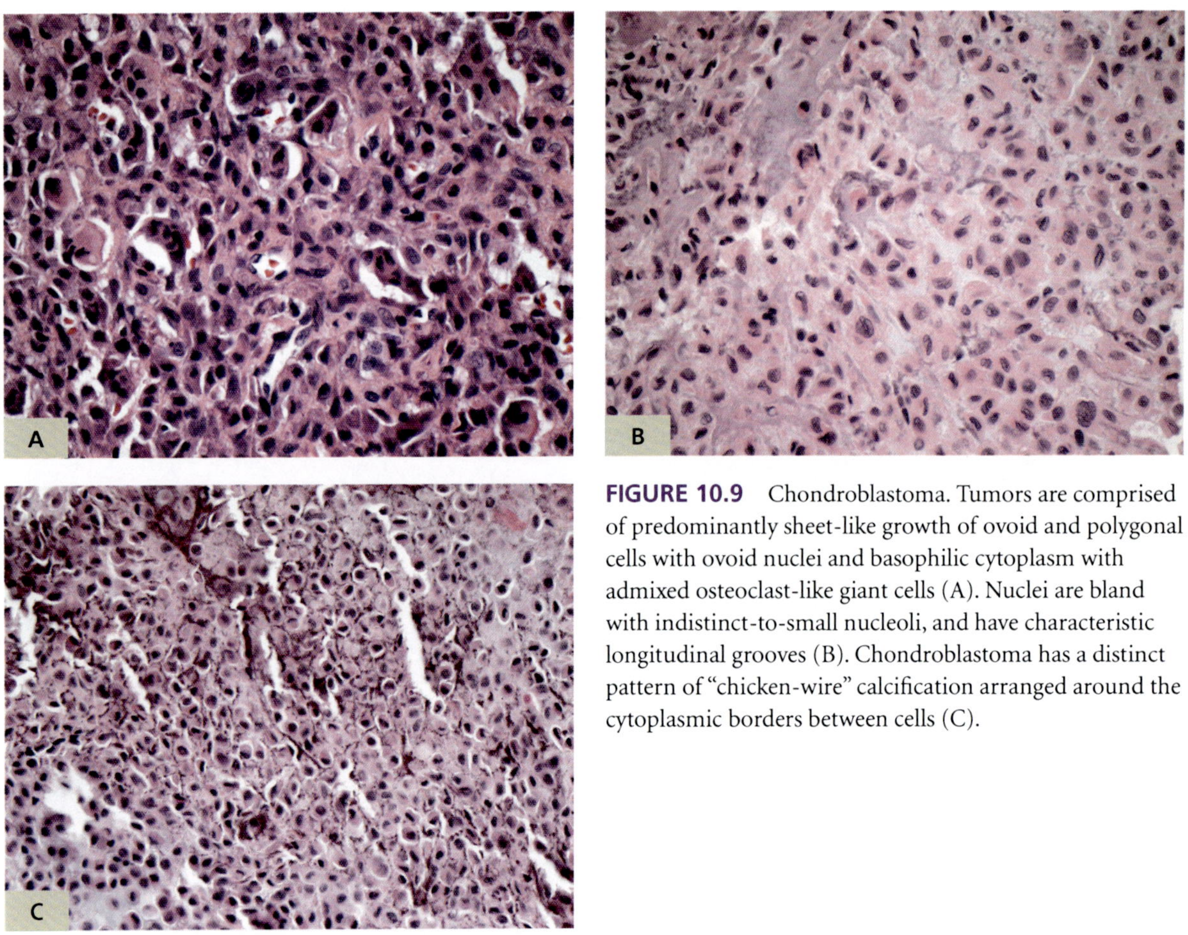

FIGURE 10.9 Chondroblastoma. Tumors are comprised of predominantly sheet-like growth of ovoid and polygonal cells with ovoid nuclei and basophilic cytoplasm with admixed osteoclast-like giant cells (A). Nuclei are bland with indistinct-to-small nucleoli, and have characteristic longitudinal grooves (B). Chondroblastoma has a distinct pattern of "chicken-wire" calcification arranged around the cytoplasmic borders between cells (C).

A distinct pattern of "chicken-wire" calcifications, in which calcifications follow the cytoplasmic borders between tumors cells, is seen in chondroblastoma (**Figure 10.9C**). Osteoclast-like giant cells are often present. Chondroblastoma is a benign neoplasm that may recur locally and occasionally show aggressive growth. Rare cases metastasize, most commonly to the lungs.

Chondroblastoma may mimic benign entities such as giant cell tumor of bone and chondromyxoid fibroma, as well as chondrosarcoma. While giant cell tumor of bone also occurs in epiphyseal locations, these occur in an older patient population after closure of the epiphyseal plates (see Chapter 8). Giant cell tumor lacks the chicken-wire calcification pattern, and tumor cells typically lack nuclear grooves. Chondromyxoid fibroma occurs in older patients in metaphyseal locations. The radiographic and morphologic features of chondroblastoma may mimic the rare clear cell variant of chondrosarcoma, which also occurs at the ends of long bones with a well-circumscribed and occasional sclerotic rim. Clear cell chondrosarcoma is multilobulated, with multinucleated giant cells clustered at the edges of lobules and osteoid formation in the center; tumor cells have a distinct cytomorphologic appearance with central round nuclei with prominent nucleoli and well-defined cytoplasmic borders (**Figure 10.10**).

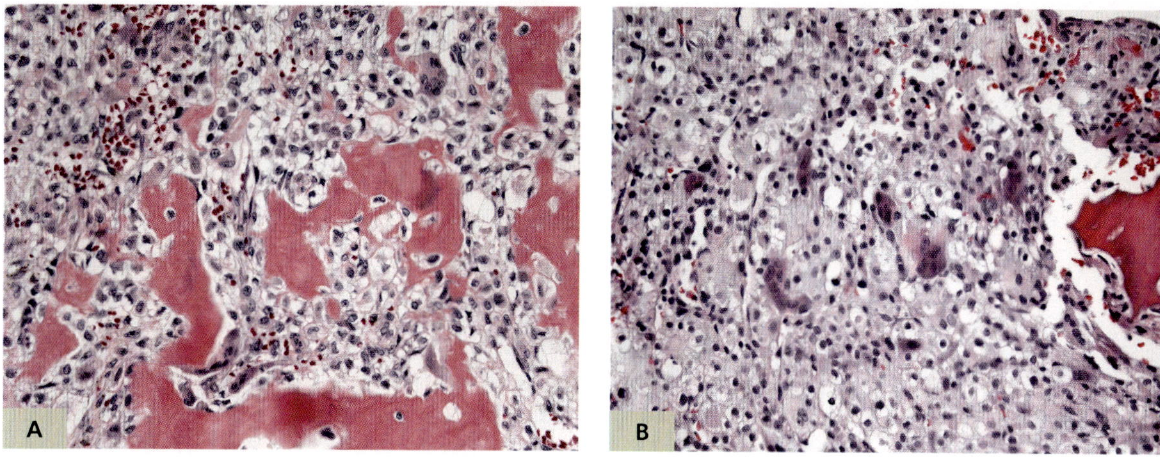

FIGURE 10.10 The clear cell variant of chondrosarcoma shows reactive osteoid formation admixed with large polygonal tumor cells that have central round nuclei with prominent nucleoli (A) and variably pale or granular cytoplasm with well-defined cell borders (B).

BIZARRE PAROSTEAL OSTEOCHONDROMATOUS PROLIFERATION

Bizarre parosteal osteochondromatous proliferation (BPOP), also discussed in Chapter 8, is a benign osteochondromatous neoplasm that affects young adults, most commonly in the digits and long bones. Tumors are attached to the underlying cortex by a bony stalk and lobulated cartilaginous cap. BPOP is characterized by the translocation t(1;17)(q32;q21) (336,338). Microscopically, BPOP shows a haphazard, disorganized arrangement of a bland spindle cell population intermixed with bony trabeculae and hypercellular cartilaginous islands (**Figure 10.11**). The hypercellular and occasionally atypical cartilage have a distinctive appearance, with blue-tinted mineralization often referred to as "blue bone." Recurrences of BPOP are common.

The hypercellular islands of cartilage with cytologic atypia may resemble chondrosarcoma. However, most primary chondrosarcomas arise in older adults and are extremely rare in the small bones of the hands and feet. Radiographic studies of BPOP do not show aggressive features, and the distinct dark blue tinctorial quality of the cartilage and the maturation of cartilage into bone are helpful diagnostic features of BPOP.

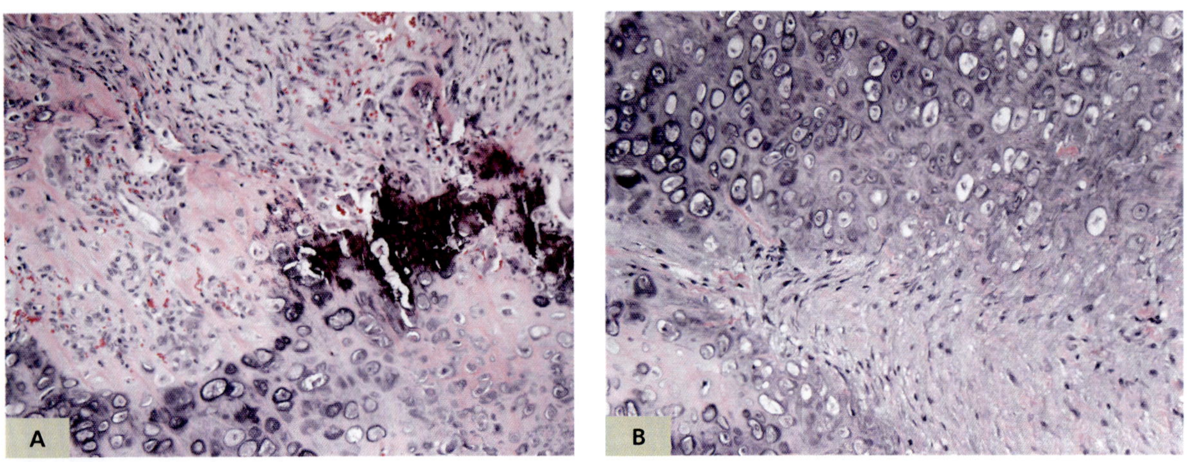

FIGURE 10.11 Bizarre parosteal osteochondromatous proliferation is comprised of a haphazard, disorganized arrangement of a bland spindle cell population intermixed with bony trabeculae and hypercellular cartilaginous islands (A). The hypercellular and occasionally atypical cartilage has a distinctive blue-tinted mineralization (B).

SYNOVIAL CHONDROMATOSIS

Synovial chondromatosis is a benign neoplasm that most commonly involves the knee joint (but has been reported in all joints and in extra-articular sites) in adult patients. Men are more commonly affected than women. Radiologic studies show small round and calcified masses within the joint space, often associated with an effusion. Grossly, nodules are predominantly embedded in the synovium and are comprised of hyaline cartilage in which chondrocytes are arranged in clusters (**Figure 10.12A**). Chondrocytes, which are arranged in clusters, are occasionally binucleated and may show nuclear enlargement, mild pleomorphism, and myxoid degeneration (**Figure 10.12B**). Recurrent translocations of chromosome 6 have been identified in synovial chondromatosis (352). Up to a fifth of cases show local recurrence, and rare cases of malignant transformation to chondrosarcoma have been reported (353).

While synovial chondromatosis may mimic chondrosarcoma, it is also important to distinguish synovial chondromatosis from osteocartilaginous loose bodies (ie, in degenerative joint disease). Total synovectomy is performed for synovial chondromatosis, given the risk of recurrence and malignant progression, while treatment of the underlying disease is necessary

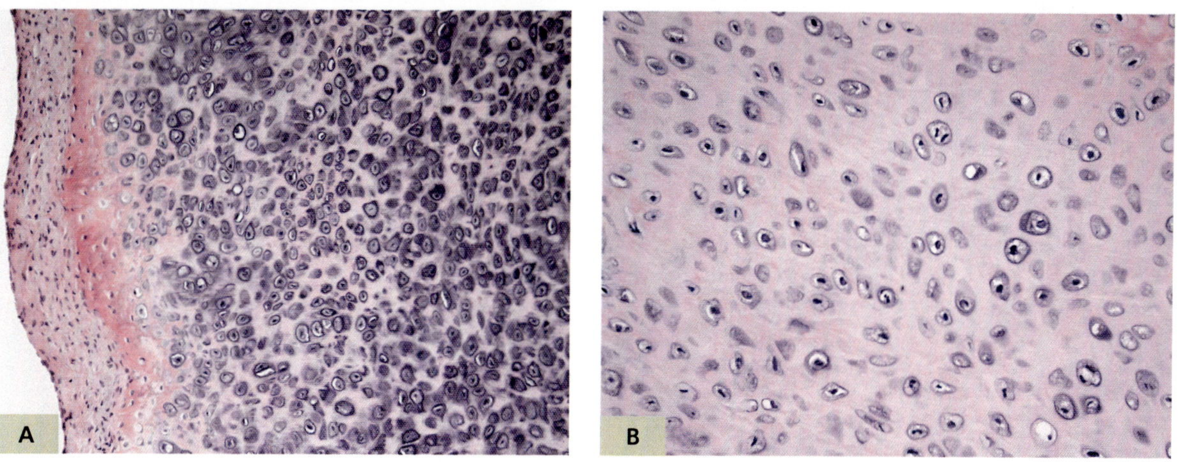

FIGURE 10.12 Synovial chondromatosis is comprised of nodules (often embedded in synovium) of hyaline cartilage in which chondrocytes are arranged in clusters (A). Chondrocytes may be binucleated and may show nuclear enlargement and mild pleomorphism (B).

for loose bodies. Loose bodies are comprised of nonneoplastic cartilage free-floating in the joint space, with chondrocytes arranged in concentric layers (**Figure 10.13**).

Synovial chondromatosis may be difficult to distinguish from chondrosarcoma, as the former shows binucleated chondrocytes with frequent enlarged nuclei having mild pleomorphism. The diagnosis of chondrosarcoma should be made when there is necrosis, extensive myxoid matrix, sheets of atypical chondrocytes, mitotic activity, and spindled cells at the periphery of nodules.

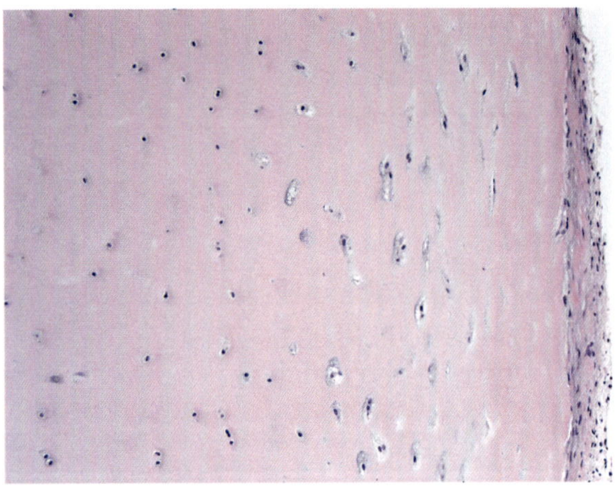

FIGURE 10.13 Osteocartilaginous loose bodies, which arise secondary to degenerative joint disease, are composed of nonneoplastic cartilage with frequent concentric arrangement of chondrocytes.

References

1. Ackerman LV. *Surgical Pathology*. 3rd ed. St. Louis, MO: CV Mosby; 1964:407–408.
2. Birch-Hirschfeld A. Die Krankheiten der Orbita. In: Graefe A, Saemisch T, eds. *Handbuch der Gesamten Augenheilkunden*. Vol 9. part 1. Berlin: Springer-Verlag; 1930:111–130.
3. Garner A. Pathology of "pseudotumors" of the orbit: a review. *J Clin Pathol*. 1973;26:639–648.
4. Umiker WO, Iverson L. Postinflammatory "tumors" of the lung. *J Thorac Surg*. 1954;28:55–63.
5. Kuzela DC. Ultrastructural study of a postinflammatory "tumor" of the lung. *Cancer*. 1975;36:149–156.
6. Makela V, Mattila S, Makinen J. Plasma cell granuloma (histiocytoma) of the lung and pleura. *Arch Pathol Microbiol Scand (A)*. 1972;80:634–640.
7. Bahadori M, Liebow AA. Plasma cell granulomas of the lung. *Cancer*. 1973;31:191–208.
8. Alvarez-Fernandez E, Escalona-Zapata J. Pulmonary plasma cell granuloma: an electron microscopic and tissue culture study. *Histopathology*. 1983;7:279–286.
9. Warter A, Satge D, Roeslin N. Angioinvasive plasma cell granulomas of the lung. *Cancer*. 1987;59:435–443.
10. Sherwin RP, Kern WH, Jones JC. Solitary mast cell granuloma (histiocytoma) of the lung. *Cancer*. 1965;18:634–641.
11. Scott HW, Morrow AG, Payne TPB. Solitary xanthoma of the lung. *Thorac Surg*. 1948;17:821–825.
12. Titus JL, Harrison EG Jr, Clagett AT, Anderson MV, KuaffL Y. Xanthomatous and inflammatory pseudotumor of the lung. *Cancer*. 1962;15:522–538.
13. Wentworth P, Lynch MJ, Fallis JC, et al. Xanthomatous pseudotumor of lung. *Cancer*. 1968;22:345–355.
14. Buell R, Want N, Seemayer TA, Ahmed MN. Endobronchial plasma cell granuloma (xanthomatous pseudotumor): a light and electron microscopic study. *Hum Pathol*. 1976;7:411–426.
15. Alegre JA, Deust J. Xanthogranuloma as a coin lesion of the lung. *Dis Chest*. 1958;33:427–431.
16. Spencer H. The pulmonary plasma cell-histiocytoma complex. *Histopathology*. 1984;8:903–916.
17. Liebow AA, Hubbel DS. Sclerosing hemangioma (histiocytoma, xanthoma) of the lung. *Cancer*. 1956;9:53–75.
18. Jensen PS, Putnam CE. Hemophilic pseudotumor: diagnosis, treatment, and complications. *Am J Dis Child*. 1975;129:717–719.
19. Hermann G, Yeh HC, Gilbert MS. Computed tomography and ultrasonography of the hemophilic pseudotumor and their use in surgical planning. *Skel Radiol*. 1986;15:123–128.
20. Kelly IM, Lees WR, Russell RC. Tumefactive biliary sludge: a sonographic pseudotumor appearance in the common bile duct. *Clin Radiol*. 1993;47:251–254.
21. Bellamy PR. The mucosal rosette: a periampullary pseudotumor within a duodenal diverticulum. *Clin Radiol*. 1993;47:117–118.
22. Coenen L, Biltjes I. Pseudotumor of the palm due to an anomalous flexor digitorum superficialis muscle belly. *J Hand Surg*. 1991;16A:1046–1051.

23. Meier S, Cagle O. Rounded atelectasis. *Surg Rounds*. 1986;8:85–90.
24. Inoshita T, Boyd W. Rounded atelectasis shown by computed tomography. *South Med J*. 1986;79:764–767.
25. Stark P. Round atelectasis: another pulmonary pseudotumor. Am *Rev Resp Dis*. 1982;125:248–250.
26. Tallroth K, Kiviranta K. Round atelectasis. *Respiration*. 1984;45:71–77.
27. Wick MR, Swanson PE. *Cutaneous Adnexal Tumors: A Guide to Pathologic Diagnosis*. Chicago, IL: ASCP Press; 1991:28.
28. Goldstein N. Ephidrosis (local hyperhidrosis): nevus sudoriferus. *Arch Dermatol*. 1967;96:67–71.
29. Kin JH, Hur H, Lee CW, Kim YT. Apocrine nevus. *J Am Acad Dermatol*. 1988;18:579–581.
30. Amazon K, Robinson MD, Rywlin AM. Ferrugination caused by Monsel's solution: clinical observations and experimentations. *Am J Dermatopathol*. 1980;2:197–205.
31. Olmstead PM, Lund HZ, Leonard DD. Monsel's solution: a histologic nuisance. *J Am Acad Dermatol*. 2980;3:492–498.
32. Tschen JA, Fechner RE. The juxtaoral organ of Chievitz. *Am J Surg Pathol*. 1979;3:147–154.
33. Danforth RA, Baughman RA. Chievitz's organ: a potential pitfall in oral cancer diagnosis. *Oral Surg*. 1979;48:231–235.
34. Ide F, Mishima K, Saito I. Juxtaoral organ of Chievitz presenting clinically as a tumor. *J Clin Pathol*. 2003;56:789–790.
35. Pantanowitz L, Tschen JA. Organ of Chievitz. *Ear Nose Throat J*. 2004;83:230.
36. Kusafuka K, Kameya T. Juxtaoral organ of Chievitz, radiologically suspicious for invasion of lingual squamous cell carcinoma. *Pathol Int*. 2007;57:754–756.
37. McBroom JM, Ramsay AD. The clinicopathological meeting: a means of auditing diagnostic performance. *Am I Surg Pathol*. 1993;17:75–80.
38. Pettinato G, Manivel JC, DeRosa N, Dehner LP. Inflammatory myofibroblastic tumor (plasma cell granuloma): clinicopathologic study of 20 cases with immunohistochemical and ultrastructural observations. *Am J Clin Pathol*. 1990;94:538–546.
39. Berardi RS, Lee SS, Chen HP, Stines GJ. Inflammatory pseudotumors of the lung. *Surg Gynecol Obstet*. 1983;156:89–96.
40. Barbareschi M, Ferrero S, Aldovini D, et al. Inflammatory pseudotumor of the lung: immunohistochemical analysis on four new cases. *Histol Histopathol*. 1990;5:205–211.
41. Cotelingam J, Jaffe ES. Inflammatory pseudotumor of the spleen. *Am J Surg Pathol*. 1984;8:375–380.
42. Monforte-Munoz H, Ro JY, Manning JT Jr, et al. Inflammatory pseudotumor of the spleen: report of two cases with a review of the literature. *Am J Clin Pathol*. 1991;96:491–495.
43. Perrone T, DeWolf-Peeters C, Frizzera G. Inflammatory pseudotumor of lymph nodes: a distinctive pattern of nodal reaction. *Am J Surg Pathol*. 1988;12:351–361.
44. Isaacson P, Buchanan R, Mepham BL. Plasma cell granuloma of the stomach. *Hum Pathol*. 1978;9:355–358.
45. Abrebanel P, Sarfaty S, Gal R, Chaimoff C, Kessler E. Plasma cell granuloma of the pancreas. *Arch Pathol Lab Med*. 1984;108:531–532.
46. Wu JP, Yunis EJ, Fetterman G, et al. Inflammatory pseudotumors of the abdomen: plasma cell granulomas. *J Clin Pathol*. 1973;26:943–948.
47. Day DL, Sane S, Dehner LP. Inflammatory pseudotumor of the mesentery and small intestine. *Pediatr Radiol*. 1986;16:210–215.
48. Chen KTK. Inflammatory pseudotumor of the liver. *Hum Pathol*. 1984;15:694–696.
49. Shek TW, Ng IO, Chan KW. lnflammatory pseudotumor of the liver: report of four cases and review of the literature. *Am J Surg Pathol*. 1993;17:231–238.
50. Fish AE, Brodey PA. Plasma cell granuloma of the kidney. *Urology*. 1976;8:89–91.
51. Nochomovitz LE, Orenstein JM. Inflammatory pseudotumor of the urinary bladder: possible relationship to nodular fasciitis. *Am J Surg Pathol*. 1985;9:366–373.

52. Dietrick DD, Kabalin IN, Daniels GF Jr, et al. Inflammatory pseudotumor of the bladder. *J Urol.* 1992;148:141–144.
53. Yapp R, Linder J, Schenker JR, Karrer FW. Plasma cell granuloma of the thyroid. *Hum Pathol.* 1985;16:848–850.
54. Earl PD, Lowry JC, Sloan P. Intraoral inflammatory pseudotumor. *Oral Surg Oral Med Oral Pathol.* 1993;76:279–283.
55. Hytiroglou P, Brandwein MS, Strauchen JA, et al. Inflammatory pseudotumor of the parapharyngeal space. *Head & Neck.* 1992;14:230–234.
56. Pettinato G, Manivel JC, Insabato L, et al. Plasma cell granuloma (inflammatory pseudotumor) of the breast. *Am J Clin Pathol.* 1988;90:627–632.
57. Eimoto T, Yanaka M, Kurosawa M, Ikeya F. Plasma cell granuloma (inflammatory pseudotumor) of the spinal cord and meninges. *Cancer.* 1978;41:1929–1936.
58. Sitton IE, Harkin IC, Gerber MA. Intracranial inflammatory pseudotumor. *Clin Neuropathol.* 1992;11:36–40.
59. Chang Y, Horoupian DS, Lane B, et al. Inflammatory pseudotumor of the choroid plexus in Sjogren's disease. *Neurosurgery.* 1991;29:287–290.
60. Valdeeswar P, Patwardhan AM, Sathe PA. Cardiac valvular inflammatory pseudotumor. *J Cardiothorac Surg.* 2008;3:53.
61. Tomiyama M, Nakatani S, Ishibashi-Ueda H, Yutani C, Yamagishi M. Inflammatory pseudotumor of the heart. *Ann Intern Med.* 2007;147:351–352.
62. Matsubara O, Tan-Liu NS, Kenney RM, Mark EJ. Inflammatory pseudotumor of the lung: progression from organizing pneumonia to fibrous histiocytoma or to plasma cell granuloma in 32 cases. *Hum Pathol.* 1988;19:807–814.
63. Yi E, Aubry MC. Pulmonary pseudoneoplasms. *Arch Pathol Lab Med.* 2010;134:417–426.
64. Bastlein C, Burlefinger R, Holzberg E, et al. Common variable immunodeficiency syndrome and nodular lymphoid hyperplasia in the small intestine. *Endoscopy.* 1988;20:272–275.
65. Bejaoui M, Guezmir M, Hamdi M, et al. Lymphoid hyperplasia of the intestine in children: 15 cases. *Ann Pediatrics (Paris).* 1992;39:359–364.
66. Colarian I, Calzada R, Iaszewski R. Nodular lymphoid hyperplasia of the colon in adults: is it common? *Gastrointest Endosc.* 1990;36:421–422.
67. Franchi LM, Chin TW, Nussbaum E, et al. Familial pulmonary nodular lymphoid hyperplasia. *J Pediatrics.* 1992;121:89–92.
68. Brodell RT, Santa Cruz DI. Cutaneous pseudolymphomas. *Dermatol Clin.* 1985;3:719–734.
69. Hammer E, Sangueza O, Suwanjindar P, et al. Immunophenotypic and genotypic analysis in cutaneous lymphoid hyperplasias. *J Am Acad Dermatol.* 1993;28:426–433.
70. Takano Y, Kato Y, Sugano H. Histopathological and immunohistochemical study of atypical lymphoid hyperplasia and benign lymphoid hyperplasia of the stomach. *Jpn J Cancer Res.* 1992;83:288–293.
71. Samoszuk M, Ramzi E, Ravel I. Disseminated persistent lymphoid hyperplasia containing Epstein-Barr virus and clonal rearrangements of DNA. *Diagn Mol Pathol.* 1993;2:57–60.
72. Cheuk W, Chan JKC. IgG4-related sclerosing disease: a critical appraisal of an evolving clinicopathologic entity. *Adv Anat Pathol.* 2010;17:303–332.
73. Slootweg PI, Panders AK, Nikkels PG. Psammomatoid ossifying fibroma of the paranasal sinuses. *J Craniomaxillofac Surg.* 1993;21:294–297.
74. Chan KW, Khoo US, Ho CM. Fibroosseous pseudotumor of the digits: report of a case with immunohistochemical and ultrastructural studies. *Pathology.* 1993;25:193–196.
75. Bosse A, Niesert W, Wuisman P, Roessner A. Fibrous dysplasia versus osteofibrous dysplasia: morphological, differential diagnostic, and clinical aspects. Experiences from the Westfalen bone tumor registry. *Z Orthop Ihre Grenzgeb.* 1993;131:42–50.
76. Kearns D, McGill T, Potsic W. Fibrous dysplasia. *Head & Neck.* 1992;14:510–512.
77. Betts NI, Stewart IC, Fonseca RI, Scott RF. Multiple central giant cell lesions with a Noonan-like phenotype. *Oral Surg Oral Med Oral Pathol.* 1993;76:601–607.

78. Wallis MG, Devakumar R, Hosie KB, et al. Complex sclerosing lesions (radial scars) of the breast can be palpable. *Clin Radiol.* 1993;48:319–320.
79. Anderson TI, Battersby S. Radial scars of benign and malignant breasts: comparative features and significance. *J Pathol.* 1985;147:23–32.
80. Farshid G, Rush G. Assessment of 142 stellate lesions with imaging features suggestive of radial scar discovered during population-based screening for breast cancer. *Am J Surg Pathol.* 2004;28:1626–1631.
81. Sohn VY, Causey MW, Steele SR, Keylock JB, Brown TA. The treatment of radial scars in the modern era—surgical excision is not required. *Am Surg.* 2010;76:522–525.
82. Walker AN, Fechner RE, Mills SE, Perry JM. Epidlelial polyps of the prostatic urethra: a light microscopic and immunohistochemical study. *Am J Surg Pathol.* 1983;7:351–356.
83. Natsheh A, Prat O, Shenfield OZ, Reinus C, Chertin B. Fibroepithelial polyp of the bladder neck in children. *Pediatr Surg Int.* 2008;24:613–615.
84. Frankendlaler R, Batsakis IG, Suarez PA. Tumefactive fibroinflammatory lesions of the head and neck. *Ann Otol Rhinol Laryngol.* 1993;102:481–482.
85. Savage PD, Wick MR, Thompson RC, Skubitz KM. Tumefactive fibroinflammatory lesion of the extremity. *Arch Pathol Lab Med.* 1991;115:230–232.
86. Klein MH, Rosenberg ZS, Lehman WB. Nonossifying fibroma of bone: a case report. *Bull Hosp Jt Dis Orthop Inst.* 1990;50:64–69.
87. Selby S. Metaphyseal cortical defects in tubular bones of growing children. *J Bone Joint Surg.* 1961;43A:395–404.
88. Bertoni F, Bacchini P, Capartna R, et al. Solid variant of aneurysmal bone cyst. *Cancer.* 1993;71:729–734.
89. Dahlin DC, McLeod RA. Aneurysmal bone cyst and other non-neoplastic conditions. *Skel Radiol.* 1982;8:243–250.
90. Salzer-Kuntschik M. Pitfalls and typical false interpretations in bone tumors, from the viewpoint of long-term consultation. *Pathologe.* 1996;17:1–5.
91. Sun ZJ, Zhao YF, Yang RL, Zwahlen RA. Aneurysmal bone cysts of the jaws: analysis of 17 cases. *J Oral Maxillofac Surg.* 2010;68:2122–2128.
92. Brastianos P, Gokasian Z, McCarthy EF. Aneurysmal bone cysts of the sacrum: a report of ten cases and review of the literature. *Iowa Orthop J.* 2009;29:74–78.
93. Smidl J, Yuppa F, Watson RC. Primary tumors and tumor-like conditions of die clavicle. *Skel Radiol.* 1988;17:235–246.
94. Dahlin DC, Unni KK. *Bone Tumors.* 4th ed. Springfield, IL: Charles C Thomas; 1986:406–481.
95. Jelsma F, Ross PJ. Tumor-like lesions of the calvaria, due to general disease processes. *Am Surg.* 1963;29:247–255.
96. Dromer C, Caulier M, LeGuennec P, et al. Tumor-like bone dystrophy and peripheral joint fusion in a patient with Paget's disease of bone. *Rev Rheum* (Engl Ed). 1995;62:142–146.
97. Hunter SB, Ballinger WE Jr, Rubin II. Multiple sclerosis mimicking primary brain tumor. *Arch Pathol Lab Med.* 1987;111:464–468.
98. Takeuchi T, Ogura M, Sato M, et al. Late-onset tumefactive multiple sclerosis. *Radiat Med.* 2008;26:549–552.
99. Chebel S, Rekik O, Boughammoura-Bouatay A, Frih-Ayed M. Pseudotumoral presentation of multiple sclerosis. *Neurochirurgie.* 2007;53:379–382.
100. Caroli E, Salvati M, Ferrante L. Tumor-like multiple sclerosis: report of four cases and literature review. *Tumori.* 2006;92:559–562.
101. Woolner LB, McConahey WM, Beahrs OH. Stroma lymphomatosa (Hashimoto's thyroiditis) and related disorders. *J Clin Endocrinol Metab.* 1959;19:53–83.
102. LiVolsi VA. The thyroid and parathyroid. In: Sternberg SS, ed. *Diagnostic Surgical Pathology.* 2nd ed. New York, NY: Lippincott-Williams & Wilkins; 1994:523–560.
103. Wick MR, Mills SE, Ritter JH, Lind AC. Postoperative/posttraumatic spindle-cell nodule of the skin: the dermal analogue of nodular fasciitis. *Am J Dermatopathol.* 1999;21:220–224.

104. Stanley MW, Skoog L, Tani EM, Horwitz CA. Nodular fasciitis: spontaneous resolution following diagnosis by fine needle aspiration. *Diagn Cytopathol.* 1993;9:322–324.
105. Lundgren L, Kindblom LG, Willems J, et al. Proliferative myositis and fasciitis: a light and electron microscopic, cytologic, DNA-cytometric and immunohistochemical study. *APMIS.* 1992;100:437–448.
106. Sarangarajan R, Dehner LP. Cranial and extracranial fasciitis of childhood: a clinicopathologic and immunohistochemical study. *Hum Pathol.* 1999;30:87–92.
107. Silva P, Bruce IA, Malik T, Homer J, Banerjee S. Nodular fasciitis of the head and neck. *J Laryngol Otol.* 2005;119:8–11.
108. Flury D, Von Hochstetter AR, Landolt U, Schmid S. Proliferative myositis: a little-known pseudomalignant lesion. *Schweiz Med Wochenschr.* 1993;123:29–34.
109. Jaffe HL. Giant cell reparative granuloma, traumatic bone cyst, and fibrous (fibro-osseous) dysplasia of the jawbones. *Oral Surg.* 1953;6:159–175.
110. Lorenzo IC, Dorfman HD. Giant cell reparative granuloma of short tubular bones of the hands and feet. *Am J Surg Pathol.* 1980;4:551–563.
111. Sass SM, Pinto MC, Jebahi Y, Bortolon L. Giant cell reparative granuloma in the mandible. *Braz J Otorhinolaryngol.* 2010;76:273.
112. Giusto TJ. Peripheral giant cell granuloma: report of two cases. *J NJ Dent Assoc.* 2010;81:22–24.
113. Hillerdal G. Asbestos-related pleural disease. *Semin Respir Med.* 1987;9:65–74.
114. Stephens M, Gibbs AR, Pooley FD, Wagner JC. Asbestos-induced pleural fibrosis: pathology and mineralogy. *Thorax.* 1987;42:583–588.
115. Howard TJ, Bennion RS, Thompson JE Jr. Xanthogranulomatous cholecystitis: a chronic inflammatory pseudotumor of the gallbladder. *Am Surg.* 1991;57:821–824.
116. Dao AH, Wong SW, Adkins RB Jr. Xanthogranulomatous cholecystitis: a clinical and pathologic study of twelve cases. *Am Surg.* 1989;55:32–35.
117. Malek RS, Elder JS. Xanthogranulomatous pyelonephritis: a critical analysis of 26 cases and of the literature. *J Urol.* 1978;119:589–595.
118. Kuo CC, Wu CF, Huang CC, et al. Xanthogranulomatous pyelonephritis: critical analysis of 30 patients. *Int Urol Nephrol.* 2010. In press.
119. Bair MJ, Lin IT, Chen HL, Wu CH. Xanthogranulomatous pyelonephritis. *Am J Med Sci.* 2010;339:574.
120. Rao RV, Kumar A, Sikora SS, Saxena R, Kapoor VK. Xanthogranulomatous cholecystitis: differentiation from associated gallbladder carcinoma. *Trop Gastroenterol.* 2005;26:31–33.
121. Sommerville J. Pseudoepitheliomatous hyperplasia. *Acta Dermatoven.* 1953;33:236–245.
122. Winer LH. Pseudoepitheliomatous hyperplasia. *Arch Dermatol Syphilol.* 1940;42:856–863.
123. Yi JU, Lee CW. Acroangiodermatitis: a clinical variant of stasis dermatitis. *Int J Dermatol.* 1990;29:515–516.
124. Ackerman LV. Extraosseous localized non-neoplastic bone and cartilage formation (so-called myositis ossificans): clinical and pathological confusion with malignant neoplasms. *J Bone Joint Surg.* 1958;40A:79–298.
125. Goldman AB. Myositis ossificans circumscripta: a benign lesion with a malignant differential diagnosis. *AJR.* 1976;126:32–40.
126. Montgomery EA, Meis JM, Mitchell MS, Enzinger FM. Atypical decubital fibroplasia: a distinctive fibroblastic pseudotumor occurring in debilitated patients. *Am J Surg Pathol.* 1992;16:708–715.
127. Fukunaga M. Atypical decubital fibroplasia with unusual histology. *APMIS.* 2001;109:631–635.
128. Ilaslan H, Joyce M, Bauer T, Sundaram M. Decubital ischemic fasciitis: clinical, pathologic, and MRI features of pseudosarcoma. *Am J Roentgenol.* 2006;187:1338–1341.
129. Liegl B, Fletcher CDM. Ischemic fasciitis: analysis of 44 cases indicating an inconsistent association with immobility or debilitation. *Am J Surg Pathol.* 2008;32:1546–1552.
130. Murphy FP, Dahlin DC, Sullivan CR. Articular synovial chondromatosis. *J Bone Joint Surg.* 1962;44A:77–86.

131. Gad A, Willen H, Willen R, et al. Necrotizing sialometaplasia of the lip simulating squamous cell carcinoma. *Histopathology*. 1980;4:111–118.
132. Pagni F, Zarate AF, Urbanski SJ. Necrotizing sialometaplasia of bronchial mucosa. *Int J Surg Pathol*. 2010;18:64–65.
133. Carlson DL. Necrotizing sialometaplasia: a practical approach to the diagnosis. *Arch Pathol Lab Med*. 2009;133:692–698.
134. Parisi JE, Scheithauer BW. Glial tumors. In: Nelson JS, Parisi JE, Schochet SS, eds. *Principles and Practice of Neuropathology*. St. Louis, MO: CV Mosby; 1993:123–183.
135. Young RH, Scully RE. Nephrogenic adenoma: a report of 15 cases. *Am J Surg Pathol*. 1986;10:268–275.
136. Saul SH. Inflammatory cloacogenic polyp. *Hum Pathol*. 1987;18:1120–1125.
137. Herman AH, Nabseth DC. Colitis cystica profunda: localized, segmental, and diffuse. *Arch Surg*. 1973;106:337–341.
138. Rosai J, Dehner LP. Nodular mesothelial hyperplasia in hernia sacs: a benign reactive condition simulating a neoplastic process. *Cancer*. 1975;35:165–175.
139. Cagle PT, Churg A. Differential diagnosis of benign and malignant mesothelial proliferations on pleural biopsies. *Arch Pathol Lab Med*. 2005;129:1421–1427.
140. Lee A, Baloch ZW, Yu G, Gupta PK. Mesothelial hyperplasia with reactive atypia: diagnostic pitfalls and role of immunohistochemical studies. *Diagn Cytopathol*. 2000;22:113–116.
141. Henderson DW, Shilkin KB, Whitaker D. Reactive mesothelial hyperplasia vs. mesothelioma, including mesothelioma in-situ: a brief review. *Am J Clin Pathol*. 1998;110:397–404.
142. Gambill EE. Pancreatitis associated with pancreatic carcinoma: a study of 26 cases. *Mayo Clin Proc*. 1971;46:174–177.
143. Bostwick DG, Egbert BM, Fajardo CF. Radiation injury of the normal and neoplastic prostate. *Am J Surg Pathol*. 1982;6:541–551.
144. Magi-Galluzzi C, Sanderson H, Epstein JI. Atypia in non-neoplastic prostate glands after radiotherapy for prostate cancer: duration of atypia and relation to type of radiotherapy. *Am J Surg Pathol*. 2003;27:206–212.
145. Civantos F. Difficulties in interpreting specimens after neoadjuvant hormonal therapy and radiation with illustration of neuroendocrine differentiation. *Mol Urol*. 2000;4:117–121.
146. Gaudin PB, Zelefsky MJ, Leibel SA, Fuks Z, Reuter VE. Histopathologic effects of three-dimensional conformal external beam radiation therapy on benign and malignant prostate tissues. *Am J Surg Pathol*. 1999;23:1021–1031.
147. Lane Z, Epstein JI. Polypoid/papillary cystitis: a series of 41 cases misdiagnosed as papillary urothelial neoplasia. *Am J Surg Pathol*. 2008:32;758–764.
148. Bonneau R, Brochu P. Neuromuscular choristoma. *Am J Surg Pathol*. 1983;7:521–528.
149. Daroca PJ Jr, Reed RI, Love GL, Kraus SO. Myoid hamartoma of the breast. *Hum Pathol*. 1985;16:212–219.
150. McDonald JR, Harrington SW, Clagett OT. Hamartoma (often called chondroma) of the lung. *J Thorac Surg*. 1945;14:128–143.
151. Takeyama J, Hayashi T, Sanada T, Shimanuki Y, Saito M, Shirane R. Rhabdomyomatous mesenchymal hamartoma associated with nasofrontal meningocele and dermoid cyst. *J Cutan Pathol*. 2005;32:310–313.
152. Cummings TJ, George TM, Fuchs HE, McLendon RE. The pathology of extracranial scalp and skull masses in young children. *Clin Neuropathol*. 2004;23:34–43.
153. Ferran M, Tribo MJ, Gonzalez-Rivero MA, Alameda F, Pujol RM. Congenital hamartoma of the scalp with meningothelial, sebaceous, muscular, and immature glandular components. *Am J Dermatopathol*. 2007;29:568–572.
154. Merchant WJ, Gale J. Intestinal metaplasia in stilbestrol-induced vaginal adenosis. *Histopathology*. 1993;23:373–376.
155. Antonioli DA, Burke L. Vaginal adenosis: analysis of 325 biopsy specimens from 100 patients. *Am J Clin Pathol*. 1975;64:625–638.

156. Robboy SJ, Hill EC, Sandberg EC, Czernobilsky B. Vaginal adenosis in women born prior to the diethylstilbestrol era. *Hum Pathol.* 1986;17:488–492.
157. Jones MA, Andrews J, Tarraza HM. Mesonephric remnant hyperplasia of the cervix: a clinicopathologic analysis of 14 cases. *Gynecol Oncol.* 1993;49:41–47.
158. Goldman RL. Hamartomatous polyp of Brunner's glands. *Gastroenterology.* 1963;44:57–62.
159. Sibley DA, Cooper PH. Rudimentary meningocele: a variant of "primary cutaneous meningioma." *J Cutan Pathol.* 1989;16:72–82.
160. Karma P, Rasanen O, Karja J. Nasal gliomas: a review and report of two cases. *Laryngoscope.* 1977;87:1169–1179.
161. McCall T, Chin SS, Salzman KL, Fults DW. Tuberous sclerosis: a syndrome of incomplete tumor suppression. *Neurosurg Focus.* 2006;20:E3.
162. Pritchard JE. Fibrous dysplasia of the bones. *Am J Med Sci.* 1951;222:313–332.
163. Regezi JA. Odontogenic cysts, odontogenic tumors, fibroosseous, and giant cell lesions of the jaws. *Mod Pathol.* 2002;15:331–341.
164. Dobbie JW. Adrenal cortical nodular hyperplasia: the aging adrenal. *J Pathol.* 1969;99:1–18.
165. Jones EC, Clement PB, Young RH. Sclerosing adenosis of the prostate gland: a clinicopathological and immunohistochemical study of 11 cases. *Am J Surg Pathol.* 1991;15:1171–1180.
166. Epstein J, Armas OA. Atypical basal cell hyperplasia of the prostate. *Am J Surg Pathol.* 1992;16:1205–1214.
167. Wanless IR, Mawdsley C, Adams R. The pathogenesis of focal nodular hyperplasia of the liver. *Hepatology.* 1985;5:1194–1200.
168. Kim T, Hori M, Onishi H. Liver masses with central or eccentric scars. *Semin Ultrasound CT MR.* 2009;30:418–425.
169. Yan BC, Hart JA. Recent developments in liver pathology. *Arch Pathol Lab Med.* 2009;133:1078–1086.
170. Boss JH, Scully RE, Wegner KH, et al. Structural variations in the adult ovary: clinical significance. *Obstet Gynecol.* 1965;25:747–763.
171. Silverberg SO. Arias-Stella phenomenon in spontaneous and therapeutic abortion. *Am J Obstet Gynecol.* 1972;112:777–780.
172. Nucci MR. Tumor-like glandular lesions of the uterine cervix. *Int J Gynecol Pathol.* 2002;21:347–359.
173. Arias-Stella J. The Arias-Stella reaction: facts and fancies four decades after. *Adv Anat Pathol.* 2002;12–23.
174. Yokota N, Kuribayashi T, Nagamine M, et al. Paraplegia caused by brown tumor in primary hyperparathyroidism: case report. *J Neurosurg.* 1989;71:446–448.
175. Bassler T, Wong ET, Brynes RK. Osteitis fibrosa cystica simulating metastatic tumor: an almost-forgotten relationship. *Am J Clin Pathol.* 1993;100:697–700.
176. Verlaan L, van der Wal B, de Maat GJ, Walemkamp G, Nollen-Lopez L, van Ooij A. Primary hyperparathyroidism and pathological fractures: a review. *Acta Orthop Belg.* 2007;73:300–305.
177. Triantaffillidou K, Zouloumis L, Karakinaris G, Kalimeras E, Iordanidis F. Brown tumors of the jaws associated with primary or secondary hyperparathyroidism: a clinical study and review of the literature. *Am J Otolaryngol.* 2006;27:281–286.
178. Al-Gahtany M, Cusimano M, Singer W, Bilbao J, Kovacs K, Marotta T. Brown tumors of the skull base: case report and review of the literature. *J Neurosurg.* 2003;98:417–420.
179. Leslie KO, Silverberg SO. Microglandular hyperplasia of the cervix. *Pathol Annu.* 1982;17:95–114.
180. Proppe KH, Scully RE, Rosai J. Postoperative spindle cell nodules of genitourinary tract resembling sarcomas: a report of eight cases. *Am J Surg Pathol.* 1984;8:101–108.
181. Young RH. Spindle cell lesions of the urinary bladder. *Histol Histopathol.* 1990;5:505–512.

182. Garijo MF, Val-Bernal JF, Vega A, Val D. Postoperative spindle-cell nodule of the breast: pseudosarcomatous myofibroblastic proliferation following endosurgery. *Pathol Int.* 2008;58:787–791.
183. Lott S, Lopez-Beltran A, Maclennan GT, Montironi R, Cheng L. Soft tissue tumors of the urinary bladder, part I: myofibroblastic proliferations, benign neoplasms, and tumors of uncertain malignant potential. *Hum Pathol.* 2007;38:807–823.
184. Micci F, Haugom L, Abeler VM, Bjerkehagen B, Heim S. Trisomy 7 in postoperative spindle cell nodules. *Cancer Genet Cytogenet.* 2007;174:147–150.
185. Spiess PE, Tuziak T, Tibbs RF, et al. Pseudosarcomatous and sarcomatous proliferations of the bladder. *Hum Pathol.* 2007;38:753–761.
186. Harik LR, Merino C, Coindre JM, Amin MB, Pedeutour F, Weiss SW. pseudosarcomatous myofibroblastic proliferations of the bladder: a clinicopathologic study of 42 cases. *Am J Surg Pathol.* 2006;30:787–794.
187. Sencer SF, Haake RI, Weisdorf DJ. Hemorrhagic cystitis after bone marrow transplantation: risk factors and complications. *Transplantation.* 1993;56:875–879.
188. Murray M. Non-neoplastic alterations of the mammary epithelium can mimic atypia. *Arch Pathol Lab Med.* 2009;133:722–728.
189. Young RH. Tumor-like lesions of the urinary bladder. *Mod Pathol.* 2009;22(suppl 2):S37–S52.
190. Nash G, Said JW, eds. *Pathology of AIDS and HIV infection.* Philadelphia, PA: WB Saunders; 1992:5–25.
191. Umlas J, Federman M, Crawford C, et al. Spindle cell pseudotumor due to *Mycobacterium avium-intracellulare* in patients with acquired immunodeficiency syndrome (AIDS). *Am J Surg Pathol.* 1991;15:1181–1187.
192. Wood C, Nickoloff BJ, Todes-Taylor NR. Pseudotumor resulting from atypical mycobacterial infection: a "histoid" variety of *Mycobacterium avium-intracellulare* complex infection. *Am J Clin Pathol.* 1985;83:524–527.
193. Chen KTK. Mycobacterial spindle cell pseudotumor of lymph nodes. *Am J Surg Pathol.* 1992;16:276–281.
194. Wagner M, Rose VA, Linder R, Schulze HJ, Krueger GR. Human pathogenic virus-associated pseudolymphomas and lymphomas with primary cutaneous manifestation in humans and animals. *Clin Infect Dis.* 1998;27:1299–1308.
195. Chalvardjian A, Picard L, Shaw R, et al. Malakoplakia of the female genital tract. *Am J Obstet Gynecol.* 1980;138:391–394.
196. Lioy-Lupis MT, Quintana RM, Monsalve J, Iotti RM. Testicular malakoplakia. *Arch Esp Urol.* 1993;46:822–824.
197. Kohl SK, Hans CP. Cutaneous malakoplakia. *Arch Pathol Lab Med.* 2008;132:113–117.
198. Yousef GM, Naghibi B, Hamodat MM. Malakoplakia outside the urinary tract. *Arch Pathol Lab Med.* 2007;131:297–300.
199. Srigley JR. Benign mimickers of prostatic adenocarcinoma. *Mod Pathol.* 2004;17:328–348.
200. Mansfield RE. Histoid leprosy. *Arch Pathol.* 1969;87:580–585.
201. Triscott JA, Nappi O, Ferrara G, Wick MR. "Pseudoneoplastic" leprosy. Leprosy revisited. *Am J Dermatopathol.* 1995;17:297–302.
202. Vantrappen G, Agg HO, Geboes K, Ponette E. Yersinia enteritis. *Med Clin North Am.* 1982;66:639–653.
203. Hostein I, Pelmus M, Aurias A, et al. Evaluation of MDM2 and CDK4 amplification by real-time PCR on paraffin wax-embedded material: a potential tool for the diagnosis of atypical lipomatous tumours/well-differentiated liposarcomas. *J Pathol.* 2004;202:95–102.
204. Binh MB, Sastre-Garau X, Guillou L, et al. MDM2 and CDK4 immunostainings are useful adjuncts in diagnosing well-differentiated and dedifferentiated liposarcoma subtypes: a comparative analysis of 559 soft tissue neoplasms with genetic data. *Am J Surg Pathol.* 2005;29:1340–1347.

205. Weaver J, Goldblum JR, Turner S, et al. Detection of MDM2 gene amplification or protein expression distinguishes sclerosing mesenteritis and retroperitoneal fibrosis from inflammatory well-differentiated liposarcoma. *Mod Pathol.* 2009;22:66–70.
206. Beham A, Fletcher CD. Intramuscular angioma: a clinicopathological analysis of 74 cases. *Histopathology.* 1991;18:53–59.
207. Emory TS, Monihan JM, Carr NJ, et al. Sclerosing mesenteritis, mesenteric panniculitis and mesenteric lipodystrophy: a single entity? *Am J Surg Pathol.* 1997;21:392–398.
208. Farshid G, Weiss SW. Massive localized lymphedema in the morbidly obese: a histologically distinct reactive lesion simulating liposarcoma. *Am J Surg Pathol.* 1998;22:1277–1283.
209. Schmack I, Patel RM, Folpe AL, et al. Subconjunctival herniated orbital fat: a benign adipocytic lesion that may mimic pleomorphic lipoma and atypical lipomatous tumor. *Am J Surg Pathol.* 2007;31:193–198.
210. Bishop E, Eble JN, Cheng L, et al. Adrenal myelolipomas show nonrandom X-chromosome inactivation in hematopoietic elements and fat: support for a clonal origin of myelolipomas. *Am J Surg Pathol.* 2006;30:838–843.
211. Ida CM, Wang X, Erickson-Johnson MR, et al. Primary retroperitoneal lipoma: a soft tissue pathology heresy?: report of a case with classic histologic, cytogenetics, and molecular genetic features. *Am J Surg Pathol.* 2008;32:951–954.
212. Macarenco RS, Erickson-Johnson MR, Wang X, et al. Retroperitoneal lipomatous tumors without cytologic atypia: are they lipomas? A clinicopathologic and molecular study of 19 cases. *Am J Surg Pathol.* 2009;33:1470–1476.
213. Maggiani F, Debiec-Rychter M, Vanbockrijck M, et al. Cellular angiofibroma: another mesenchymal tumour with 13q14 involvement, suggesting a link with spindle cell lipoma and (extra)-mammary myofibroblastoma. *Histopathology.* 2007;51:410–412.
214. Flucke U, van Krieken JH, Mentzel T. Cellular angiofibroma: analysis of 25 cases emphasizing its relationship to spindle cell lipoma and mammary-type myofibroblastoma. *Mod Pathol.* 2011;24:82–89.
215. Chen BJ, Marino-Enriquez A, Fletcher CD, et al. Loss of retinoblastoma protein expression in spindle cell/pleomorphic lipomas and cytogenetically related tumors: an immunohistochemical study with diagnostic implications. *Am J Surg Pathol.* 2012;36:1119–1128.
216. Maire G, Forus A, Foa C, et al. 11q13 alterations in two cases of hibernoma: large heterozygous deletions and rearrangement breakpoints near GARP in 11q13.5. *Genes Chromosom Cancer.* 2003;37:389–395.
217. Furlong MA, Fanburg-Smith JC, Miettinen M. The morphologic spectrum of hibernoma: a clinicopathologic study of 170 cases. *Am J Surg Pathol.* 2001;25:809–814.
218. Bartuma H, Domanski HA, Von Steyern FV, et al. Cytogenetic and molecular cytogenetic findings in lipoblastoma. *Cancer Genet Cytogenet.* 2008;183:60–63.
219. Yoshida H, Miyachi M, Ouchi K, et al. Identification of COL3A1 and RAB2A as novel translocation partner genes of PLAG1 in lipoblastoma. *Genes Chromosom Cancer.* 2014;53:606–611.
220. Coffin CM, Lowichik A, Putnam A. Lipoblastoma (LPB): a clinicopathologic and immunohistochemical analysis of 59 cases. *Am J Surg Pathol.* 2009;33:1705–1712.
221. Crozat A, Aman P, Mandahl N, et al. Fusion of CHOP to a novel RNA-binding protein in human myxoid liposarcoma. *Nature.* 1993;363:640–644.
222. Matsuyama A, Hisaoka M, Hashimoto H. PLAG1 expression in mesenchymal tumors: an immunohistochemical study with special emphasis on the pathogenetical distinction between soft tissue myoepithelioma and pleomorphic adenoma of the salivary gland. *Pathol Int.* 2012;62:1–7.
223. Erickson-Johnson MR, Chou MM, Evers BR, et al. Nodular fasciitis: a novel model of transient neoplasia induced by MYH9-USP6 gene fusion. *Lab Invest.* 2011;91:1427–1433.

224. Macchia G, Trombetta D, Moller E, et al. FOSL1 as a candidate target gene for 11q12 rearrangements in desmoplastic fibroblastoma. *Lab Invest.* 2012;92:735–743.
225. Carlson JW, Fletcher CD. Immunohistochemistry for beta-catenin in the differential diagnosis of spindle cell lesions: analysis of a series and review of the literature. *Histopathology.* 2007;51:509–514.
226. Montgomery EA, Meis JM, Mitchell MS, et al. Atypical decubital fibroplasia. A distinctive fibroblastic pseudotumor occurring in debilitated patients. *Am J Surg Pathol.* 1992;16:708–715.
227. Liegl B, Fletcher CD. Ischemic fasciitis: analysis of 44 cases indicating an inconsistent association with immobility or debilitation. *Am J Surg Pathol.* 2008;32:1546–1552.
228. Nishio J, Iwasaki H, Nagatomo M, et al. Fibroma of tendon sheath with 11q rearrangements. *Anticancer Res.* 2014;34:5159–5162.
229. Merchant NB, Lewis JJ, Woodruff JM, et al. Extremity and trunk desmoid tumors: a multifactorial analysis of outcome. *Cancer.* 1999;86:2045–2052.
230. Cates JM, Stricker TP. Surgical resection margins in desmoid-type fibromatosis: a critical reassessment. *Am J Surg Pathol.* 2014;38:1707–1714.
231. Lazar AJ, Tuvin D, Hajibashi S, et al. Specific mutations in the beta-catenin gene (CTNNB1) correlate with local recurrence in sporadic desmoid tumors. *Am J Pathol.* 2008;173:1518–1527.
232. Salas S, Chibon F, Noguchi T, et al. Molecular characterization by array comparative genomic hybridization and DNA sequencing of 194 desmoid tumors. *Genes Chromosom Cancer.* 2010;49:560–568.
233. Miyaki M, Konishi M, Kikuchi-Yanoshita R, et al. Coexistence of somatic and germ-line mutations of APC gene in desmoid tumors from patients with familial adenomatous polyposis. *Cancer Res.* 1993;53:5079–5082.
234. Cook JR, Dehner LP, Collins MH, et al. Anaplastic lymphoma kinase (ALK) expression in the inflammatory myofibroblastic tumor: a comparative immunohistochemical study. *Am J Surg Pathol.* 2001;25:1364–1371.
235. Patel AS, Murphy KM, Hawkins AL, et al. RANBP2 and CLTC are involved in ALK rearrangements in inflammatory myofibroblastic tumors. *Cancer Genet Cytogenet.* 2007;176:107–114.
236. Marino-Enriquez A, Wang WL, Roy A, et al. Epithelioid inflammatory myofibroblastic sarcoma: an aggressive intra-abdominal variant of inflammatory myofibroblastic tumor with nuclear membrane or perinuclear ALK. *Am J Surg Pathol.* 2011;35:135–144.
237. Harik LR, Merino C, Coindre JM, et al. Pseudosarcomatous myofibroblastic proliferations of the bladder: a clinicopathologic study of 42 cases. *Am J Surg Pathol.* 2006;30:787–794.
238. Hirsch MS, Dal Cin P, Fletcher CD. ALK expression in pseudosarcomatous myofibroblastic proliferations of the genitourinary tract. *Histopathology.* 2006;48:569–578.
239. Pedeutour F, Simon MP, Minoletti F, et al. Translocation, t(17;22)(q22;q13), in dermatofibrosarcoma protuberans: a new tumor-associated chromosome rearrangement. *Cytogenet Cell Genet.* 1996;72:171–174.
240. Patel KU, Szabo SS, Hernandez VS, et al. Dermatofibrosarcoma protuberans COL1A1-PDGFB fusion is identified in virtually all dermatofibrosarcoma protuberans cases when investigated by newly developed multiplex reverse transcription polymerase chain reaction and fluorescence in situ hybridization assays. *Hum Pathol.* 2008;39:184–193.
241. Chmielecki J, Crago AM, Rosenberg M, et al. Whole-exome sequencing identifies a recurrent NAB2-STAT6 fusion in solitary fibrous tumors. *Nat Genet.* 2013;45:131–132.
242. Robinson DR, Wu YM, Kalyana-Sundaram S, et al. Identification of recurrent NAB2-STAT6 gene fusions in solitary fibrous tumor by integrative sequencing. *Nat Genet.* 2013;45:180–185.
243. Yoshida A, Tsuta K, Ohno M, et al. STAT6 immunohistochemistry is helpful in the diagnosis of solitary fibrous tumors. *Am J Surg Pathol.* 2014;38:552–559.
244. Doyle LA, Vivero M, Fletcher CD, et al. Nuclear expression of STAT6 distinguishes solitary fibrous tumor from histologic mimics. *Mod Pathol.* 2014;27:390–395.

245. Cranshaw IM, Gikas PD, Fisher C, et al. Clinical outcomes of extra-thoracic solitary fibrous tumours. *Eur J Surg Oncol.* 2009;35:994–998.
246. Wilky BA, Montgomery EA, Guzzetta AA, et al. Extrathoracic location and "borderline" histology are associated with recurrence of solitary fibrous tumors after surgical resection. *Ann Surg Oncol.* 2013;20:4080–4089.
247. Pauwels P, Sciot R, Croiset F, et al. Myofibroblastoma of the breast: genetic link with spindle cell lipoma. *J Pathol.* 2000;191:282–285.
248. Chen E, Fletcher CD. Cellular angiofibroma with atypia or sarcomatous transformation: clinicopathologic analysis of 13 cases. *Am J Surg Pathol.* 2010;34:707–714.
249. Hornick JL, Fletcher CD. Soft tissue perineurioma: clinicopathologic analysis of 81 cases including those with atypical histologic features. *Am J Surg Pathol.* 2005;29:845–858.
250. Doyle LA, Moller E, Dal Cin P, et al. MUC4 is a highly sensitive and specific marker for low-grade fibromyxoid sarcoma. *Am J Surg Pathol.* 2011;35:733–741.
251. Panagopoulos I, Storlazzi CT, Fletcher CD, et al. The chimeric FUS/CREB3l2 gene is specific for low-grade fibromyxoid sarcoma. *Genes Chromosom Cancer.* 2004;40:218–228.
252. Guillou L, Benhattar J, Gengler C, et al. Translocation-positive low-grade fibromyxoid sarcoma: clinicopathologic and molecular analysis of a series expanding the morphologic spectrum and suggesting potential relationship to sclerosing epithelioid fibrosarcoma: a study from the French Sarcoma Group. *Am J Surg Pathol.* 2007;31:1387–1402.
253. Arbajian E, Puls F, Magnusson L, et al. Recurrent EWSR1-CREB3L1 gene fusions in sclerosing epithelioid fibrosarcoma. *Am J Surg Pathol.* 2014;38:801–808.
254. Delaney D, Diss TC, Presneau N, et al. GNAS1 mutations occur more commonly than previously thought in intramuscular myxoma. *Mod Pathol.* 2009;22:718–724.
255. Knezevich SR, McFadden DE, Tao W, et al. A novel ETV6-NTRK3 gene fusion in congenital fibrosarcoma. *Nat Genet.* 1998;18:184–187.
256. West RB, Rubin BP, Miller MA, et al. A landscape effect in tenosynovial giant-cell tumor from activation of CSF1 expression by a translocation in a minority of tumor cells. *Proc Natl Acad Sci U S A.* 2006;103:690–695.
257. Cupp JS, Miller MA, Montgomery KD, et al. Translocation and expression of CSF1 in pigmented villonodular synovitis, tenosynovial giant cell tumor, rheumatoid arthritis and other reactive synovitides. *Am J Surg Pathol.* 2007;31:970–976.
258. Jaffer S, Ambrosini-Spaltro A, Mancini AM, et al. Neurothekeoma and plexiform fibrohistiocytic tumor: mere histologic resemblance or histogenetic relationship? *Am J Surg Pathol.* 2009;33:905–913.
259. Enzinger FM, Zhang RY. Plexiform fibrohistiocytic tumor presenting in children and young adults. An analysis of 65 cases. *Am J Surg Pathol.* 1988;12:818–826.
260. Remstein ED, Arndt CA, Nascimento AG. Plexiform fibrohistiocytic tumor: clinicopathologic analysis of 22 cases. *Am J Surg Pathol.* 1999;23:662–670.
261. Fletcher C, Bridge J, Hogendoorn P, et al, eds. *WHO Classification of Tumours of Soft Tissue and Bone. Pathology and Genetics of Tumours of Soft Tissue and Bone.Â.* Lyon: IARC Press; 2013.
262. Deyrup AT, Lee VK, Hill CE, et al. Epstein-Barr virus-associated smooth muscle tumors are distinctive mesenchymal tumors reflecting multiple infection events: a clinicopathologic and molecular analysis of 29 tumors from 19 patients. *Am J Surg Pathol.* 2006;30:75–82.
263. Jones D, Bhatia VK, Krausz T, et al. Crystal-storing histiocytosis: a disorder occurring in plasmacytic tumors expressing immunoglobulin kappa light chain. *Hum Pathol.* 1999;30:1441–1448.
264. Lebeau A, Zeindl-Eberhart E, Muller EC, et al. Generalized crystal-storing histiocytosis associated with monoclonal gammopathy: molecular analysis of a disorder with rapid clinical course and review of the literature. *Blood.* 2002;100:1817–1827.
265. Fairweather PM, Williamson R, Tsikleas G. Pulmonary extranodal marginal zone lymphoma with massive crystal storing histiocytosis. *Am J Surg Pathol.* 2006;30:262–267.

266. Mosquera JM, Sboner A, Zhang L, et al. Recurrent NCOA2 gene rearrangements in congenital/infantile spindle cell rhabdomyosarcoma. *Genes Chromosom Cancer.* 2013;52:538–550.
267. Agaram NP, Chen CL, Zhang L, et al. Recurrent MYOD1 mutations in pediatric and adult sclerosing and spindle cell rhabdomyosarcomas: evidence for a common pathogenesis. *Genes Chromosom Cancer.* 2014;53:779–787.
268. Nascimento AF, Raut CP, Fletcher CD. Primary angiosarcoma of the breast: clinicopathologic analysis of 49 cases, suggesting that grade is not prognostic. *Am J Surg Pathol.* 2008;32:1896–1904.
269. McMenamin ME, Fletcher CD. Reactive angioendotheliomatosis: a study of 15 cases demonstrating a wide clinicopathologic spectrum. *Am J Surg Pathol.* 2002;26:685–697.
270. Brenn T, Fletcher CD. Cutaneous epithelioid angiomatous nodule: a distinct lesion in the morphologic spectrum of epithelioid vascular tumors. *Am J Dermatopathol.* 2004;26:14–21.
271. Sangueza OP, Walsh SN, Sheehan DJ, et al. Cutaneous epithelioid angiomatous nodule: a case series and proposed classification. *Am J Dermatopathol.* 2008;30:16–20.
272. Rosen PP, Ridolfi RL. The perilobular hemangioma. A benign microscopic vascular lesion of the breast. *Am J Clin Pathol.* 1977;68:21–23.
273. Montgomery E, Epstein JI. Anastomosing hemangioma of the genitourinary tract: a lesion mimicking angiosarcoma. *Am J Surg Pathol.* 2009;33:1364–1369.
274. Kryvenko ON, Gupta NS, Meier FA, et al. Anastomosing hemangioma of the genitourinary system: eight cases in the kidney and ovary with immunohistochemical and ultrastructural analysis. *Am J Clin Pathol.* 2011;136:450–457.
275. Lin J, Bigge J, Ulbright TM, et al. Anastomosing hemangioma of the liver and gastrointestinal tract: an unusual variant histologically mimicking angiosarcoma. *Am J Surg Pathol.* 2013;37:1761–1765.
276. Pansuriya TC, van Eijk R, d'Adamo P, et al. Somatic mosaic IDH1 and IDH2 mutations are associated with enchondroma and spindle cell hemangioma in Ollier disease and Maffucci syndrome. *Nat Genet.* 2011;43:1256–1261.
277. Kurek KC, Pansuriya TC, van Ruler MA, et al. R132C IDH1 mutations are found in spindle cell hemangiomas and not in other vascular tumors or malformations. *Am J Pathol.* 2013;182:1494–1500.
278. Errani C, Zhang L, Sung YS, et al. A novel WWTR1-CAMTA1 gene fusion is a consistent abnormality in epithelioid hemangioendothelioma of different anatomic sites. *Genes Chromosom Cancer.* 2011;50:644–653.
279. Antonescu CR, Le Loarer F, Mosquera JM, et al. Novel YAP1-TFE3 fusion defines a distinct subset of epithelioid hemangioendothelioma. *Genes Chromosom Cancer.* 2013;52:775–784.
280. Antonescu CR, Chen HW, Zhang L, et al. ZFP36-FOSB fusion defines a subset of epithelioid hemangioma with atypical features. *Genes Chromosom Cancer.* 2014;53:951–959.
281. Brenn T, Fletcher CD. Radiation-associated cutaneous atypical vascular lesions and angiosarcoma: clinicopathologic analysis of 42 cases. *Am J Surg Pathol.* 2005;29:983–996.
282. Patton KT, Deyrup AT, Weiss SW. Atypical vascular lesions after surgery and radiation of the breast: a clinicopathologic study of 32 cases analyzing histologic heterogeneity and association with angiosarcoma. *Am J Surg Pathol.* 2008;32:943–950.
283. Gengler C, Coindre JM, Leroux A, et al. Vascular proliferations of the skin after radiation therapy for breast cancer: clinicopathologic analysis of a series in favor of a benign process: a study from the French Sarcoma Group. *Cancer.* 2007;109:1584–1598.
284. Mentzel T, Schildhaus HU, Palmedo G, et al. Postradiation cutaneous angiosarcoma after treatment of breast carcinoma is characterized by MYC amplification in contrast to atypical vascular lesions after radiotherapy and control cases: clinicopathological, immunohistochemical and molecular analysis of 66 cases. *Mod Pathol.* 2012;25:75–85.
285. Guo T, Zhang L, Chang NE, et al. Consistent MYC and FLT4 gene amplification in radiation-induced angiosarcoma but not in other radiation-associated atypical vascular lesions. *Genes Chromosom Cancer.* 2011;50:25–33.

286. Nascimento AF, Fletcher CD. The controversial nosology of benign nerve sheath tumors: neurofilament protein staining demonstrates intratumoral axons in many sporadic schwannomas. *Am J Surg Pathol.* 2007;31:1363–1370.
287. McMenamin ME, Fletcher CD. Expanding the spectrum of malignant change in schwannomas: epithelioid malignant change, epithelioid malignant peripheral nerve sheath tumor, and epithelioid angiosarcoma: a study of 17 cases. *Am J Surg Pathol.* 2001;25:13–25.
288. Smith K, Mezebish D, Williams JP, et al. Cutaneous epithelioid schwannomas: a rare variant of a benign peripheral nerve sheath tumor. *J Cutan Pathol.* 1998;25:50–55.
289. Kindblom LG, Meis-Kindblom JM, Havel G, et al. Benign epithelioid schwannoma. *Am J Surg Pathol.* 1998;22:762–770.
290. Saad AG, Mutema GK, Mutasim DF. Benign cutaneous epithelioid Schwannoma: case report and review of the literature. *Am J Dermatopathol.* 2005;27:45–47.
291. Rezanko T, Sari AA, Tunakan M, et al. Epithelioid schwannoma of soft tissue: unusual morphological variant causing a diagnostic dilemma. *Ann Diagn Pathol.* 2012;16:521–526.
292. Jo VY, Fletcher CD. Epithelioid malignant peripheral nerve sheath tumor: clinicopathologic analysis of 63 cases. *Am J Surg Pathol.* 2015;39:673–682.
293. Hornick JL, Bundock EA, Fletcher CD. Hybrid schwannoma/perineurioma: clinicopathologic analysis of 42 distinctive benign nerve sheath tumors. *Am J Surg Pathol.* 2009;33:1554–1561.
294. Harder A, Wesemann M, Hagel C, et al. Hybrid neurofibroma/schwannoma is overrepresented among schwannomatosis and neurofibromatosis patients. *Am J Surg Pathol.* 2012;36:702–709.
295. Crew AJ, Clark J, Fisher C, et al. Fusion of SYT to two genes, SSX1 and SSX2, encoding proteins with homology to the Kruppel-associated box in human synovial sarcoma. *EMBO J.* 1995;14:2333–2340.
296. Liegl B, Hornick JL, Corless CL, et al. Monoclonal antibody DOG1.1 shows higher sensitivity than KIT in the diagnosis of gastrointestinal stromal tumors, including unusual subtypes. *Am J Surg Pathol.* 2009;33:437–446.
297. Demetri GD, von Mehren M, Antonescu CR, et al. NCCN Task Force report: update on the management of patients with gastrointestinal stromal tumors. *J Natl Compr Canc Netw.* 2010;8(Suppl 2):S1–41; quiz S42–4.
298. Miettinen M, Sobin LH, Lasota J. Gastrointestinal stromal tumors of the stomach: a clinicopathologic, immunohistochemical, and molecular genetic study of 1765 cases with long-term follow-up. *Am J Surg Pathol.* 2005;29:52–68.
299. Miettinen M, Makhlouf H, Sobin LH, et al. Gastrointestinal stromal tumors of the jejunum and ileum: a clinicopathologic, immunohistochemical, and molecular genetic study of 906 cases before imatinib with long-term follow-up. *Am J Surg Pathol.* 2006;30:477–489.
300. Dwight T, Benn DE, Clarkson A, et al. Loss of SDHA expression identifies SDHA mutations in succinate dehydrogenase-deficient gastrointestinal stromal tumors. *Am J Surg Pathol.* 2013;37:226–233.
301. Miller K, Goodlad JR, Brenn T. Pleomorphic dermal sarcoma: adverse histologic features predict aggressive behavior and allow distinction from atypical fibroxanthoma. *Am J Surg Pathol.* 2012;36:1317–1326.
302. Medeiros F, Erickson-Johnson MR, Keeney GL, et al. Frequency and characterization of HMGA2 and HMGA1 rearrangements in mesenchymal tumors of the lower genital tract. *Genes Chromosom Cancer.* 2007;46:981–990.
303. McCluggage WG, Connolly L, McBride HA. HMGA2 is a sensitive but not specific immunohistochemical marker of vulvovaginal aggressive angiomyxoma. *Am J Surg Pathol.* 2010;34:1037–1042.
304. Hornick JL, Dal Cin P, Fletcher CD. Loss of INI1 expression is characteristic of both conventional and proximal-type epithelioid sarcoma. *Am J Surg Pathol.* 2009;33:542–550.
305. Doyle LA, Fletcher CD. Metastasizing "benign" cutaneous fibrous histiocytoma: a clinicopathologic analysis of 16 cases. *Am J Surg Pathol.* 2013;37:484–495.

306. Antonescu CR, Dal Cin P, Nafa K, et al. EWSR1-CREB1 is the predominant gene fusion in angiomatoid fibrous histiocytoma. *Genes Chromosom Cancer*. 2007;46:1051–1060.
307. Shadan FF, Mascarello JT, Newbury RO, et al. Supernumerary ring chromosomes derived from the long arm of chromosome 12 as the primary cytogenetic anomaly in a rare soft tissue chondroma. *Cancer Genet Cytogenet*. 2000;118:144–147.
308. Dahlen A, Mertens F, Rydholm A, et al. Fusion, disruption, and expression of HMGA2 in bone and soft tissue chondromas. *Mod Pathol*. 2003;16:1132–1140.
309. Folpe AL, Fanburg-Smith JC, Billings SD, et al. Most osteomalacia-associated mesenchymal tumors are a single histopathologic entity: an analysis of 32 cases and a comprehensive review of the literature. *Am J Surg Pathol*. 2004;28:1–30.
310. Bahrami A, Weiss SW, Montgomery E, et al. RT-PCR analysis for FGF23 using paraffin sections in the diagnosis of phosphaturic mesenchymal tumors with and without known tumor induced osteomalacia. *Am J Surg Pathol*. 2009;33:1348–1354.
311. Lee JC, Jeng YM, Su SY, et al. Identification of a novel FN1-FGFR1 genetic fusion as a frequent event in phosphaturic mesenchymal tumour. *J Pathol*. 2015;235:539–545.
312. Hornick JL, Fletcher CD. Cellular neurothekeoma: detailed characterization in a series of 133 cases. *Am J Surg Pathol*. 2007;31:329–340.
313. Liegl B, Hornick JL, Fletcher CD. Primary cutaneous PEComa: distinctive clear cell lesions of skin. *Am J Surg Pathol*. 2008;32:608–614.
314. Hantschke M, Mentzel T, Rutten A, et al. Cutaneous clear cell sarcoma: a clinicopathologic, immunohistochemical, and molecular analysis of 12 cases emphasizing its distinction from dermal melanoma. *Am J Surg Pathol*. 2010;34:216–222.
315. Zucman J, Delattre O, Desmaze C, et al. EWS and ATF-1 gene fusion induced by t(12;22) translocation in malignant melanoma of soft parts. *Nat Genet*. 1993;4:341–345.
316. Antonescu CR, Tschernyavsky SJ, Woodruff JM, et al. Molecular diagnosis of clear cell sarcoma: detection of EWS-ATF1 and MITF-M transcripts and histopathological and ultrastructural analysis of 12 cases. *J Mol Diagn*. 2002;4:44–52.
317. Hornick JL, Fletcher CD. Myoepithelial tumors of soft tissue: a clinicopathologic and immunohistochemical study of 101 cases with evaluation of prognostic parameters. *Am J Surg Pathol*. 2003;27:1183–1196.
318. Brandal P, Panagopoulos I, Bjerkehagen B, et al. Detection of a t(1;22)(q23;q12) translocation leading to an EWSR1-PBX1 fusion gene in a myoepithelioma. *Genes Chromosom Cancer*. 2008;47:558–564.
319. Antonescu CR, Zhang L, Chang NE, et al. EWSR1-POU5F1 fusion in soft tissue myoepithelial tumors. A molecular analysis of sixty-six cases, including soft tissue, bone, and visceral lesions, showing common involvement of the EWSR1 gene. *Genes Chromosom Cancer*. 2010;49:1114–1124.
320. Flucke U, Palmedo G, Blankenhorn N, et al. EWSR1 gene rearrangement occurs in a subset of cutaneous myoepithelial tumors: a study of 18 cases. *Mod Pathol*. 2011;24:1444–1450.
321. Agaram NP, Chen HW, Zhang L, et al. EWSR1-PBX3: a novel gene fusion in myoepithelial tumors. *Genes Chromosom Cancer*. 2015;54(2):63–71.
322. Brandal P, Panagopoulos I, Bjerkehagen B, et al. t(19;22)(q13;q12) translocation leading to the novel fusion gene EWSR1-ZNF444 in soft tissue myoepithelial carcinoma. *Genes Chromosom Cancer*. 2009;48:1051–1056.
323. Huang SC, Chen HW, Zhang L, et al. Novel FUS-KLF17 and EWSR1-KLF17 fusions in myoepithelial tumors. *Genes Chromosom Cancer*. 2015;54(5):267–275.
324. Puls F, Arbajian E, Magnusson L, et al. Myoepithelioma of bone with a novel FUS-POU5F1 fusion gene. *Histopathology*. 2014;65:917–922.
325. Gleason BC, Fletcher CD. Myoepithelial carcinoma of soft tissue in children: an aggressive neoplasm analyzed in a series of 29 cases. *Am J Surg Pathol*. 2007;31:1813–1824.
326. Gebre-Medhin S, Nord KH, Moller E, et al. Recurrent rearrangement of the PHF1 gene in ossifying fibromyxoid tumors. *Am J Pathol*. 2012;181:1069–1077.

327. Graham RP, Weiss SW, Sukov WR, et al. PHF1 rearrangements in ossifying fibromyxoid tumors of soft parts: a fluorescence in situ hybridization study of 41 cases with emphasis on the malignant variant. *Am J Surg Pathol.* 2013;37:1751–1755.
328. Antonescu CR, Katabi N, Zhang L, et al. EWSR1-ATF1 fusion is a novel and consistent finding in hyalinizing clear-cell carcinoma of salivary gland. *Genes Chromosom Cancer.* 2011;50:559–570.
329. Attwooll C, Tariq M, Harris M, et al. Identification of a novel fusion gene involving hTAFII68 and CHN from a t(9;17)(q22;q11.2) translocation in an extraskeletal myxoid chondrosarcoma. *Oncogene.* 1999;18:7599–7601.
330. Panagopoulos I, Mertens F, Isaksson M, et al. Molecular genetic characterization of the EWS/CHN and RBP56/CHN fusion genes in extraskeletal myxoid chondrosarcoma. *Genes Chromosom Cancer.* 2002;35:340–352.
331. Foo WC, Cruise MW, Wick MR, et al. Immunohistochemical staining for TLE1 distinguishes synovial sarcoma from histologic mimics. *Am J Clin Pathol.* 2011;135:839–844.
332. Deshpande A, Nelson D, Corless CL, et al. Leiomyoma of the gastrointestinal tract with interstitial cells of Cajal: a mimic of gastrointestinal stromal tumor. *Am J Surg Pathol.* 2014;38:72–77.
333. Conner JR, Hornick JL. SATB2 is a novel marker of osteoblastic differentiation in bone and soft tissue tumours. *Histopathology.* 2013;63:36–49.
334. Paparella ML, Olvi LG, Brandizzi D, et al. Osteosarcoma of the jaw: an analysis of a series of 74 cases. *Histopathology.* 2013;63:551–557.
335. Oliveira AM, Perez-Atayde AR, Inwards CY, et al. USP6 and CDH11 oncogenes identify the neoplastic cell in primary aneurysmal bone cysts and are absent in so-called secondary aneurysmal bone cysts. *Am J Pathol.* 2004;165:1773–1780.
336. Zambrano E, Nose V, Perez-Atayde AR, et al. Distinct chromosomal rearrangements in subungual (Dupuytren) exostosis and bizarre parosteal osteochondromatous proliferation (Nora lesion). *Am J Surg Pathol.* 2004;28:1033–1039.
337. Storlazzi CT, Wozniak A, Panagopoulos I, et al. Rearrangement of the COL12A1 and COL4A5 genes in subungual exostosis: molecular cytogenetic delineation of the tumor-specific translocation t(X;6)(q13–14;q22). *Int J Cancer.* 2006;118:1972–1976.
338. Nilsson M, Domanski HA, Mertens F, et al. Molecular cytogenetic characterization of recurrent translocation breakpoints in bizarre parosteal osteochondromatous proliferation (Nora's lesion). *Hum Pathol.* 2004;35:1063–1069.
339. Bovee JV, Cleton-Jansen AM, Wuyts W, et al. EXT-mutation analysis and loss of heterozygosity in sporadic and hereditary osteochondromas and secondary chondrosarcomas. *Am J Hum Genet.* 1999;65:689–698.
340. Wuyts W, Van Hul W, De Boulle K, et al. Mutations in the EXT1 and EXT2 genes in hereditary multiple exostoses. *Am J Hum Genet.* 1998;62:346–354.
341. Mejia-Guerrero S, Quejada M, Gokgoz N, et al. Characterization of the 12q15 MDM2 and 12q13-14 CDK4 amplicons and clinical correlations in osteosarcoma. *Genes Chromosom Cancer.* 2010;49:518–525.
342. Dujardin F, Binh MB, Bouvier C, et al. MDM2 and CDK4 immunohistochemistry is a valuable tool in the differential diagnosis of low-grade osteosarcomas and other primary fibro-osseous lesions of the bone. *Mod Pathol.* 2011;24:624–637.
343. Tarkkanen M, Bohling T, Gamberi G, et al. Comparative genomic hybridization of low-grade central osteosarcoma. *Mod Pathol.* 1998;11:421–426.
344. Yoshida A, Ushiku T, Motoi T, et al. Immunohistochemical analysis of MDM2 and CDK4 distinguishes low-grade osteosarcoma from benign mimics. *Mod Pathol.* 2010;23:1279–1288.
345. Evans HL, Ayala AG, Romsdahl MM. Prognostic factors in chondrosarcoma of bone: a clinicopathologic analysis with emphasis on histologic grading. *Cancer.* 1977;40:818–831.
346. Gelderblom H, Hogendoorn PC, Dijkstra SD, et al. The clinical approach towards chondrosarcoma. *Oncologist.* 2008;13:320–329.

347. Schmale GA, Conrad EU, 3rd, Raskind WH. The natural history of hereditary multiple exostoses. *J Bone Joint Surg Am.* 1994;76:986–992.
348. Wicklund CL, Pauli RM, Johnston D, et al. Natural history study of hereditary multiple exostoses. *Am J Med Genet.* 1995;55:43–46.
349. Legeai-Mallet L, Munnich A, Maroteaux P, et al. Incomplete penetrance and expressivity skewing in hereditary multiple exostoses. *Clin Genet.* 1997;52:12–16.
350. Amary MF, Bacsi K, Maggiani F, et al. IDH1 and IDH2 mutations are frequent events in central chondrosarcoma and central and periosteal chondromas but not in other mesenchymal tumours. *J Pathol.* 2011;224:334–343.
351. Romeo S, Duim RA, Bridge JA, et al. Heterogeneous and complex rearrangements of chromosome arm 6q in chondromyxoid fibroma: delineation of breakpoints and analysis of candidate target genes. *Am J Pathol.* 2010;177:1365–1376.
352. Buddingh EP, Krallman P, Neff JR, et al. Chromosome 6 abnormalities are recurrent in synovial chondromatosis. *Cancer Genet Cytogenet.* 2003;140:18–22.
353. Davis RI, Hamilton A, Biggart JD. Primary synovial chondromatosis: a clinicopathologic review and assessment of malignant potential. *Hum Pathol.* 1998;29:683–688.

Index